A Textbook of Community Nursing

A Textbook of Community Nursing is a comprehensive and evidence-based introduction covering the full range of professional topics, including professional approaches to care, public health, eHealth, therapeutic relationships and the role of community nursing in mental health. The new edition has been updated throughout, including new guidelines and policies. It also provides a stronger focus on evidence-based practice.

This user-friendly and accessible textbook includes the following:

- Current theory, policy and guidelines for practice. All chapters are underpinned by a strong evidence base.
- Learning objectives are provided for each chapter, plus exercises and activities to test current understanding, promote reflective practice and encourage further reading.
- Case studies and examples from practice which draw on all branches of community nursing are provided to illustrate practical application of theory.

This is an essential text for all pre-registration nursing students, students in specialist community nursing courses and qualified nurses entering community practice for the first time.

Sue Chilton, Senior Lecturer/Academic Course Leader in the School of Health and Social Care, University of Gloucestershire, Gloucester, UK

Heather Bain, Academic Strategic Lead: Academic Programmes, School of Nursing and Midwifery, Robert Gordon University, Aberdeen

A Textbook of Community Nursing

Edited by
SUE CHILTON and HEATHER BAIN

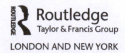

Routledge
Taylor & Francis Group

LONDON AND NEW YORK

First published 2018
by Routledge
2 Park Square, Milton Park, Abingdon, Oxon OX14 4RN

and by Routledge
711 Third Avenue, New York, NY 10017

Routledge is an imprint of the Taylor & Francis Group, an informa business

British Library Cataloguing-in-Publication Data
A catalogue record for this book is available from the British Library

---

Library of Congress Cataloging-in-Publication Data

Names: Chilton, Sue, editor. | Bain, Heather, editor.
Title: A textbook of community nursing / edited by Sue Chilton and Heather Bain.
Description: 2. | Abingdon, Oxon ; New York, NY : Routledge, 2018. | Includes bibliographical references and index.
Identifiers: LCCN 2017015104| ISBN 9781138068247 (hbk) | ISBN 9781498725378 (pbk) | ISBN 9781315157207 (ebk)
Subjects: | MESH: Community Health Nursing
Classification: LCC RT98 | NLM WY 106 | DDC 610.73/43--dc23
LC record available at https://lccn.loc.gov/2017015104

ISBN: 978-1-138-06824-7 (hbk)
ISBN: 978-1-4987-2537-8 (pbk)
ISBN: 978-1-315-15720-7 (ebk)

Typeset in Minion 10 pts by
diacriTech, Chennai
Printed in Great Britain by Ashford Colour Press Ltd

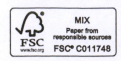

MIX
Paper from
responsible sources
FSC® C011748

CONTRIBUTORS

Fiona Baguley MSc PgCert HELT
School of Nursing and Midwifery
Robert Gordon University
Aberdeen, Scotland

Heather Bain EdD PgCert HELT BA DipDN RGN
School of Nursing and Midwifery
Robert Gordon University
Aberdeen, Scotland

Julie Bliss MSc PGCE BSc RGN DN FHEA QN
Florence Nightingale Faculty of Nursing and Midwifery
King's College London
London, England

Debbie Brown PgDip BSc (Hons) SRN
Department of Primary Care/ANP Burnt Ash Surgery
NHS Lewisham Clinical Commissioning Group
London, England

Nicola Brownie MSc PGCert HELT
School of Nursing and Midwifery
Robert Gordon University
Aberdeen, Scotland

Sue Chilton MSc PGCHE BNurs RN DN HV DNT
School of Health and Social Care
University of Gloucestershire
Gloucester, United Kingdom

Ann Clarridge MSc BSc (Hons) Dip Th PCCEA RN DN
Holy Trinity Church
Northwood, Diocese of Londonformerly Principal Lecturer
London South Bank University
London, United Kingdom

Jacqueline Corbett MSc BSc (Hons)
University of South Wales
Glyntaff, United Kingdom

Fiona Couper MA BA (Hons) SRN RMN Dip Nurse Education Lecturer
Florence Nightingale Faculty of Nursing and Midwifery
King's College London
London, England

Caroline A.W. Dickson PhD MSc PG Cert Prof Ed BA RN Dip DN RNT
SPQ Community Nursing in the Home/District Nursing, Division of Nursing
Occupational Therapy and Arts Therapies, School of Health Sciences
Queen Margaret University
Edinburgh, Scotland

Helen Gough MEd PgC BSc DN RGN FHEA
School of Health and Life Sciences
Glasgow Caledonian University
Glasgow, Scotland

Jill Y Gould MSc BSc (Hons) RGN DN CPT QN SF HEA
University of Derby
Derby, United Kingdom

Sue Harness PGCE BSc (Hons) SFHEA DN QN RGN
Programme Lead Community Specialist Practice
University of Cumbria
Carlisle, England

Gina King RN DN BSc (Palliative Care) PGCHE Dip Reflexology
Quality Improvement Lead for End of Life Care
South West Strategic Clinical Network
Bristol, United Kingdom

Helen McVeigh MA BSc (Hons) RNT RGN
Leicester School of Nursing and Midwifery
De Montfort University
Leicester, England

Sue Miller RGN RSCN DN Cert Ed BSc (Hons) MSc

Jayne Murphy MA BSc (Hons) DipHE, RN (Adult) SFHEA QN
University of Wolverhampton
Wolverhampton, West Midlands, England

Lois Seddon, RN MSc PGCE RNT DN SCPHN (HV) QN
Nursing Specialist Practice Programmes
University of Suffolk
Ipswich, England

Jo Skinner
London Metropolitan University
London, England

Anne Smith MSc BSc (Hons) (Dist Nurs) PGCHE QN RN
University of Reading
Berkshire, England

Debra Smith MA BSc (Hons) DN RN
University of Wolverhampton
West Midlands, England

Sally Sprung MA BSc (Hons) DN RNT RGN FHEA QN
School of Nursing and Allied Health
Liverpool John Moores University
Liverpool, England

Patricia Wilson PhD MSc BED (Hons) RN NDN
Primary Care Unit Centre for Health Service Studies
University of Kent
Canterbury, Kent, England

FOREWORD

All four countries of the United Kingdom recognize that nurses are leading and supporting the implementation of the shared policy imperative for more care to be delivered in or closer to the home.

This comprehensive book confirms the critical and evolving role of the nurse in the community in supporting individuals, families and carers at every stage of their lives.

The themes of each chapter illustrate both the rapidly changing policy context of care in the community and the political, economic, scientific and technical developments that have influenced and supported the growth of the nurse's role.

There could not be a better time to work in the community, as this book illustrates so clearly; autonomous roles, leadership of teams and the potential to care for acutely ill patients in their own homes are just some examples which demonstrate the range of advanced level, specialized skills now required.

There is also a clear recognition that with this responsibility there is a need for the underpinning high level of nursing knowledge which includes asset- and strength-based approaches to care, a demonstration of cultural competence and a considerable level of understanding concerning the social determinants of health.

In the world of healthcare today, there is an expectation that people will take a greater part in decisions about their health and in managing their healthcare. Consideration of what it is to be a professional in this current context is therefore important – but also serves as a reminder of the privilege of working with individuals and communities and the trusting, often long-term therapeutic relationships that are developed and maintained.

For those who are new to nursing in the community there is a coverage of holistic assessments, a nursing practice that involves a person-centred, partnership approach and includes addressing the spiritual needs of patients. The central role of carers and the nurses' role in supporting adult and young carers are given a high profile. This is significant as carers frequently provide the majority of care for patients, and yet their role so often goes unrecognized.

Collaborative working has always been important to nurses working in the community. There is now an imperative to working with colleagues in the voluntary, social and healthcare systems in a more integrated way. New service models provide many opportunities for this and nurses are experts at building relationships with others to the benefit of the patient, family and carers.

With people living increasingly longer lives – which is a cause for celebration – there is a consequent increase in those living with long-term conditions. It is excellent to see a focus on the principles of long-term condition management within the current policy context and the pivotal role of the nurse in the community setting.

A focus on the nurse's central role and the skills required to provide high-quality care in the home at the end of life is given the attention it rightly deserves. There is an often forgotten army of nurses who provide a critical service in the co-ordination and delivery of care for patients at the end of their lives, every day. This happens in every village, town and city around the United Kingdom and yet is rarely given the attention it deserves in the media.

The ways in which nursing is embracing technology to enhance patient care are illustrated in their leadership of new ways of working and a nuanced understanding of patients' responses to such opportunities.

Reading this cleverly woven set of chapters provides a reminder of the unique combination of autonomous and team working that is the joy of serving a community as a highly skilled, creative and resourceful nurse. It provides essential reading to those who are new to a rewarding nursing career in the community and a welcome invigoration for those nurses who have been privileged to serve their communities for many years.

Dr Crystal Oldman
Chief Executive
The Queen's Nursing Institute

INTRODUCTION

Sue Chilton and Heather Bain

This book has been designed to support staff who may be new to working in a community setting and is an essential guide to practice. We envisage that it will be useful for pre-registration students on community placement, community staff nurses and nurses moving from an acute work environment to take up a community post. The aim of the book is to develop and support nurses to work safely and effectively in a range of community locations.

Community nurses work in a great diversity of roles and a variety of settings – including schools, the workplace, health clinics and the home (Naidoo and Wills, 2016). They empower individuals, families and communities to have control over their health and to improve their wellbeing. They also work across the lifespan, and with a range of social groups that include those who are vulnerable, experience inequalities and are socially excluded. Not only do community nurses work autonomously in leading, managing and providing acute and long-term health and social care, anticipatory care and palliative care, but they also have a public health remit. They have a pivotal role in health protection, ill-health prevention and health improvement.

Community practice is dynamic, forever changing and in a constant state of flux. Baguley et al. (2010) have conceptualized community nursing in Figure I.1, which illustrates that, in the promotion of optimum health and wellbeing, community

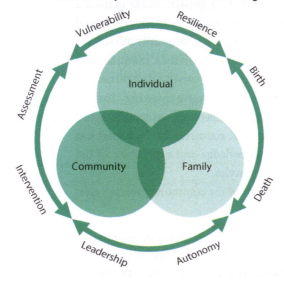

FIGURE I.I Promotion of optimum health and well-being. (Reproduced from Baguley et al., *Concept of Community Nursing*, Aberdeen: Robert Gordon University, 2010.)

The editors would like to thank colleagues from the Association of District Nurse Educators (ADNE), many of whom have contributed to the book. The ADNE (www.adne.co.uk) is committed to raising the profile of district nursing and its purpose is the educational preparation and support of district nurses and other health professionals working in primary and community care across the United Kingdom.

Within each chapter, further readings and resources are suggested. We hope you find this book informative and inspirational in developing your professional practice.

REFERENCES

taken place across the United Kingdom in recent years. In England, for example, general practitioner (GP) fundholding was replaced by primary care groups, which then developed into primary care trusts (DH, 1997). Further changes quickly followed with the largest structural reorganisation of the National Health Service (NHS) since its inception in 1948, involving the development of GP consortia (DH, 2010a), which have wide-ranging responsibilities for commissioning services and manage the vast majority of the NHS budget. Over the last few months, there has been the development of 'Sustainability and Transformation Plans' (STPs) which involve partners working together in 'place-based systems of care' to transform health and social care delivery within local populations. These plans are focused on improving quality and developing new ways of working; improving health and well-being; and improving the efficiency of services in hospitals and the community (Alderwick et al., 2016). Political analysts have recognised the potential value of STPs in supporting new care models and promoting collaboration between key stakeholders but also advise caution and the need for close monitoring and evaluation in testing whether service changes and related financial plans are viable (King's Fund, 2017).

Although, from an academic perspective, the notion of 'community' has been discussed widely across a range of disciplines, including sociology and anthropology (Cohen, 1985), clarity with regard to a definitive definition eludes us.

<table>
<tr><td>**ACTIVITY 1.1**</td><td>**Reflection point**
Compile a list of words that helps to define 'community' for you. Identify any recurring themes that emerge when considering different types of communities or different contexts within which the term is used.</td></tr>
</table>

Laverack (2009) offers four key characteristics of a 'community' which help to summarise many of the definitions found in the literature. These are as follows:

- Spatial dimension – referring to a place or location
- Interests, issues or identities that heterogeneous groups of people share
- Social interactions that are often powerful in nature and tie people into relationships or strong bonds with each other
- Shared needs and concerns that can be addressed by collective and collaborative actions

Although the essence of 'community' is difficult to capture within a definition, the word itself largely conveys a positive impression conjuring up feelings of harmony and co-operation. It is unsurprising to find that it is a word used frequently by politicians within government documents to create just that effect.

The uncertainty with regard to the true meaning of the word 'community' also applies within community nursing (Hickey and Hardyman, 2000). It is pivotal (Carr, 2001) that the context within which care takes place, including physical and social aspects among many others, is considered alongside the geographical

CHAPTER

I

Nursing in a communit environment

Sue Chilton

LEARNING OUTCOMES

- Compare and contrast definitions of 'community', exploring the c
  in which the term is used and, specifically, how it is interpreted wit
  community nursing.
- Explore the environmental, social, economic, professional and politi
  factors influencing the delivery of community healthcare services an
  critically appraise ways in which local services aim to be responsive t
  specific needs of their population.
- Develop insight into the complex nature of the environment of comm
  healthcare.
- Identify the skills and qualities required of nurses working in communit
  settings.

INTRODUCTION

This chapter considers the complex environment within which community nu
practice and offers some definitions of 'community' and ways in which the tern
used. It explores the wide range of factors impacting upon the services commun
nurses provide for patients and discusses ways of tailoring care to respond
local needs. Key skills and qualities currently required by community nurses ar
identified and discussed.

DEFINITIONS OF 'COMMUNITY'

Changes in terms of the location and nature of community nursing care provision
have occurred over the years in response to a variety of influencing factors. More
recently, we have seen a distinct shift of services from the hospital setting to primary
care and community locations (Turnbull, 2017; McGarry, 2003). Current health and
social care policy directives indicate that still more services will be provided within
the community context in the future (Scottish Government, 2013; Welsh Assembly
Government, 2013; Scottish Government, 2010; DHSSPSSNI, 2011; NHS England,
2014). In order to provide the required administrative and managerial infrastructure
to accommodate these changes, several major organisational reconfigurations have

location of care. By attempting to include the wide array of elements involved, the true complexity of nursing within the community begins to emerge. Although some of the challenges, such as interacting with patients and families in their own homes, are acknowledged within the literature (Luker et al., 2000; Quaile, 2016a), the meaning of 'community' within community nursing is often assumed and taken for granted (St John, 1998).

St John (1998: 63) interviewed community nurses who explained the nature of the communities they worked within in terms of 'geography; provision of resources; a network and target groups'. Some nurses described their communities as a 'client' or an entity, particularly where members of the community were connected. If a population was not connected, nurses defined community as the next largest connected element such as a group or family.

It would appear, therefore, that definitions of community often include the dimensions of people, geography or space and shared elements, relationships or interests and incorporate some form of interaction. Many of these common themes are captured in the following definition of 'community' as

> ... a social group determined by geographical boundaries and/or common values and interests. Its members know and interact with each other. It functions within a particular social structure and exhibits and creates certain norms, values and social institutions.
>
> (*WHO, 1974*)

Awareness of the networks that exist within a community helps in identifying opportunities or strategies to engage 'hidden' members of the population. 'Social capital' is a term used to explain networks and shared norms that form an essential component of effective community development (Wills, 2009). It is proposed that poor health is linked to low social capital and social exclusion where poverty or discrimination exist (Wilkinson, 2005). According to the National Occupational Standards in Community Development Work, the main aim of community development work is

> collectively to bring about social change and justice by working with communities to identify their needs, opportunities, rights and responsibilities; plan, organise and take action and evaluate the effectiveness and impact of the action all in ways which challenge oppressions and tackle inequalities.
>
> (*Lifelong Learning UK, 2009*)

Community development work is inclusive, empowering and collaborative in nature and is underpinned by the principles of equality and anti-discrimination, social justice, collective action, community empowerment and working and learning together.

A study by McGarry (2003) identifies the central position of the home and relationships that take place within it in defining the community nurse's role. Four key themes emerging from her research are 'being a guest' within the home, the maintenance of personal-professional boundaries, notions of holistic care and professional definitions of community. The findings highlight the tensions for nurses in embracing their personal perceptions of community nursing while trying to work effectively within the constraints of organisational and professional boundaries.

Kelly and Symonds (2003), in their exploration of the social construction of community nursing, discuss three key perspectives of the community nurse as carer, the community nurse as an agent of social control and community nursing as a unified discipline. The authors discuss the proposition that community nurses are still reliant on others to present the public image of community nursing that is portrayed. They argue, interestingly, that community nurses may not possess enough autonomy to define their own constructs and articulate these to others.

Community Links is a charitable organisation which, through its national work, shares lessons with government and community groups across the country to achieve social change. The charity's chief executive, Blake, believes the concept of community has become more complex and that a top-down or narrow definition may not be useful and can, in certain instances, have negative consequences. According to Blake (2013), community is a 'fluid, chaotic thing' and defining the concept is not essential and adds that 'It's the doing something together that is important'. People can belong to many different communities whether based on geography, ethnicity, religion, interest or other social factors such as disability or refugee status and this notion of multiple communities can strengthen and add value to communities. In addition, communities are not static and can change over time, presenting challenges to service providers who may need to adapt their interventions depending on the expressed needs of a community at any one time (Niven, 2013).

Niven (2013) interviewed five community leaders from different charitable and voluntary organisations and found that, although community identity is difficult to conceptualise, these leaders sensed that a strong desire from the public to be part of a community is returning.

FACTORS INFLUENCING THE DELIVERY OF COMMUNITY HEALTHCARE SERVICES

Community nurses face many challenges within their evolving roles. The transition from working in an institutional setting to working in the community can be somewhat daunting at first (Sines et al., 2013a). As a student on community placement or a newly employed staff nurse, it soon becomes apparent that there is a wide range of factors influencing the planning and delivery of community healthcare services. Within the home/community context, those issues that impact upon an individual's health are more apparent. People are encountered in their natural habitats rather than being isolated within the hospital setting. Assessment is so much more complex in the community, as the nurse must consider the interconnections between the various elements of a person's lifestyle. Chapter 7 explores the concept of assessment in more detail. In addition, community nurses are often working independently, making complex clinical decisions without the immediate support of the wider multidisciplinary team or access to a range of equipment and resources as would be the case in a hospital or other institutional healthcare environment. It is recognised, for example, that district nurses are frequently challenged with managing very complex care situations which require advanced clinical skills, sophisticated decision making and expert care planning (Quaile, 2016a). Ford (2016) also acknowledges the need for specialist district nurse practitioners to have expert knowledge and advanced clinical skills as well as highly developed interpersonal skills and a clear understanding of a whole systems approach.

Defining health is complex as it involves multiple factors. According to Blaxter (1990), health can be defined from four different perspectives: an absence of disease, fitness, ability to function and general well-being. The concept of health has many dimensions such as physical, mental, emotional, social, spiritual and societal. All aspects of health are interdependent in a holistic approach. It is prudent to view individuals within their wider context, when considering issues relating to their health and well-being to ensure that relevant social determinants are taken into account (Figure 1.1).

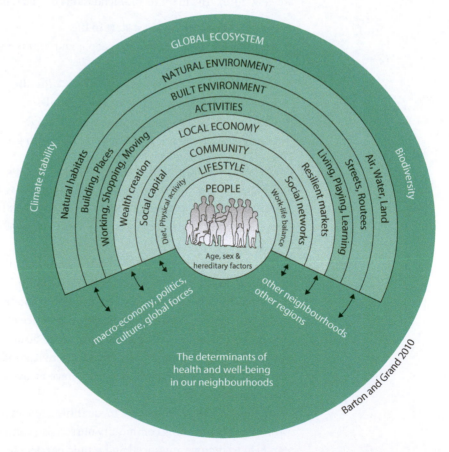

Figure 1.1 The health map. (From Barton H and Grant M., *Journal of the Royal Society for the Promotion of Health*, 126, 152–253, 2006.) The determinants of health and well-being in our neighbourhoods.

There are acknowledged inequalities in health status between different people within society and major determinants include social class, culture, occupation, income, gender and geographical location. Health inequalities were highlighted and 'put on the map' in the Black Report of 1980 (DHSS, 1980) and relate to the difference between groups or populations defined socially and demographically that are unfair, avoidable and remedial rather than innate differences between groups (Gillam et al., 2012). Several reports have been published since the 1980s, across the countries making up the United Kingdom, providing comprehensive reviews of the literature/research available on inequalities in health (DHSS, 1980; Acheson Report, 1998; *Marmot Review*, 2010; Welsh Government, 2014 DHSSPSNI, 2014; Scottish Government, 2016). Although these documents have sought to inform the national public health agenda of the day, the reality is that unacceptable inequalities remain.

Health inequalities are not random but related to the 'social gradient' in health: geographical locations with high levels of income deprivation typically have lower life expectancy. This relationship is referred to as the 'Marmot Curve' in the independent and influential report in England, *Fair Society, Healthy Lives* (*Marmot Review*, 2010). The main recommendations of this report are as follows:

- Giving every child the best start in life
- Enabling all children, young people and adults to maximise their capabilities and have control over their lives
- Creating fair employment and good work for all
- Ensuring a healthy standard of living for all
- Creating and developing healthy and sustainable places and communities
- Strengthening the role and impact of ill-health prevention

Disadvantaged children in Britain continue to experience poorer health outcomes than their wealthier counterparts, including increased levels of obesity and mental health conditions, and, according to child health experts, their future health and happiness are in jeopardy as a result (Royal College of Paediatrics and Child Health, 2017).

The *Marmot Review* (2010) states that people living in more disadvantaged communities die 7 years earlier on average than people living in more prosperous communities. Those in the poorest neighbourhoods will also experience more of their lives with a disability – an average difference of 17 years.

Bambra (2016), a leading expert in public health, draws on case studies from across the world to examine the social, environmental, economic and political causes of health inequalities, how they have evolved over time and what they are like today.

In order to improve health inequalities, Marmot (2010) suggests that health professionals, including community nurses, can contribute in three ways. First, they can help to remove any social and ethnic barriers to receiving healthcare. Second, they should act as advocates for their service users and work in collaboration with other health and social care providers. Finally, they should base health improvement initiatives/best practice on rigorous evidence and research so that strategies used are effective and replicable. In response to this, the DH (2010b) recognises that disadvantaged areas face the toughest challenges and are set to receive greater rewards for any health improvements made.

Buck and Maguire (2015) advocate a more nuanced and integrated policy response and state that, although there is some evidence of integration, an approach to health inequalities delivered through population health systems that clearly integrate NHS services with other public health services and public health initiatives is required.

Although there is some evidence of positive findings over the 2000s, continuing austerity will inevitably have consequences for health inequalities. In addition, it is essential that the implementation of policy at community level needs to reflect local knowledge, history and experience if it is to be realistic and effective (Buck and Maguire, 2015).

Chapter 2 explores key concepts relating to public health and health inequalities in greater detail.

The increased emphasis lately on the development of a primary care–led NHS has come about in response to demographic, technological, political and financial influences, among others. An increasing population of older people, shorter hospital stays, improvements in technology and patient preference have all contributed to the advocated movement of resources from the acute to the primary care sector.

The development of new competencies to provide services away from hospital settings means that an increasing number of people with both acute and long-term conditions will eventually receive care at home or in a range of other locations within the community. It is envisaged that hospitals will mainly provide diagnostic and specialist services in the future (NHS England, 2014).

If the aims of current policy directives are to be realised, plans to address the 'triple fragmentation' – between health and social care, primary and secondary care and physical and mental health services – as described by Stevens (2016) will need to be a priority (King's Fund, 2017).

MEETING THE NEEDS OF THE LOCAL POPULATION

Community nurses can identify the needs of their given population by conducting a health needs assessment, which is a process of gathering information from a variety of sources in order to assist the planning and development of services. As society is constantly changing, health needs assessment is not a static exercise.

The National Institute for Health and Care Excellence (NICE, 2017) defines 'health needs assessment' as

> A systematic process used by NHS organisations and local authorities to assess the health problems facing a population. This includes determining whether certain groups appear more prone to illness than others and pinpointing any inequalities in terms of service provision. It results in an agreed list of priorities to improve healthcare in a particular area.

Buck and Gregory (2013) recognise the need for a clear purpose and 'robust local framework based on outcomes-focused partnerships and commitment to systematic health impact assessment' to improve the public's health and tackle health inequalities. To this end, information is required regarding disease patterns (epidemiology) and public health in a particular area (locality/community/neighbourhood) as well as data regarding local environmental factors/resources (knowledge base/experience of community service providers), in other words, a combination of 'hard' (statistical/ research-based/quantitative) data and 'soft' (experiential/anecdotal/qualitative) data.

Qualitative information may include newspapers; meetings of agencies; diaries, meeting notes of local workers; projects undertaken by students on programmes of study; photographs and videos. Quantitative data will be obtained from a variety of sources but will consist mainly of statistical evidence and research-based studies (Hawtin and Percy-Smith, 2007).

Three key approaches to health needs assessment described by Coles and Porter (2008) are epidemiological, comparative and corporate. A comprehensive assessment would normally incorporate more than one of these approaches.

ACTIVITY 1.2

Reflection point
Consider the area/team within which you are working at present. What sources of information would help inform you of the specific needs of your client group/population? Make a list and try to divide the information into either 'hard' or 'soft' data.

Explore the different sources of data available to inform a health and social needs assessment of your local community. Much information can be obtained from the local council, libraries and Internet sources (see Further Resources list).

In capturing the 'essence' of a locality, the term 'community profile' is frequently used to describe an area in relation to its amenities, demography (characteristics of the population), public services, employment, transport and environment. Traditionally, health visitors, in particular, have been required to produce community profiles as a form of assessment during their training.

'Community profiling' can be defined as

> a comprehensive description of the needs of a population that is defined, or defines itself, as a community and the resources that exist within that community, carried out with the active involvement of the community itself, for the purpose of developing an action plan or other means of improving the quality of life of the community.
>
> *(Hawtin and Percy-Smith, 2007: 10)*

There are three interacting levels identified within profiling, which are

• Community – Assessment of need within a locality/neighbourhood
• Practice – Assessment of need within a GP practice
• Caseload – Assessment of need within a health professional's caseload

Any attempt to analyse the series of complex processes that makes up a living community without the participation of local residents/consumers is a fairly fruitless exercise. In gathering information from a large community population, a variety of methods may prove useful. An approach entitled Participatory Rapid Appraisal has been described elsewhere (Coles and Porter, 2008) and involves community members in the collection of information and related decision making. Originally used in developing countries to assess need within poor rural populations, it has been employed in deprived urban areas. A wide variety of data-collection methods is used and Participatory Rapid Appraisal involves local agencies and organisations working together. By working in partnership with local residents, action is taken by community members who have identified issues of local concern/interest and discussed potential solutions. Clearly, Participatory Rapid Appraisal could be used to help tackle specific issues as well as large-scale assessments.

Current government policy (DH, 2010a,b) stresses the importance of a localised approach to community healthcare service provision. Each locality is different in terms of its characteristics, which might include its demography, geographical location, environment, amenities, transport systems, unemployment levels, deprivation scores, work opportunities and access to services, for example. As a result of these potential variations, it is important to interpret national guidelines according to local needs. Each locality will have its own individualised local targets for public health tailored to the specific requirements of the local population. Such targets are usually chosen following an examination of local information sources, such as epidemiological data collected by the relevant Public Health Department, general practice profiles and caseload analysis data obtained from local healthcare practitioners, for example. Roberson (2016), following a comprehensive review of the literature relating to caseload management by district nursing teams, concludes that effective and efficient caseload management is essential in improving the quality of care to patients, and ensuring that limited valuable resources are used in the most appropriate way.

By systematically reviewing local information sources and working within government/professional guidelines, community nurses have an opportunity to develop practice and more collaborative ways of working.

Example 1.1

From general practice profile information, one locality identified a significantly high percentage of the older population with dementia. As a result, the community psychiatric nurse team working with older people in the locality liaised with the district nurses and practice nurses across the identified GP practices with a view to discussing the provision of support for the carers involved.

DH (2010a) highlights the importance of frontline staff taking responsibility for implementing changes in the NHS. This will involve community nurses becoming more actively involved in health needs assessment. Within the public health reports from the four countries across the United Kingdom, it has been recognised that there are populations whose healthcare needs are unmet, which presents community nurses with the challenge of redefining their services to more accurately respond to the needs of their particular patient group. Responding more appropriately is not an easy task as many of these unmet needs often require seeking out and might exist within the more disadvantaged sectors of society. It is not unreasonable to assume that many community nurses will require a greater understanding of different cultural issues and social value systems before they are able to identify specific unmet needs. The inverse care law means that, ironically, the more advantaged people in society tend to receive better healthcare services (Acheson, 1998; *Marmot Review*, 2010). Current NHS policy is attempting to rectify this anomaly and end the 'postcode lottery', which suggests you are able to determine your health status from the place where you live.

Although National Service Frameworks (NSFs) are national guidelines produced to encourage the dissemination of best practice in relation to particular conditions or client groups, it is the responsibility of frontline staff to implement them locally and interpret them according to local conditions.

ACTIVITY 1.3

Action point
In relation to the locality in which you are based within the community, find out about ways in which the NSFs are being implemented at a local level. Gather information regarding local initiatives and examples of any community nurses working in collaboration with other individuals/organisations/agencies in addressing the NSF guidelines.

THE COMPLEX NATURE OF THE ENVIRONMENT OF COMMUNITY HEALTHCARE

Kelly and Symonds (2003) discuss how community nurses have been obliged to conform to current views and power structures since the beginning of the nineteenth century. Even the caring nature of their role has been often overlooked as a result of influence from more powerful groups to conform to more stereotypical female roles and medical models of care. Recent shifts into community and primary healthcare have prompted community nurses to re-examine their position, which has involved empowering the more disadvantaged groups within society in the form of 'social support'. However, the development of the caring aspect of community nursing has been compromised by models of primary healthcare delivery in favour of activity that is more medically rather than socially focused.

An understanding of community care as a 'process' rather than a 'context' is proposed to enable us to value community nursing as advanced specialist practice in its own right rather than as institutional or acute care nursing in another setting. Appreciation of the true complexity of meeting the health and social care needs of service users in the community only really becomes evident with experience. Eng et al. (1992) encourage an 'understanding that a community is a "living" organism with interactive webs of ties among organisations, neighbourhoods, families and friends'. Recent research by

Jackson et al. (2015), using the Cassandra Matrix activity tool, indicates that their methodology has significant potential to measure the complexity of nursing work in community settings. This pioneering research may be able to help community nurses articulate the qualitative nature of more personalised, highly complex approaches to care in community settings rather than rely on measures that have traditionally only been able to capture more restricted task-based, quantitative activities.

ACTIVITY 1.4

Reflection point

Reflect on a health problem/issue that you or a family member or friend may have experienced. Consider the effects of this experience on everybody involved and the health and social care needs that resulted.

- Make a list of the identified health and social care needs of all those people involved.
- Were all of the needs addressed or met? If not, why not?
- Who was involved in meeting these needs?
- Consider the different sources of support, information, care, treatment and advice offered and given. Was the overall package of care well co-ordinated?
- Were there other potential sources of help that were untapped at the time?
- Were sources of care and support readily available or did they need seeking out?
- Were self-care strategies employed in any way?
- With hindsight, how would you rate the quality of care and support received/ obtained?
- What do you consider to be the most important elements of high-quality care provision?

On reflecting on the above activity, you may have identified service providers from statutory, voluntary or charitable agencies and organisations. Individuals responsible for assessing, planning, delivering and evaluating care based on apparent needs may have been professionally qualified or not. Sources of support may have come from recognised services or consisted of more informal networks. Information to help you make sense of the experience could be accessed in a variety of ways. Frustrations, concerns and reassurance at the time will probably have linked to a range of factors – such as interpersonal communication, transport, accessibility of services, effectiveness of treatment, information available and financial issues, for example.

The National Nursing Research Unit (NNRU, 2011) has conducted research measuring patient experience in the primary care sector that included patients with different illnesses/conditions. Generic themes that were important to patients included being treated as a person; staff who listen and spend time; individualised treatment and no labelling; feeling informed, receiving information and given options; patient involvement in care-efficient processes; and emotional and psychological support. The authors highlight the need for policy makers to start to consider the relational aspects of a patient's experience more – such as compassion, empathy and emotional support – as well as the functional aspects of service provision – such as access, waiting and food. Such information can only be collected from patients and carers themselves.

The community environment is a fascinating yet complicated matrix of elements. There are myriad individuals, groups, agencies and organisations involved in the delivery of health and social care. Potential barriers to effective co-ordination of services and support include different management systems and ways of working between organisations, conflicting ideologies or philosophies of care of service providers, a variety of communication networks and channels, and power differentials and stereotyping between different groups in society.

COMMUNITY NURSES: KEEPING THE FOCUS ON PERSON-CENTRED CARE

Clearly, there are differences between communities in terms of the locations in which community healthcare services are offered to service users. Provision will vary considerably between a very rural community as opposed to an urban one. For example, in a rural location, there might tend to be more community hospitals, providing more accessible local services that are not of a specialist nature whereas walk-in centres, for example, tend to be located in more densely populated areas such as city centres and airports.

Community nursing takes place in a wide variety of settings.

ACTIVITY 1.5

Action point
From personal or professional experience, list as many different locations as you can where community nurses provide care. This might help you to identify a wide range of community nursing roles.

In the early 1990s, the United Kingdom Central Council for Nursing, Midwifery and Health Visiting United Kingdom Central Council for Nursing, Midwifery and Health Visiting (UKCC) conducted the PREP project to clarify the future training requirements for post-registration nurses in terms of education and practice. At the time, eight community specialist practice disciplines were identified and included occupational health nursing, community children's nursing, community nursing learning disability, community mental health nursing, general practice nursing, school nursing, health visiting and district nursing. The UKCC (1994) proposed a common core-centred course for all specialities, which was to be at first degree level at least and 1 year in length. According to the UKCC (1994), the remit of community specialist practice embraces 'clinical nursing care, risk identification, disease prevention, health promotion, needs assessment and a contribution to the development of public health services and policy'. Clearly, a higher level of decision making is involved in specialist community nursing practice.

A brief synopsis of each of the eight community specialist practice nursing roles is offered below. For a more detailed discussion of the roles of these community nurses, please refer to Sines et al. (2013b).

Occupational health nursing

Occupational health nursing is a relatively new nursing discipline that has developed from its origins in 'industrial nursing' in the mid-nineteenth century when the role was mainly curative rather than preventative.

Occupational health nurses are in charge of safeguarding public health in the workplace setting and their role is varied (RCN, 2017).

Occupational health nurses (OHNs) work within the wider occupational health services and engage in preventative activities to advise employers, employees and their representatives on health and safety issues in the working environment and the adaptation of the working environment to the capabilities of the employees (RCN, 2017).

Key skills of the OHN include risk assessment, health surveillance and health promotion and health protection. Attendance management and the use of strategies to enable a successful return to work following an accident or serious illness are seen as important elements of the role of the OHN (The Council for Work and Health, 2016).

OHNs holding an appropriate qualification are eligible for registration on the third part of the Nursing and Midwifery Council (NMC) register for Specialist Community Public Health Nursing (SCPHN), which was established in 2004.

O'Reilly (2015) provides an interesting discussion of recent developments in health and well-being at work, reviewing the latest research of relevance, and considers the role of OHNs in the future.

Community children's nursing

Over the past decade, there has been a rapid expansion of community children's nursing (CCN) services and this development has been supported by a number of pertinent government reports.

There are three key elements within the delivery of CCN services, which are (1) first contact/acute assessment, diagnosis, treatment and referral of children; (2) continuing care, chronic disease management and meeting the imperatives of the Children's National Service Framework; and (3) public health/health protection and promotion programmes – working with children and families to improve health and reduce the impact of illness and disability (RCN, 2014a). The role of the community children's nurse encompasses education, training, emotional support and expert clinical care and requires high-order cognitive skills in relation to decision making, problem solving and solution finding (Carter et al., 2009).

The CCN works with children, young people, their parents/carers and families alongside the wider children's workforce across health, education and social care and should be able to engage and communicate with children and young people in shared decision making (Carter et al., 2009).

The required educational preparation to become an advanced community children's nurse practitioner (RCN, 2014b) – with the required skills to work across a range of situations and environments for children and young people with acute, long-term, continuing and palliative care nursing needs – has been under discussion more recently and professional guidance is offered by the RCN (2014c).

Community nursing learning disability

According to Barr (2009), in the mid-1970s there was recognition of the need for more community-based services to be provided for people with learning disabilities living at home and their families. Around this time, different models of service were developing around the notion of 'normalisation', which is the underlying philosophy of many of the services provided for people with learning disabilities. Normalisation may be defined as 'a complex system which sets out to value positively devalued individuals and groups' (Race, 1999).

Service principles for learning disability services should place people with learning disabilities at the centre of care; provide care in an attractive environment; have clear arrangements for safeguarding; provide access to independent advocacy services; be open to internal and external scrutiny; and have comprehensive training in place for staff (RCN, 2014d).

The role of community nurses for people with learning disabilities (CNLDs) has changed markedly over the past few years. It is becoming more health focused and a particular emphasis in the future will be with people who have increasingly complex physical and mental health needs.

A study by Mafuba and Gates (2015) demonstrates the valuable role of the community learning disability nurses in health surveillance, health promotion, health facilitation, health prevention and protection, health education and healthcare delivery.

Concern has been expressed recently about the dwindling numbers of CNLDs and reduction of students undertaking specialist programmes of study for this discipline.

Jukes and Aspinall (2015) assert that

> What is clear within learning disability nursing and services is the demand for leadership in the quest for improving the quality and effectiveness of services across health and social care.

The authors discuss the need to pursue a framework- such as the Promoting Action on Research Implementation in Health Services (PARiHS) model – that promotes and focuses on integrating knowledge transfer into services for people with a learning disability and the inherent challenges.

Community mental health nursing

The community mental health nursing (CMHN) service has been well documented since its inception in the mid-1950s. The expertise of the CMHN lies in assessing the mental health of an individual within a family and social context. CMHNs may be located in health centres, GP practices, voluntary organisations and accident and emergency departments. They represent people with mental health needs and provide high-quality therapeutic care. Five elements underpin the professional practice of CMHNs (McLaughlin and Long, 2009). First, a guiding paradigm within CMHN involves respecting, valuing and facilitating the growth unique within each individual (Rogers, 1990). Second, therapeutic presence is needed to restore clients' dignity and worth as healthy, unique human beings. Third, the therapeutic encounter is essential for healing and growth. Fourth, the principles of CMHN include the search for recognised and unrecognised mental health needs; the prevention of a disequilibrium in mental health; the facilitation of mental health–enhancing activities; therapeutic approaches to mental healthcare and influences on policies affecting mental health, and, finally, the National Service Framework (DH, 1999).

CMHNs work with individuals and groups of people across the lifespan responding to the current needs of the young (Pym, 2016) as well as the older population (DH, 2016).

Although several models are emerging in the organisation, delivery and evaluation of community mental health services, the guiding principles remain the same. Collaboration between government, local authorities, the voluntary and statutory services, and community groups both nationally and locally is pivotal in improving the nation's mental health as we strive to achieve 'parity of esteem' between mental and physical health and related services (NHS England, 2016).

General practice nursing

Nurses have been working in general practice for over 100 years (Sines et al., 2013a). Since the early 1990s, the number of practice nurses has grown considerably in response to the demands of general practice.

Practice nurses frequently fulfil the role of 'gatekeeper' and are relatively easily accessible and acceptable to patients as they are located within GP surgeries. The role of the practice nurse is wide ranging and covers all age groups within the practice population. Three key aspects of the role are first contact, public health and long-term condition management (Sines et al., 2013a). Practice nurses have become involved in the implementation of NSF guidelines at a local level and often play a key role in establishing nurse-led clinics to tackle public health targets.

In order to develop innovative ways of delivering services with a changing skill mix within general practice, practice nurses will require well-developed leadership and management skills in the future (QNI, 2015) in responding to the well-documented pressures in general practice (Baird et al., 2016).

In England, clear guidance is now available for general practice nurses following the development and publication of the General Practice Nursing Service Education and Career Framework by Health Education England (HEE) (2015). Alongside this, the Queen's Nursing Institute (QNI) and QNI Scotland are currently updating the standards for General Practice Nursing Education and Practice.

School nursing

School nurses have been employed within the school health service for more than 100 years and are seen as central to child-focused public health practice (Jameson and Thurtle, 2009).

Key aspects of the school nurse's role include the assessment of health needs of children and school communities, agreement of individual and school plans and delivery of these through multidisciplinary partnerships; playing a key role in immunisation and vaccination programmes; contributing to personal and health and social education and to citizenship training; working with parents to promote positive parenting; offering support and counselling, promoting positive mental health in young people and advising and co-ordinating healthcare to children with medical needs.

School nurses holding an appropriate qualification are eligible for registration on the third part of the NMC register for SCPHN:

> With the development of children's trusts and the provision of statutory guidance on interagency working and co-operation to improve the well-being of children and young people, school nurses need to work hard to build links with education and social care teams.
>
> *(Sines et al., 2013a)*

Health visiting

The health visiting service has been in existence for more than 100 years and has its roots in public health and concern about poor health. The overall aim of the service is the promotion of health and the prevention of ill health. According to the Council for the Education and Training of Health Visitors (CETHV, 1977), the four main elements of the health visitor's (HV) role include the search for health needs; stimulation of awareness of health needs; influence on policies affecting health; and facilitation of health-enhancing activities.

HVs holding an appropriate qualification are eligible for registration on the third part of the NMC register for SCPHN.

HVs need to engage actively in public health work, with individuals, families, groups and communities working collaboratively with the full range of community services (Sines et al., 2013b). Recent government directives (DH, 2010a) have highlighted the need for HVs to maintain a focus on children and families. At the same time, the profession is keen to develop their future roles in consultation with the public they serve.

District nursing

District nurses (DNs) can trace their roots back to the mid-1800s at least, and the historical development of the service is well recorded. They used to work in relative isolation but are more likely nowadays to work within a team. The role of the district nurse has evolved over time in response to political influences and the changing needs of the populations served. Although it is acknowledged that the role of the district nursing service is not clearly defined, it involves the assessment, organisation and delivery of care to support people living in their own homes. Current research, however, by Jackson et al. (2015), using the Cassandra Matrix Activity tool, has the potential to assist community and district nurses in demonstrating the complex nature of their work in the near future. The current work of the district nurse includes responsibility for providing pathways of nursing care during acute, long-term (Carrier and Newbury, 2016) and terminal illness and is detailed in the new vision and model for district nursing (DH/NHS/QNI, 2013). The majority of people on the district nurse's caseload tend to be from the older generation – an often vulnerable and marginalised group of people within society.

Again, like their GPN colleagues, DNs have clear guidance in England, following the development and publication of the District Nursing Service Education and Career Framework by Health Education England (HEE, 2015). In addition, the Queen's Nursing Institute (QNI) and QNI Scotland have developed and published updated Voluntary Standards for District Nurse Education and Practice (QNI/QNIS, 2015).

With the current pressures on health and social care, there has been renewed attention on the pivotal role of the DN in leading and managing complex care at home (Chalk and Legg, 2017). The value of the DN's role in caring for patients at home, avoiding unnecessary hospital admissions, cannot be underestimated. Equally, DNs are central to ensuring effective discharge planning (QNI, 2016). The King's Fund Report entitled 'Understanding Quality in District Nursing Services' (Maybin et al., 2016) highlights the dissonance between the policy incentive to promote care in community settings and the capacity problems being experienced in district nursing services, and, among its recommendations, proposes the development of a rigorous framework to assess and monitor the quality of care in the community (Quaile, 2016b). Ongoing work by the QNI on what constitutes a safe caseload to protect staff well-being while also ensuring high-quality and safe patient care – comprising holistic care and care continuity – within current resources will further inform the debate (While, 2016).

In addition to the community specialist practitioner nursing roles identified above, there are, of course, many other community nursing roles. Numerous specialist nurses work within the community environment and these include roles that link specifically to a particular condition or illness (such as the specialist nurse for diabetes) or to a group of conditions, such as long-term conditions (Community Matron). Other community nurses work with specific client groups, such as homeless or older people. A range of different titles exists for various roles and often the terms 'specialist' or 'advanced' practitioner are applied. Such a plethora of titles can cause confusion and form part of the wider ongoing specialist-generalist debate within community nursing circles.

Begley et al. (2014) conclude from their research that healthcare policy makers believe that specialists and advanced practitioners contribute to higher quality patient/client care, particularly at a strategic level, and could make an important contribution to future health service developments, particularly in relation to long-term conditions management and community care, where more advanced practitioner posts are required.

THE FUTURE VISION

In order to provide high-quality care to patients, community nurses need the necessary skills, knowledge and expertise, and it is the responsibility of individual practitioners and their employing authority to ensure that appropriate preparatory education and training are organised.

Workforce planning assists employing authorities in predicting future demand in terms of recruitment and education of new staff and the continuing professional development of existing staff. In addition, employers develop and update policies and procedures in relation to the clinical responsibilities of community nurses, and these should relate to the latest benchmarking criteria and government/professional guidelines. The views of service users and carers should influence the preparation of health and social care service providers (NNRU, 2011) and evidence will be required that this is the case in the future (NHS England, 2014). 'The Five Year Forward View' in England states the need to capture 'the renewable energy represented by patients and communities' and 'engage with communities and citizens in new ways, involving them directly in decisions about the future of health and care services'. Seale (2016) explores innovative ideas on establishing more collaborative relationships among professionals, patients, carers and communities based on project work conducted by the King's Fund.

Recent government reforms in terms of the structures and systems that form the NHS (NHS England, 2014) have led to an acknowledgement by community nurses that their roles and responsibilities need to be examined and redefined in preparation for the new challenges ahead. Leadership, practice development and partnership working are key elements within the roles of all community nurses.

As far back as 1995, Hyde stated that applying the concept 'community nurse' across all the different disciplines was unhelpful and confusing and that the concept has become popular as a result of the following myths, which still largely hold true today:

- Community nursing is the same as hospital nursing: skills are simply transferred to a different setting.
- Community nursing is peripheral to the centrality of hospital nursing.
- Community nursing is primarily about visiting the sick.
- All community nurses share a unified vision of the nature of care.

(Hyde, 1995: 2)

It is important for community nurses to critically examine the concept of 'community nurse' and how it has evolved over time if they are to influence their future professional development and emphasise their caring role.

At present, the future educational preparation of many community nursing disciplines is under review by the government, relevant professional bodies and community nurses themselves. In England, recent concerns regarding ongoing problems recruiting to specialist post-registration educational programmes have prompted Health Education England, in collaboration with Public Health England, to set up a review into the educational preparation of community nurses and how this is commissioned. The issues involved relate to health visitors, district nurses and school nurses, in particular, with a suggestion that practice nursing courses are expected to attract more registrants than planned. HEE has identified the need for new models of training to develop the community workforce to meet the demand from their ever-changing local populations and this will also involve community learning disability nursing (Merrifield, 2017).

At a time of qualified staff reductions due to the economic climate, increasing demand for health services is leading to an emphasis on improving productivity by changing the skill mix within community nursing teams and working in different ways. Many community nurses are fearful that care will be compromised if person-centred approaches are replaced by task allocation models of care. Concerns revolve around the potential loss of a holistic approach, which would lead to fragmentation of care, lack of continuity and poorer quality services.

Recent reports (Care Quality Commission, 2016: Nuffield Trust and King's Fund, 2016: Triggle and Rhodes, 2016) have highlighted the current state of our health and social care services and the very real challenges they face.

In response, priorities for the future have been identified by the King's Fund (2017) and include supporting new care models centred on the needs of patients; strengthening and implementing collaborative ways of working; improving productivity and delivering better value; developing and strengthening leadership at all levels and securing adequate funding for health and social care.

Many community nurses are concerned that this situation will worsen if community nurses are not adequately prepared for their demanding and challenging roles and more collaborative relationships are not established between professionals, patients, carers and communities. Interestingly, Community Links (2011) has produced a literature review of the role of effective relationships in public services entitled *Deep Value*. This review describes the value created when relationships in public services are effective, including both improved service outcomes and wider benefits for service users. It concludes that improving the effectiveness of relationships is therefore an important strategy for improving quality and performance.

Baird, who is currently developing a vision for the future of community-based health services, founded on an evidence-based UK-wide and international review of best practice models of service, states that:

> …people increasingly live with long-term conditions for a significant part of their lives and need good-quality care where they live. If the ambition is to move from high-cost, reactive and bed-based care to care that is preventive, proactive and based closer to people's homes, then health and care leaders at all levels must ensure that there is upfront investment in community services and that those services are clearly explained, visible and easily accessible. (Baird, 2017: 2)

FURTHER RESOURCES

www.ons.gov.uk – Independent information to improve our understanding of the UK's economy and society

www.neighbourhood.statistics.gov.uk – Detailed statistics within specific geographical areas

www.imd.communities.gov.uk

www.census.gov.uk – Index of Multiple Deprivation – statistics available at ward level

www.poverty.org.uk – UK site for statistics on poverty and social exclusion

www.direct.gov.uk – Public services all in one place – according to postcode

www.ic.nhs.uk – NHS Information Centre for health and social care

www.qof.ic.nhs.uk – Quality and Outcomes Framework – GP practice results database

www.marmotreview.org – Baseline figures for some key indicators of the social determinants of health, health outcomes and social inequalities for specific geographical areas

http://content.digital.nhs.uk/social-care – Information on adult social care for planning, delivering and monitoring services

www.hse.gov.uk/Statistics/industry/healthservices/index.htm – Health and Safety Executive – Health and Social Care sectorhttps://digital.nhs.uk/ – New name for Health and Social Care Information Centre

www.ninis2.nisra.gov.uk/public/Theme.aspx?themeNumber=134 – Statistics and information on public health, health services, social care and health and safety at work in Northern Ireland

www.gov.scot/Topics/Statistics/Browse/Health – Range of information on health and social care – Scottish Government

https://statswales.gov.wales/catalogue/Health-and-Social-care – Comprehensive set of information on health, health services and social services in Wales

REFERENCES

Acheson D (1998) *Independent Inquiry into Inequalities in Health Report*. London: The Stationery Office.

Alderwick H, Dunn P, McKenna H et al. (2016) *Sustainability and transformation plans in the NHS: How are they being developed in practice?*, London: King's Fund

Barr O (2009) Community nursing learning disability. In: Sines D, Saunders M and Forbes–Burford J (eds) *Community Health Care Nursing*, 4th edn. Chichester: Wiley–Blackwell.

Baird B, Charles A, Honeyman M, et al. (2016) *Understanding Pressures in General Practice*. London: King's Fund

Baird B (2017) *A Vision for the Future of Community-based Health Services*. London: King's Fund. https://www.kingsfund.org.uk/blog/2017/01/taking-right-approach-community-based-health-services, Accessed January 18, 2017.

Bambra C (2016) *Health Divides: Where You Live Can kill You*, Bristol: Policy Press.

Barton H and Grant M (2006) A health map for the local human habitat. The Journal of the *Royal Society for the Promotion of Health* 126:252–3.

Begley C, Murphy K, Higgins A and Cooney A (2014) Policy makers' views on impact of specialist and advanced practitioner roles in Ireland: The SCAPE study. *Journal of Nursing Management* 22:40 pp, 410–22.

Blake G (2013) cited in: Niven, (2013) The complexity of defining community, Guardian newspaper (Accessed 18 January 2017) https://www.theguardian.com/voluntary-sector-network/2013/may/03/community-spurs-fans.

Blaxter M (1990) *Health and Lifestyles*. London: Routledge.

Buck D and Gregory S (2013) *Improving the Public's Health: A Resource for Local Authorities*. London: King's Fund.

Buck D and Maguire D (2015) *Inequalities in Life Expectancy*. London: King's Fund.

Care Quality Commission (2016) *The State of Health Care and Adult Social Care in England 2015/16*, London: CQC

Carr S (2001) Nursing in the community—Impact of context on the practice agenda. *Journal of Clinical Nursing* 10: 330–6.

Carrier J and Newbury G (2016) Managing long-term conditions in primary and community care. *British Journal of Community Nursing* 21(10):504–8.

Carter B, Coad J, Goodenough T, Anderson C and Bray L (2009) *Community Children's Nursing in England: An Appreciative Review of CCNs*. Department of Health in collaboration with the University of Lancashire and the University of the West of England.

Cohen AP (1985) *The Symbolic Construction of Community*. London: Routledge.

Coles L and Porter E (eds) (2008) *Public Health Skills: A Practical Guide for Nurses and Public Health Practitioners*. Oxford: Blackwell Publishing.

Community Links (2011) *Deep Value. A Literature Review of the Role of Effective Relationships in Public Services*. London: Community Links.

Council for the Education and Training of Health Visitors (CETHV) (1977) *An Investigation into the Principles of Health Visiting*. London: CETHV.

The Council for Work and Health (2016) Planning the future: Implications for occupational health; delivery and training. http://www.councilforworkandhealth.org.uk/images/uploads/library/Final%20Report%20-%20Planning%20the%20Future%20-%20Implications%20for%20OH%20-%20Proof%202.pdf, Accessed January 23, 2017.

Department of Health (DH) (1997) *The New NHS: Modern, Dependable*. London: HMSO.

DH (1999) *National Service Framework for Mental Health: Modern Standards and Service Models*. London: Department of Health.

DH (2010a) *Equity and Excellence: Liberating the NHS*. London: HMSO.

DH (2010b) *Healthy Lives, Healthy People*. London: HMSO. Department of Health/Department for Education and Skills (DH/DfES) (2004) *National Service Framework for Children, Young People and Maternity Services: Core Standards*. London: The Stationery Office.

DH/NHS/QNI (2013) *Care in Local Communities: A New Vision and Model for District Nursing*, London: DH/NHS/QNI.

DH (2016) *Making a Difference in Dementia: Nursing vision and strategy*. London: DH.

Department of Health and Social Security (DHSS) (1980) *Inequalities in Health (The Black Report)*. London: HMSO.

DHSSPS (2010) *Healthy Futures 2010–2015: The Contribution of Health Visitors and School Nurses in Northern Ireland*. Belfast: DHSSPSNI.

Department of Health, Social Services and Public Safety (DHSSPSNI) (2011) Transforming Your Care. A review of Health and Social care in Northern Ireland. http://www.transformingyourcare.hscni.net/wp-content/uploads/2012/10/Transforming-Your-Care-Review-of-HSC-in-NI.pdf, Accessed January 18, 2017.

DHSSPSNI (2014) *Making Life Better: A Whole System Strategic Framework for Public Health 2013-2023*. Belfast: DHSSPSNI.

Eng E, Salmon ME and Mullan F (1992) Community empowerment: the critical base for primary health care. *Family and Community Health* 15:1–12.

Ford, S (2016) All district nurses 'should have specialist qualification', Nursing Times. (Accessed 20 January 2017) http://www.nursingtimes.net/news/community/all-district-nurses--should-have-specialist-qualification/7005789.fullarticle.

Gillam, S, Yate, J and Badrinath, P (2012) *Essential Public Health: Theory and Prcatice*, 2nd edn. New York, NY: Cambridge University Press.

Hawtin M and Percy-Smith J (2007) *Community Profiling: A Practical Guide*. Milton Keynes: Open University Press.

Health Education England (2015) *District Nursing and General Practice Nursing Service Education and Career Framework*. London: HEE.

Hickey G and Hardyman R (2000) Using questionnaires to ask nurses about working in the community: Problems of definition. *Health and Social Care in the Community* 8:70–8.

Hyde V (1995) Community nursing: a unified discipline? In Cain P, Hyde V and Howkins É (eds) *Community Nursing: Dimensions and Dilemmas*. London: Arnold.

Jameson M and Thurtle V (2009) School nursing. In Sines D, Saunders M and Forbes–Burford J (eds) *Community Health Care Nursing*, 4th edn. Chichester: Wiley–Blackwell.

Jackson, C, Leadbetter, T, Manley, K, Martin, A and Wright, T (2015), Making the complexity of community nursing visible: the Cassandra project. *British Journal of Community Nursing* 20(3):126–33.

Jukes, M and Asinall, SL (2015), Leadership and learning disability nursing. *British Journal of Nursing* 24(18):912–16.

Kelly A and Symonds A (2003) *The Social Construction of Community Nursing*. Basingstoke: Palgrave Macmillan.

King's Fund (2017) *Priorities for the NHS and Social Care in 2017*. London: King's Fund

Laverack G (2009) *Public Health. Power, Empowerment and Professional Practice*. Basingstoke: Palgrave Macmillan.

Lifelong Learning UK (2009) *National Occupational Standards for Community Development*. London: Lifelong Learning UK.

Luker K, Austin L, Caress A and Hallett C (2000) The importance of 'knowing the patient': Community nurses' constructions of quality in providing palliative care. *Journal of Advanced Nursing* 31:775–82.

Mafuba, K and Gates, B (2015), An investigation into the public health roles of community learning disability nurses. *British ournal of Learning Disability* 43(1):1–7.

Marmot Review (2010) *Fair Society, Healthy Lives: Strategic Review of Health Inequalities in England Post–2010*. London: The Marmot Review.

Maybin, J, Charles, A, and Honeyman, M (2016) *Understanding Quality in District Nursing Services*. London: King's Fund.

McGarry J (2003) The essence of 'community' within community nursing: a district nursing perspective. *Health and Social Care in the Community* 11:423–30.

McLaughlin D and Long A (2009) Community mental health nursing. In Sines D, Saunders M and Forbes–Burford J (eds) *Community Health Care Nursing*, 4th edn. Chichester: Wiley–Blackwell.

Merrifield, N (2017), Ongoing problems with filling community nurse training course places spark national review, *Nursing Times News*—6 January 2017.

National Institiute for Health and Care Excellence (2017) *Glossary.* London: NICE.

National Nursing Research Unit (NNRU) (2011) *Measuring Patient Experience in the Primary Care Sector: Does a Patient's Condition Influence What Matters?* London: NNRU.

NHS England (2014) Five Year Forward View. (Accessed 18 January 2017) https://www.england.nhs.uk/wp-content/uploads/2014/10/5yfv-web.pdf.

NHS England (2016) *The Five year Forward View for Mental Health.* London: NHS England.

Niven (2013) The complexity of defining community, Guardian newspaper. (Accessed 18 January 2017) https://www.theguardian.com/voluntary-sector-network/2013/may/03/community-spurs-fans.

Nuffield Trust/King's Fund (2016) *Social Care for Older People: Home Truths.* London: Nuffield Trust/King's Fund.

O'Reilly, N (2015) Evolution of occupational health 2: Occupational health at the crossroads. *Occupational Health* 67(10).

Parliamentary and Health Service Ombudsman (2011) *Care and Compassion? Report of the Health Service Ombudsman on Ten Investigations into NHS Care of Older People.* London: The Stationery Office.

Pym, H (2016) Mental health survey reveals pressure on young, BBC news (Health)—29 September 2017.

Quaile A (2016a) Ensuring the district nursing role does not die out. *British Journal of Community Nursing* 21(9): 430–32.

Quaile A (2016b) Demand on district nursing services leaving staff 'on their knees' says King's Fund. *British Journal of Community Nursing* 21(10): 490–1.

Queen's Nursing Institute (2015) *General Practice Nursing in the 21st Century: A Time of Opportunity.* London:QNI.

QNI/QNIS (2015) *The QNI/QNIS Voluntary Standards for District Nurse Education and Practice.* London/Edinburgh: QNI/QNIS.

QNI (2016). *Discharge Planning: Best Practice in Transitions of Care.* London: QNI.

Race DG (1999) *Social Role Valorisation and the English Experience.* London: Whiting and Birch.

Rogers CR (1990) *Client Centred Therapy.* London: Constable.

Roberson C (2016) Caseload management methods for use with district nursing teams: A literature review. *British Journal of Community Nursing*21(5):248–55.

Royal College of Nursing (2014a) *Children and Young People's Nursing: A Philosophy of Care.* London: RCN.

Royal College of Nursing (2014b) *The Future for Community Children's Nursing: Challenges and Opportunities.* London: RCN.

Royal College of Nursing (2014c) *Specialist and Advanced Practice for Children and Young People.* London: RCN.

Royal College of Nursing (2014d) *Learning from the Past—Setting out the Future: Developing Learning Disability Nursing in the UK. An RCN Position Statement on the Role of the Learning Disability Nurse.* London: RCN.

Royal College of Nursing (RCN) (2017) Occupational Health Nursing. (Accessed 23 January 2017) https://www.rcn.org.uk/clinical-topics/public-health/specialist-areas/occupational-health.

Royal College of Paediatrics and Child Health (2017) *State of Child Health Report*. London: RCPCH

Scottish Government (2010) *The Healthcare Quality Strategy for NHS Scotland*. Edinburgh: Scottish Government.

Scottish Government (2013) A route map to the 2020 vision for Health and Social Care. (Accessed 18 January 2017) http://www.gov.scot/Resource/0042/00423188.pdf.

Scottish Government (2016) *2015 Review of Public Health in Scotland: Strengthening the Function and Refocusing Action for a Healthier Scotland*. Edinburgh: Scottish Government.

Seale, B (2016) *Patients as Partners: Building Collaborative Relationships Among Professionals, Patients, Carers and Communities*. London: King's Fund.

Sines D, Saunders M and Forbes–Burford J (2013a) (eds) *Community Health Care Nursing*, 4th edn. Chichester: Wiley–Blackwell.

Sines, D, Aldridge-Bent, S, Fanning, A, Farrelly, P, Potter, K and Wright, J (eds) (2013b), *Community and Public Health Nursing*, 5th edn. Chichester: Wiley-Blackwell

Smith A (2010) District nursing: An endangered species? *Journal of Community Nursing* 24:44.

St John W (1998) Just what do we mean by community? Conceptualisations from the field. Health and Social Care in the Community 6:63–70.

Stevens, S (2016) Keynote Lecture at QNI conference in London—September 2016.

Triggle, N and Rhodes, D (2016), Elderlyfailed by 'shameful' care system, BBC News—17 November 2016.

Turnbull, A (2017) More care must be in homes, says chief nursing officer. http://www.independentnurse.co.uk/news-ezine/More-care-must-be-in-homes-says-chief-nursing-officer/149732/298809/, Accessed January 18, 2017.

UKCC (1994) *Standards for Specialist Education and Practice*. London: UKCC.

Welsh Assembly Government (2013) Delivering safe care, compassionate care. (Accessed 18 January 2017) http://gov.wales/docs/dhss/report/130710safecarefen.pdf.

Welsh Government (2014) *Listening to You—Your Health Matters*. Cardiff: Welsh Government.

While A (2016), Quality versus quantity in district nursing. *British Journal of Community Nursing* 21(11): 586.

Wilkinson R (2005) *The Impact of Inequality. How to Make Sick Societies Healthier*. London: Routledge.

Wills J (2009) Community development. In Sines D, Saunders M and Forbes–Burford J (eds) *Community Health Care Nursing*, 4th edn. Chichester: Wiley–Blackwell.

World Health Organization (WHO) Expert Committee on Community Health Nursing (1974) *Community Health Nursing, Report of a WHO Expert Committee* (Technical Report Series no. 558). Geneva: World Health Organization.

Public health and the promotion of well-being

Fiona Baguley

LEARNING OUTCOMES

- Examine the principles of public health, health and well-being.
- Explore the relevance of public health to community nursing.
- Appraise the concept of health and ways of determining health need.
- Critically analyse opportunities for nurses to positively influence health and well-being of populations, families and individuals in the community setting.

INTRODUCTION

This chapter explores public health, identifies the relationship between health and well-being and discusses the relevance to community nursing. The intention is to reaffirm the importance and highlight the opportunities nurses have to positively influence the health of the public and to promote well-being at individual or community (population) levels.

Throughout the chapter there are activities presented to support learning and development; they are also intended to act as a catalyst to foster a deeper understanding of public health through reflection and informed discussion.

HEALTH AND WELL-BEING

As healthcare practitioners who foster a holistic approach to care assessment and delivery it is important to understand what health, well-being and public health are and the differences between them. The community practitioner should also have knowledge and understanding of the relationship of cause and effect and how it impacts on care delivery, treatment and outcome.

Health

The World Health Organization (WHO) defines health as

> a state of complete physical, mental and social well-being and not merely the absence of disease or infirmity.

(WHO, 1946: 2)

While the word 'complete' might render the definition as idealistic and perhaps unattainable, the definition does acknowledge that health is a multidimensional issue, with well-being as an integral part, including the physical, mental and social aspects. Subsequent WHO publications have contextualised the definition and presented it in light of the importance of recognising underpinning health determinants and influencing factors such as income, education and social exclusion/inclusion (WHO, 2006).

According to Raymond (2005), health can be conceptualised from several perspectives as shown in Box 2.1.

Box 2.1 Concepts of health (Raymond, 2005)

- A biomedical perspective, which emphasises medical interventions to treat disease, and is mainly concerned with functional capacity
- A behavioural perspective, which emphasises individual responsibility for health-influencing behaviour
- A social perspective, which focuses on social and political determinants of health and emphasises social justice

---

In their discussion paper, Huber et al., (2011) identify the physical, mental and social aspects of health and the assessment of health. Discussion takes place around the definition of health and introduces the concept of health being the ability to change and self-direct. Concepts can be applied to individuals, groups or communities and could be seen to relate directly the concepts of empowerment and resilience on several levels.

Naidoo and Wills (2015) challenge the adequacy of the preceding perspectives and suggest that no single theory sufficiently explains the health experience. Moreover, they state that health is considered to be the unique experience of the individual while at the same time being influenced by external factors (Naidoo and Wills, 2015).

From the above it is clear that defining what health is can be complex and wider than a lack of disease.

ACTIVITY 2.1

Consider the relevance of these definitions to the role of the nurse in relation to the nurse as an
- Empowering agent
- Enabler
- Supporter of self-managed care and wellness to people in their care and people in the local community

---

Well-being

When reading the WHO definition of health above is it noteworthy that the concept of well-being is integral. Well-being as a notion applies to all individuals, regardless of their physical or psychological state (Sines et al., 2013). The term 'well-being' was analysed by the Sustainable Development Research Network (SDRN, 2005), who conclude that the term encompasses the concepts of life satisfaction (happiness, quality of life), physical health, income and wealth, relationships, work and leisure, personal stability and lack of depression. You may wish to consider at this point whether one of those mentioned is more significant to well-being than another, or whether and how they relate.

The idea of health and well-being being closely related is embedded in government policy. The Organization for Economic Co-operation and Development (OECD, 2013) report that lower income countries do well in relation to subjective perceptions of well-being and overall work-life balance, while higher income counties struggled with work-life balance and within these higher income counties poorer educated and low income populations do less well – resulting in poorer health and social isolation. Why would this be? The role of expectation and perception links clearly to the emotional well-being of populations and their emotional health. These ideas of lifestyle influence on health are discussed by Hanlon et al., (2012), who consider the challenges of modernity on well-being. For example, culture, inequality, obesity, addictions and population changes all influence well-being and health, and vice versa. Hanlon et al., in their discussion suggest well-being and the perception of it vary at an individual level, and the measurement of it often occurs at a community level to enable organisations to identify key issues and strengths that can be prioritised for the good of the majority, therefore, targeting areas of concern or priority and concentrating resources.

ACTIVITY 2.2

Using the SWOT (strengths, weaknesses, opportunities, threats) analysis tool below, consider your own health and well-being/lifestyle. What are negative and positive influencing factors?

Develop these thoughts and consider the influencing factors of income, peer group, upbringing, culture, genetics and education.

Consider your perceptions and expectations.

What do you measure yourself against?

STRENGTHS	WEAKNESSES
OPPORTUNITIES	THREATS

SOCIAL DETERMINANTS OF HEALTH

The social determinants of health are the social, economic and environmental conditions that influence the health and well-being of individuals and populations. They include the conditions of daily life and the factors that influence those conditions and subsequently determine the extent to which a person has the resources to meet needs and deal with changes to his or her circumstances (LGID, 2010).

A person's age, sex and hereditary factors are genetic or biological in nature. These are by and large fixed entities that we have no influence over; however, they lie within the wider determinants of health arising from social, environmental, economic and cultural conditions. Such factors can directly influence health, or have a bearing on the lifestyle decisions we make and our ability to make such choices. Dahlgren and Whitehead's (1991) widely accessible model introduced in Chapter 1 demonstrates how health is influenced, either positively or negatively, by a variety of factors.

In the United Kingdom, inequitable opportunities and variations in health exist between sectors of the population. This conclusion has been well documented in key studies of the nation's health identified below:

- Black Report (1980)
- Acheson Report (1998)
- Wanless Report (2004)
- Equally Well (Scottish Government, 2008)
- Marmot Review (2010)

The above reports (which are detailed below) indicate that socio-economic factors are strong indicators for health and well-being, with low socio-economic status leading to disadvantage which can take on many forms, for example, poverty of opportunity, poor education and emotional disease.

Within healthcare there is recognition and understanding of the importance of the wider determinants of health and health inequalities. There is also acknowledgement that addressing these root causes of ill health requires public health to be everyone's business and responsibility, including community services and nurses (NMC, 2015; RCN, 2012; Wilkinson and Marmot, 2003). People are presently living longer and also often living longer with one or more long-term conditions. Moreover, populations are living in the home setting and receiving care in that setting or between home, hospital or charitable organisation (Department of Health, 2014; Scottish Government, 2011), often caring for or being cared for by other family or community members (see Chapter 9) with significant consequences. For all of the above, the root cause of ill health and 'dis-ease' on several levels is significant for care managers and providers to understand.

PUBLIC HEALTH

Public health seeks to protect and improve the health of communities, identifying causes of poor health, disease and illness in populations and examining it from the wider social and economic standpoints. The four underpinning tenets of public health are health protection, health promotion, illness prevention and reducing inequalities (Skills for Health, 2008).

The concept of health and, conversely, illness has been the subject of much debate in society, both before and after the inception of the National Health Service (NHS) in 1948. In modern times the association between health and social determinants can be traced back in policy to some of the work of the early social reformers. Edwin Chadwick, one of the more well known, produced a report in 1842 entitled *Report of the Sanitary Conditions of the Labouring Population of Great Britain* (Chadwick, 1965) in which the relevance of social conditions of the poor and their ability to influence their plight were made explicit in relationship to individuals' health. This report to the poor law commissioners resulted in the first Public Health Act in 1884.

Since then public health has been part of the United Kingdom's healthcare provision. The United Kingdom has seen many different approaches to public health over the past 150 years, each reflecting a more detailed/broader understanding of health and illness in society. Activities have included interventions to address inequalities on a population level, through the provision of state education and increased employment opportunities, to programmes of illness prevention through mass vaccination of children.

Acheson (1988) defined public health as 'the science and art of preventing disease, prolonging life and promoting health through the organised efforts of society'. The vision of the collective efforts of society, empowering individuals and groups was clearly expressed in the White Paper Saving Lives: Our Healthier Nation (DH, 1999: 3), in which the strategic intent of government was set out as being to improve the health of the population as a whole by increasing the length of life and the number of years people spend free from illness; to improve the health of the worst off in society and to narrow the health gap.

Wanless (2004: 27) defines public health as 'the science and art of preventing disease, prolonging life and promoting health through the organised efforts and informed choices of society, organisation, public and private communities and individuals.' Wanless (2004) and Kerr (Scottish Executive, 2005) took the traditional view of public health further and place responsibility on society, organisations, communities and individuals to implement public health improvement through their organised efforts (Crabbe and Hemingway, 2014).

In 2007, a major criticism of contemporary healthcare provision was made by Lord Darzi, who observed that the NHS was still overwhelmingly concerned with treatment of the sick, and that it should move from a 'sickness service to a well-being service' (Darzi, 2007: 37). Importantly, this inclusion of well-being in policy encourages services to place greater emphasis on social health and emotional well-being. The emerging emphasis on personal responsibility also signified the importance of the role of the individual and not the healthcare practitioner when it comes to making lifestyle decisions.

The role of the healthcare practitioner (in this case the community nurse) can be crucial to achieving health-related goals, as community nurses are often in a position to assist individuals to either access services or support individuals, the family, groups and communities in making informed decisions about their health and well-being.

Strategy and policy

As mentioned previously Acheson (1988) and others defined public health and influenced clearly expressed goals. A strategy is a plan of action designed to achieve a long-term or overall goal. Public health strategies exist to improve and protect health and well-being in a population. The UK's Public Health Skills and Career Framework broadens this purpose and expresses that the purpose of public health should improve health and well-being in the population, prevent disease and minimise its consequences, thus prolonging valued life and reducing inequalities in health (Skills for Health, 2008). Furthermore, they consider that this is achieved through a culture which 'mobilises the organised efforts of society' (Skills for Health, 2008) by empowering individuals and by tackling the wider social, economic, environmental and biological determinants of health and well-being.

Policy is the definition and setting of goals, often made explicit in the form of written legislation. Health policy influences us, as health professionals, in terms of the institutions we work in and the practices we follow in delivering care. To act as persons' advocate we need to be aware of their rights as clarified in policy. Policy can have either a negative or positive impact on health as it has direct and indirect influence on all aspects of our lives. Public health policy is developed as a result of networks of decisions involving a wide range of people and organisations at local, national and international levels. Social policy traditionally includes public policy in the areas of welfare benefits, unemployment, the NHS, personal social services, education and training. However, despite this optimism and the inequality gap continued to widen (Smith and Eltanani, 2014).

In their UK-wide study, Smith and Eltanani (2015) suggest that knowing what works (significant for the development of policy and strategy) is complex and that there exists little agreement among researchers about to what is effective in reducing health inequalities. However, in their study they stated that there was 'consensus among researchers about the need for upstream, redistributive and public-service-orientated approaches to reducing health inequalities'.

From the above it is evident that ongoing research and partnership working are critical in the achievement of improving health and addressing inequalities. As the contribution of health professionals to public health is widely acknowledged within recent government policy across the United Kingdom, it is worth reflecting on what this means for your role as a nurse. Governments within the United Kingdom have clearly stated their commitment to public health, health and well-being in documents including, a DoH white paper (DoH, 2010a); Equally Well (Scottish Government, 2008) and Early Years Framework (Scottish Government, 2009), in which they set out strategies for improving the nation's health by taking preventative measures. They continue to build on these in more recent policies in each of the four UK Nations while staying true to the idea that promoting health and well-being through prevention of illness is achievable through the collective efforts of society.

ACTIVITY 2.3

The idea of health and well-being has been embedded in government policy for many years and continues to be. Additionally, health and well-being were identified in the Key Stage Skills Framework (2004) as a key skill area for all nurses to achieve and is reflected in the NMC Code (2015), for example, within clause 2.2 'recognise and respect the contribution that people can make to their own health and wellbeing'

Consider your own government and local policies, as well as the healthcare philosophy where you work and the education you have undertaken to date. Reflect on how they have been influenced by the concept of well-being and the prevention of ill health from pre-conception of the child until after death.

INFLUENCING FACTORS

In this section, we explore health inequality, community development and assessing population needs in more detail.

Health inequality

We already identified that there is a substantial body of evidence which indicates that individuals further down the social ladder have more disease and die earlier (Donkin et al., 2002) and this has not changed over time, despite there being an NHS free at the point of delivery in the United Kingdom. You might like to consider why this is. Several factors were considered in the Black Report (1980) including genetic factors, living and working conditions, lack of empowerment or learned behaviour (poor health literacy). Tackling these persistent health inequalities has traditionally seen government policy funnel resources towards specific individuals or groups within society through targeted services. Public health requires services to focus upon the underlying social and contextual causes of the problems, suggesting that to improve health for all of us action is needed across the social gradient (Marmot, 2010).

ACTIVITY 2.4

Box 2.2 indicates the National Statistics Socio-Economic Classification (National Statistics – The National Statistics Socio-Economic Classification, 2010). Consider where you might be on this scale. Now think of life events that might alter where you sit on the scale and the impact of those on well-being, for example, divorce or having dependents. Having read about the determinants of health and well-being; poverty and inequality you may want to continue this exercise by considering why some people are vulnerable and others are not in the same circumstances.

- Why can people be vulnerable at different times in their life?
- What makes people vulnerable?
- What are they vulnerable to?
- How is this understanding relevant to you as a nurse?
- How might vulnerability impact health, well-being and the ability to maintain some control over their lifestyle?

Box 2.2 National Statistics Socio-Economic Classification (NS-SEC, 2010)

Class 1: Higher Managerial and Professional Occupations
   1.1 Higher Managerial, e.g. Company Directors, Bank Managers, Senior Civil Servants
   1.2 Higher Professional, e.g. Doctors, Barristers and Solicitors, Teachers and Social Workers
Class 2: Lower Managerial and Professional Occupations, e.g. Nurses, Actors and Musicians, Police, Soldiers

Class 3: Intermediate Occupations, e.g. Secretaries, Clerks
Class 4: Small Employers and Own Account Workers, e.g. Publicans, Playgroup Leaders, Farmers, Taxi Drivers
Class 5: Lower Supervisory and Technical Occupations, e.g. Printers, Plumbers, Butchers, Train Drivers
Class 6: Semi-Routine Occupations, e.g. Shop Assistants, Traffic Wardens, Hairdressers
Class 7: Routine Occupations, e.g. Waiters, Road Sweepers, Cleaners, Couriers
Class 8: Never Worked and Long-Term Unemployed Office for National Statistics

Community development

The National Occupational Standards in Community Development Work (2009) (available online at: https://www.fcdl.org.uk/learning-qualifications/archive/community-development-national-occupational-standards-2009/) state that

> Community development is a long-term value based process which aims to address imbalances in power and bring about change founded on social justice, equality and inclusion.

In doing so it promotes participation and partnership working that facilitate people to

- Identify their own needs and aspirations
- Take action to exert influence on the decisions that affect their lives
- Improve the quality of their own lives, the communities in which they live and societies of which they are a part

Potter and Will (2013) identified that community development projects aim to involve vulnerable and socially excluded people in decision-making processes. In other words, it aims to promote and foster empowerment at both individual and community levels, however, projects and goals are often determined by health or political agendas as well as evidence.

Assessing population need

There are three main approaches to needs assessment in public health, characterised as epidemiological, comparative and corporate. See Box 2.3.

Stevens and Raftery (1994), recognising the limitations of each of the three approaches above, developed the pragmatic approach to needs assessment. This process combines all of the above approaches, drawing upon evidence from a variety of sources.

Identifying individual and public health needs through the use of assessment and assessment tools affords nurses the opportunity to promote health and well-being in the communities within which they work at individual and local levels, with more advanced community nurses informing at local and national levels.

Box 2.3 Approaches to Public Health Assessment

Epidemiological	The word 'epidemiology' means 'studies upon the population' (Fine, 2015). Epidemiological trends are studied and recorded and used as key drivers of change in public health and health service provision. Trends can be identified, policy influenced and services adjusted to meet future demands. An epidemiological approach to needs assessment, proposed by Williams and Wright (1998), combines the three elements of identifying health status through incidence/prevalence data, effectiveness and cost-effectiveness of interventions and the current level of service provision. The benefit of this approach is that its systematic and objective method quickly identifies specific problems; however, it can assume standardised prevalence and focus upon medical rather than social need (Haughey, 2008).
Comparative	A comparative approach can be used cross-nationally and locally and compares levels of service provision between these localities, for example, the service provision in one town compared with another of similar demography. Thus, it is often used to provide a timely and inexpensive assessment.
Corporate.	A corporate approach considers making the needs assessment responsive to local concerns. This approach collects the knowledge and views of the stakeholders of the issues being addressed in the needs assessment. The stakeholders can be a collective of practitioners, in both primary and secondary care settings, health and social care service managers, commissioners of services, experts in the field and service users.

In recent years, there has been an increased fusion between health and social care services. Generally systematic methods of identifying the health and healthcare needs of an individual or population and making recommendations for changes to meet these needs is carried out by both agencies using a tool or model that provides practitioners with a framework for undertaking this complex and important needs assessment in a structured way (Public Health England, 2013).

People, through the influence of social determinants, have measurable differences in their health status. All too often this is compounded by inequitable access to healthcare. Disadvantaged individuals and groups, despite having the greatest overall need, are the least likely to access services (Levesque, 2013). However, it is important that service delivery reaches these groups as it is generally viewed that a need, if met, will result in an improvement in people's health (Haughey, 2008); however, what constitutes need is widely contested. Needs are variable; they can be objective and measurable, obvious or hidden. Conversely, they too are subjective, personal and interchangeable according to context (Cowley, 2008a). Taxonomies of need exist, for example, Bradshaw (1972), as also discussed in Chapter 7, and are essential to improve and protect health and well-being as a result of meeting the public health agenda. From your reading and practice experience, you will have a good understanding of the importance of holistic health needs assessment in your role as a community practitioner and understand that to attain an accurate health needs assessment of a case, assessment might have to be carried out at different levels from the individual, to the family/group and the community in which the individual lives, depending on the purpose.

PROMOTING HEALTH AND WELL-BEING

ACTIVITY 2.5

Take some time to explore definitions of the following key terms:

- Demography
- Epidemiology
- Empowerment
- Social Gradient
- Equity/Equality

Health promotion

Health promotion as a concept came to the fore in the 1980s (Runciman, 2014). The WHO (1984) succinctly defined health promotion as 'the process of enabling people to increase control over and to improve their health'. This definition is still relevant today and relates to the concept of empowerment and the nurse as a leader and educator. Ewle and Simnett (2010) note that there is no single 'right' approach, activity or way of 'doing' health promotion. The definition underpins current government policy, actively placing the individual at the center of care and encouraging their involvement in the decision processes in order to take control of health decisions: 'No decision about me without me' (DH, 2010b). Public health clearly encompasses health promotion. It can be concluded that health promoters (such as community nurses) should aim to enhance participation, equity and fairness to improve the health of individuals, families and communities.

Nurses are involved in public health activity through their day-to-day contact with patients, clients, families and carers; delivering health promotion activity, planned or unplanned by providing information, education, facilitating motivation and empowerment. Community nurses are in a strong position to promote health and well-being. Their knowledge of the local community and access to clients and their families in their own homes enables community nurses to develop a deep understanding of the factors that influence the health of individuals, families and communities. Their ability to influence the care received by individuals and to influence local health policy development is high.

For community nurses (at every level) health promotion activity is now embedded in the role – often carried out in a more informal manner on a one-to-one basis. The challenge is to identify and articulate the community nurse's contribution to health promotion through effective leadership and the use of evidence-based, proactive, contemporary practice (Runciman, 2014).

Health promotion models

There are several models of health promotion, examples of which appear in Box 2.4.

Box 2.4 Health Promotion Model Examples

MODEL	
Beatie (1991)	Beatie (1991, cited in Katz et al., 2000) developed an analytical model that highlighted the interplay of intervention (authoritative or negotiated which equates to professional or client led) and the focus of intervention (individual or society). Beatie (1991, cited in Katz et al., 2000) developed an analytical model that highlighted the interplay of intervention (authoritative or negotiated which equates to professional or client led) and the focus of intervention (individual or society).
Tannahill (1985)	Tannahill identified prevention, health education and health protection in overlapping spheres to describe the services and activities that constituted health promotion practice.
Tonnes and Tilford (2001)	Tonnes and Tilford identified educational, preventative, empowerment and radical approaches but viewed empowerment as central to health promotion.
Ewles and Simnett (2003)	Ewles and Simnett proposed a model that described five approaches to health promotion: medical, behaviour change, educational, client-centred and societal change. The values which underpinned the approaches were represented in a corresponding gradient from professional-led to client-led activity. (See Box 2.5.)

Other theories that contribute towards the understanding of the effect of health promotion interventions on the client and why people seek help are the psychological theories of behaviour change which aim to explain why and how people can change their behaviour. An example is Becker's Health Belief Model (cited in Wills and Earle, 2007).

Assets approach

Demographic changes, reductions in public sector spending and the gap between the life and health outcomes of the best and the worst off have influenced recent discussion about the need for new approaches to public service delivery.

One specific model which has attracted much attention is the use of asset-based approaches to improving health.

Taking an asset-based approach involves mobilising the skills and knowledge of individuals and the connections and resources within communities and organisations, rather than focusing on problems and deficits. The approach aims to empower individuals, enabling them to rely less on public services. However, there remains a limited evidence base linking actions to strengthen individual and community assets with improved health and well-being. An asset-based approach is, therefore, one which seeks positively to mobilise the assets, capacities or resources available

Box 2.5 Approaches to Behaviour Change (Ewle and Simnett, 2010)

APPROACH	

Medical	• Based on a medical model of health
	• Aims to reduce morbidity and premature mortality (freedom from medically defined disease and disability)
	• Targets whole populations or high-risk groups
	• Values preventative medical procedures
	• Prominent in current health promotion and healthcare, but could be considered paternalistic (i.e. one person deciding what is best for another)
	• Focuses on the absence of disease rather than on promoting positive health
	• Ignores the social and environmental dimensions of health
	• Primary prevention – The goal is to protect healthy people from developing disease or injury in the first place
	  • Education – Nutrition, regular exercise, dangers of tobacco, alcohol and other drugs
	  • Legislation – Seatbelts, Health and Safety at Work Act 1974, food hygiene laws
	  • Examinations and screening tests to monitor risk factors for illness
	  • Immunisation against infectious disease
	  • Controlling potential hazards at home and work
	• Secondary prevention – Interventions after an illness or serious risk factors diagnosed
	• Goal is to halt or slow the progress of disease (if possible) in its earliest stages; in the case of injury, goals include limiting long-term disability and preventing re-injury
	• Tertiary prevention – Interventions after an illness or serious risk factors are diagnosed
	• Goal is to halt or slow the progress of disease (if possible) in its earliest stages; in the case of injury, goals include limiting long-term disability and preventing re-injury

Behaviour change	• Encourages individuals to change their behaviour and adopt healthy lifestyles • Views health as belonging to an individual, and it is the individual who chooses when he or she is ready and able to change his or her lifestyle and improve health which involves a change in attitude followed by a change in behaviour
Educational	• Provides individuals with knowledge and understanding to make well-informed choices about their health behaviour • Aim of health promoter/health professional to impart information with minimal personal values • Individual decides whether to act on the health education and any decisions reached • Can also include developing skills required for healthy living • Does *not* try to persuade or motivate change in one direction

Empowerment/ client-centred	• 'Bottom-up' approach, seeks to enable people to take control over their lives, identify their concerns and gain the skills and confidence to act on them
	• Agendas set by client(s) – Health professionals guide, support, facilitate and encourage; initiates the process then withdraws
	• Conditions for empowerment: For people to be empowered they need to
	• Recognise and understand their powerlessness; feel strongly enough about their situation to want to change it; feel capable of changing the situation by having information, support and life skills (Naidoo and Wills, 2016)
Social change	• Sometimes termed radical health promotion; recognises importance of socio-economic environment in determining health
	• Focuses at policy/environmental level
	• Tries to change physical, social and economic environments to have the effect of promoting health; i.e. focusing on changing society, not the behaviour of individuals

to individuals and communities which could enable them to gain more control over their lives and circumstances (Foot and Hopkins, 2010).

A wide range of techniques are used to take an asset-based approach, including asset mapping, co-production and various community-led, community engagement and community development methods.

Assests can be grouped into the following:

Individual assets (e.g. resilience, commitment to learning, self-esteem, sense of purpose)

Community assets (e.g. family and friendship networks, social capital, community cohesion, religious tolerance, intergenerational solidarity)

(NES, 2011).

Strengths-based approach

'Strength-based working' is a term that is heard more frequently in health and social care settings and can be seen as similar to assets approaches to promoting health behaviour change and public health outcomes. Strength-based working means viewing and treating people in a positive manner and can be aligned with the concepts of self-efficacy. Self-efficacy is identified by Borland (2013) as individuals' belief that they can facilitate change in themselves within the context of their circumstances; therefore, some people who have a high level of self-efficacy may be able to affect change with some success, whereas other people who have low self-efficacy may choose to not attempt health-improving activity or give up easily when challenges are presented. Borland (2013) suggests that self-belief if negative can get in the way of health-promoting changes in behaviour due to an unsuccessful concept or image of individuals in their mind, and this image can be changed by developing an adjusted sense of self. Upton (2013, cited Banduram 1977b: 51) identifies two particular areas from Bandura's social learning theory and suggests that in order to develop this adjusted sense of self we can look to strength-based working to support self-efficacy by influencing verbal persuasion and reduce emotional arousal. This can be achieved by identifying a genuine potential for change in individuals by recognising, naming and developing abilities, skills, expertise and social networks in the individual and by reducing the emotional arousal associated with a negative self-image. Neuroplasticity can help us consider how thinking positively about individual's strengths can change the way the individual thinks. Davidson and Begley (2012) advocate that by encouraging individuals to think positive thoughts about their abilities they can change the chemistry of their brains to become more successful in the actions they undertake.

Nursing skills

Given the complexity of concepts of health, and the interrelationship between the multiple factors that influence it, you will appreciate that a variety of approaches and methods can be utilised to promote health.

To help you clarify your own understanding of how health promotion has developed over the twentieth century, access the Ottawa Charter for Health Promotion on the WHO site.

Many of the above theories describe or analyse health promotion practice, but the skill of health promotion practice requires a deep understanding of communication and partnership working theory to achieve the goal, which is to enable people to increase control over and to improve their health (empowerment and choice). Rollnick et al., (1999) proposed a client-centred philosophy of partnership working (Motivational Interviewing) to complement Prochaska and DeClemente's (1983) Trans-theoretical (stages of change) theory. The aim was to facilitate individuals to move through the stages of precontemplation – contemplation – making changes – maintaining changes. Rollnick et al., suggested that a practitioner could reduce resistance to change by relationship building using a therapeutic approach based on trust and information exchange to negotiate the agenda and to set achievable goals based on the individual's vision of importance and their confidence to make the change. Motivational interviewing is discussed further in Chapters 8 and 13. Gallant et al., (2002) conducted a very informative concept analysis of partnership working which identified three phases to the partnership working relationship: the initiating phase, the working phase and an evaluation phase. To work in partnership one needs to build a professional therapeutic relationship based on trust. The professional must be competent and honest and display professional integrity (to work in the best interests of the client/patient) at all times and the client must be a willing partner (Potter and Wills, 2013).

ACTIVITY 2.6

Consider Box 2.5. What needs to be in place for each of these approaches to be successful? You can think of policy, legislation, attitude, values, skills, abilities, and so on. Carry out a mind map. You can use this exercise in relation to an individual or community you have been involved with clinically.

SCREENING

It is worth considering screening at this point. As a practitioner working in the community, you may well be involved in a screening programme to meet with the Public Health Domain of the Quality and Outcomes Framework (HSCIS, 2015). Screening is considered to be a preventative activity that seeks to identify an unsuspected disease or pre-disease condition. It aims to find those most at risk for which an effective intervention is available (Crichton and Mulhall, 2015). Health screening is now a widely accepted service that is largely accepted by the general public. Most people at some point in their life have undergone screening of one sort of another (for example, breast screening, cervical screening, child development screening, elderly screening; blood tests, hearing test). Although widely accepted, health screening, because it proactively seeks to detect disease before symptoms present, is often the subject of continuing ethical debate and concern around whether the most vulnerable populations are reached (Crichton and Mulhall, 2015).

CULTURAL AWARENESS

In the 1960s, culture and cultural competence were first mentioned in the nursing literature in relation to the accessibility and equity of service to populations identified as 'different' (Vandenberg, 2010). However, at that point, the focus was on race and ethnicity. Cultural competence fosters understanding of race relations, cultural practices both of the client group and importantly the practitioner and the culture that the healthcare system stems from. Cultural competence and awareness development is an ongoing process that in the nursing workforce is critical to reducing health disparities and is important when preparing nurses to deliver high-quality, person-centered care (Montenery et al., 2013).

Benkert et al., (2005) identified that cultural understanding and knowledge should further develop and be inclusive of socially constructed factors such as sexual orientation as well as the traditionally appreciated ones of race and ethnicity. Continued recognition of the disparities of care provision and access between differing cultural groups have called for care to be culturally responsive (Diaz et al., 2015). Garneau and Pepin (2015: 9–15) developed a constructivist definition of cultural competence that you may find useful:

A complex know-act grounded in critical reflection and action, which the health care professional draws upon to provide culturally safe, congruent, and effective care in partnership with individuals, families, and communities living health experiences and which takes into account the social and political dimensions of care.

The development of cultural competence for any professional is an ongoing process (Camphinha-Bacote, 2002). Camphinha-Bacote (2002) broke down cultural competence into five concepts that work together to develop the whole, and from that developed a model of cultural competence:

- Cultural desire
- Cultural awareness
- Cultural knowledge
- Cultural skill
- Cultural encounter

Examples of where cultural dimensions might occur include a person's' health and wellness belief systems; how illness, disease, and their causes are perceived; the behaviour of individuals seeking healthcare, and their attitudes toward healthcare providers; and importantly the views and values of those delivering healthcare. As Szczepura (2005) states, improved openness and understanding of the health beliefs, practices and cultural needs of individuals is essential to provide equitable and effective access to healthcare services for all populations over and above service provision.

ACTIVITY 2.7

Reflect on how you deliver sensitive care with an attitude of openness and tolerance.

This may require you to reflect on your own cultural beliefs

You may find the people whom you care for are the best source of evidence to access cultural needs and as a professional you must remain cognisant of the fact that you cannot tar everyone with the same brush. Cultural competence and safety should not just work at an individual level, but be evident at a wider level for the provision of care.

APPLYING THEORY TO PRACTICE

Many chapters in this book will support you applying theory to nursing practice in the community. Community nurses develop very complex relationships with people and often other family or group members which is discussed further in Chapter 5. For individuals who rely on their family for care the nurse must holistically assess and work with the person, being respectful of the needs of both individual and carer/family within the context that they live and the influencing factors. Chapters 7, 8 and 9 consider aspects of assessment of individuals, families and carers. Many people may also have other professionals involved in their care. Community nurses as the principal care providers in the client's home need to work in partnership with other professionals who may work for health, other statutory agencies, the voluntary or independent sectors, although this can be difficult to achieve at times. When working with other professionals in partnership the same principles of trust, which include honesty, competence and integrity, apply. Communication between professionals that is respectful, open and honest is essential to achieve the best outcomes for clients and their families. Chapter 10 explores further the benefits of collaborative working. Although health promotion is often defined in terms of work with populations and work with individuals is defined as health education, all interventions that aim to enable people to take control over their own health on an individual or population basis are considered to be health-promoting interventions (Whitehead and Irvine, 2010).

CONCLUSION

As services are redesigned to deliver care closer to home it is widely acknowledged that community environments are where there is an emphasis on health promotion and prevention of ill health. With population changes and ever-emerging challenges, for example, antibiotic resistance, it is incumbent on the current nursing workforce to develop an approach to community nursing that goes beyond the idea that nursing is no more than assessing, planning and implementing/evaluating the delivery of care associated with a set of clinical tasks. Effective community nursing must identify and engage in public health activity, inter-agency working, multi-agency working and research in order to promote health and well-being in society and for individuals.

Through the presentation of relevant underpinning theory and policy this chapter has demonstrated that public health is everyone's business and that community nurses are in a key position to enable and empower individuals and communities across all levels, from some of the hard-to-reach groups in the population, such as the housebound, to those eagerly involved with promoting their own health and improving their own sense of well-being.

You may want to conclude this chapter by considering the following:

- What support do we need in the United Kingdom to live healthier lives?
- Thinking about the future of health and social care services, where should our focus be?

FURTHER READING

Public Health England (2014) A framework for personalised and population health for nurses, midwives, health visitors and allied health professional. PHE 2014532. HYPERLINK "https://www.gov.uk/government/uploads/system/uploads/attachment_data/file/377450/Framework_for_personalised_care_and_population_health_for_nurses.pdf.

Schulte P, Guerin R, Schill AL et al., 2015 Considerations for Incorporating "Well-Being" in Public Policy for Workers and Workplaces. *American Journal of Public Health* 105(8):31–44.

REFERENCES

Acheson D (1988) *Public Health in England*. London: HMSO.

Acheson D (1998) *Independent Inquiry into Inequalities in Health*. London: HMSO.

Benkert R, Guthrie B and Pohl J (2005) Cultural competence of nurse practitioer students :A consortium's experience. *Journal of Nursing Education* 44(5):225–33.

Black Report (1980) *Inequalities in Health—Report of the Research Working Group*. London: DHSS.

Borland R (2013) *Understanding Hard to Maintain Behaviour Change: A Dual Process Approach*. Hoboken: Wiley.

Chadwick E (1965 [1842]) *Report of the Sanitary Conditions of the Labouring Population of Great Britain*. Edinburgh: Edinburgh University Press.

Camphinha-Bacote J (2002) The process of cultural competence in delivery of healthcare services: A model of care. *Journal of Transcultural Nursing* 13:181–92 from Montenery S, Jones A, Perry N, et al., 2013 Cultural competence in nursing faculty: A journey, not a destination. *Journal of Professioanl Nursing* 29(6):e51–e57.

Cowley S. (2008a) Foreword. In Coles L and Porter E (eds) (2008) *Public Health Skills: A Practical Guide for Nurses and Public Health Practitioners*. Oxford: Blackwell, p. vii.

Crabbe K and Hemingway A (2014) A matter for the midwife? *British Journal of Midwifery* 22(9):634.

Crichton N and Mulhall A (2015). Chapter 3. In Naidoo J, Wills J (eds) *Health Studies An Introduction*, 3rd ed. London: Bailliere Tindall.

Dahlgren G and Whitehead M (1991) In Acheson D (ed) (1998) *Part 1 Independent Inquiry into Inequalities in Health*. London: HMSO.

Darzi A (2007) *Our NHS Our Future: The Next Stage Review Interim Report*. London: NHS COI for the Department of Health.

Davidson R and Begley S (2012) *The Emotional Life of Your Brain: How Its Unique Patterns Affect the Way You Think, Feel, and Live-And How You Can Change Them*. London: Hachette.

Department of Health (DH) (1999) *Saving Lives: Our Healthier Nation*. London: Department of Health.

Department of Health (2010a) *Healthy Lives, Healthy People*. London: The Stationery Office.

Department of Health (2010b) *Equity and Excellence: Liberating the NHS*. London: The Stationery Office.

Donkin A, Goldblatt P and Lynch K (2002) Inequalities in life expectancy by social class 1972–1999. *Health Statistics Quarterly* 15:5–15.

Department of Health (2014) *Transforming Primary Care* London: The Stationery Office.

Diaz C, Clarke P and Gatua M (2015) Cultural competence in rural nursing education: Are we there yet? *Nursing Education Perspectives* 36(1):22–26.

Ewles L and Simnett I (2003) *Promoting Health: A Practical Guide*, 5th edn. Edinburgh: Bailliere Tindall.

Ewle L. and Simnett, I (2010) *Promoting Health: A Practical Guide*, 6th edn. Edinburgh: Bailliére Tindall.

Fine P (2015) Another defining moment for epidemiology *Lancet* 385(9965):319–20.

Foot J and Hopkins T (2010) *A Glass Half-full: How an Asset Approach Can Improve Community Health and Well-being*. London: Improvement and Development Agency.

Gallant H, Marcia C and Carnevale F (2002) Partnership: An analysis of the concept within the nurse–client relationship. *Journal of Advanced Nursing* 40:149–57.

Garneau A and Pepin J (2015) Cultural competence. A constructivist definition. *Journal of Transcultural Nursing* 26(1):9–15.

Hanlon P, Carlisle S, Hannah M and Lyon A (2012) The *Future Public Health*. Milton Keynes, England: The Open University press.

Haughey R (2008) Assessing and identifying health needs. In Coles L and Porter E (eds) *Public Health Skills: A Practical Guide for Nurses and Public Health Practitioners*. Oxford: Blackwell.

HSCIS (2015) *Quality and Outcomes Framework—Prevalence, Achievements and Exceptions Report, England 2014–15*. London: Health and Social Care Information Centre.

Huber M, Bolk L, Knottnerus A et al., (2011) Health How should we define it. *British Medical Journal* 343:235.

Katz J, Peberdy A and Douglas J (2000) *Promoting Health: Knowledge and Practice*, 2nd edn. Milton Keynes: Open University Press.

LevesqueJ-F, Harris M and Russell G (2013) Patient-centred access to health care: Conceptualising access at the interface of health systems and populations. *International Journal for Equity in Health* 12:18

Local Government Improvement and Development (LGID) (2010) *Understanding and Tackling the Wider Social Determinants of Health*. (Accessed 12 October 2010) www.idea.gov.uk/idk/core/page.do?pageId=14114189.

Marmot M (2010) *Fair Society, Healthy Lives*. (Accessed 10 June 2010) www.ucl.ac.uk/gheg/marmotreview/FairSocietyHealthyLivesExecSummary.

Montenery S, Jones A, Perry N, et al., 2013 Cultural competence in nursing faculty: A journey, not a destination. *Journal of Professionl Nursing* 29(6): e51–e57.

Naidoo J and Wills J (2015) *Health Studies An Introduction*, 3rd edn, Chap. 1. London: Bailliere Tindall

Naidoo J and Wills J (2016) *Foundations for Health Promotion*, 4th edn. London: Elsevier.

National Statistics—The National Statistics Socio-Economic Classification. (2010) *Office for National Statistics*. Basingstoke: Palgrave Mcmillan. Available at https://www.ons.gov.uk/methodology/classificationsandstandards/otherclassifications/thenationalstatisticssocioeconomicclassificationnssecrebasedonsoc2010

NHS Education Scotland (2011) *Asset-Based Approaches to Health Improvement*. Edinburgh: NES.

Nursing and Midwifery Council. (NMC) (2015). *The Code: Professional Standards of Practice and Behavior for Nurses and Midwives*. London: NMC.

OECD (2013) *How's Life? 2013 Measuring Well-Being*. Paris: OECD Publishing.

Potter K and Wills J (2013) Chapter 2. In Sines D, Aldridge-Bent S, Farrelly P, Potter K, Wright J (2013) *Community and Public Health Nursing*, 5th edn. UK: Wiley Blackwell.

Prochaska JO and DiClemente CC (1983) Stages and processes of self change of smoking: Toward an integrative model of change. *Journal of Consulting and Clinical Psychology* 51:390–5.

Public Health England (2013) *Joint Health and Social Care Self-Assessment Framework*. London: PHE

Raymond B (2005) Health needs assessment, risk assessment and public health. In Sines D, Appleby F and Frost M (eds) *Community Health Care Nursing*, 3rd edn. Oxford: Blackwell, pp. 70–88.

Rollnick S, Mason P and Butler C (1999) *Health Behaviour Change: A Guide to Practitioners*. London: Churchill Livingstone.

Royal College of Nursing (2012) *Going Upstream: Nursing's Contribution to Public Health Prevent, Promote and Protect RCN Guidance for Nurses.* London: RCN.

Runciman P (2014) The health promotion work of the district nurse: Interpreting its embeddedness. *Primary Care Research and Development* 15(1):15–25.

Szczepura A (2005) Access to health care for ethnic minority populations *Postgrad. Medical Journal* 81:141–7.

Scottish Executive (2005) *Kerr Report; Building a Health Service Fit for the Future.* Edinburgh: Scottish Government

Scottish Government (2008) *Equally Well: Report of the Ministerial Task Force on Health Inequalities.* Edinburgh: Scottish Government

Scottish Government (2009) *Early Years Framework.* Edinburgh: Scottish Government

Scottish Government (2011) *2020 Vision: Strategic Narrative—Achieving Sustainable Quality in Scotland's Healthcare.* Edinburgh: Scottish Government

Sines D, Aldridge-Bent S, Farrelly P et al., (2013) *Community and Public Health Nursing,* 5th edn. UK: Wiley Blackwell.

Skills for Health (2008) *Skills and Career Framework.* (Accessed 29 July 2016) http://www.skillsforhealth.org.uk/

Smith KE and Eltanani MK (2015) What kinds of policies to reduce health inequalities in the UK do researchers support? *Journal of Public Health* 37(1):6–17.

Stevens A and Raftery J (1994) *Introduction to Health Care Needs Assessment,* vol. 1. Oxford: Radcliffe Medical Press, pp. 1–30.

Sustainable Development Research Network (2005) *Wellbeing Concepts and Challenges: Discussion Paper* by Fiona McAllister for SDRN. DEFRA.

Tannahill A (1985) What is health promotion? *Health Education Journal* 44:167–8.

Tonnes K and Tilford S (2001) *Health Promotion Effectiveness, Efficiency and Equity,* 3rd edn. Cheltenham: Nelson Thornes.

Upton D (2013) *Introducing Psychology for Nurses and Healthcare Professionals.* Abingdon: Taylor and Francis.

Vandenberg H (2010) Culture theorizing past and present: Trends and challenges *Nursing Philosophy* 11, 238–49.

Wanless D and HM Treasury (2004) *Securing Good Health for the Whole Population: Final Report.* London: The Stationery Office.

Whitehead D and Irvine F (2010) *Health Promotion and Health Education in Nursing.* Basingstoke: Palgrave Macmillan.

Wilkinson R and Marmot M (2003) *Social Determinants of Health. The Solid Facts,* 2nd edn. Geneva: WHO Europe International Centre for Health and Society.

Williams R and Wright J (1998) Epidemiological issues in health needs assessment. *British Medical Journal* 316:1379–82.

Wills J and Earle S (2007) Theoretical perspectives on promoting public health. In Earle S, Lloyd C, Sidell M and Spurr S (eds) *Theory and Research in Promoting Public Health,* Chapter 5. Milton Keynes: Open University Press.

World Health Organization (WHO) (1946) *Constitution.* Geneva: WHO, p. 2.

WHO (1984) Health Promotion: A Discussion Document on the Concepts and Principles. Copenhagen: WHO.

WHO (2006) *Engaging for Health: A Global Health Agenda 2006–2015.* WHO Library Cataloguing-in-Publication Data.

Professional approaches to care

Jo Skinner

INTRODUCTION

The relationship between professionals and clients has been the central feature of professional practice throughout history. Professionalism has never been more important regarding public trust and care quality. The nature of professional practice in the community is particularly challenging given the complex care needs, diverse organisations and professions, as well as the need to demonstrate cost-effective health outcomes. The relationship between service users and professionals is changing radically.

This chapter explores the transition in professional practice from a traditional, hierarchical and individualistic model to a more inclusive partnership model. The partnership model includes extended service user and carer involvement, interprofessional working and a wider public health approach (see Chapters 2, 8 and 10). Throughout the chapter, issues relating to both models and ethical principles underpinning practice are highlighted; a case study and examples from different areas of community practice are used to illustrate the principles. There are three sections: the first presents an overview of the traditional model of professional practice, followed by principles informing professional practice and finally factors influencing the development of a new extended partnership model of professional practice.

CASE STUDY

Marjory Davies is 85 years old and lives alone in a three-bedroom house with four flights of stairs. Miss Davies has had a series of falls; the most recent fall required several weeks in hospital. Ahmed, her neighbour, had noticed her curtains were not drawn and he alerted Miss Davies' general practitioner (GP). Miss Davies has returned home and the district nurse has assessed Miss Davies to plan her rehabilitation. Her social worker has advised Miss Davies about her options for residential care. Miss Davies has consistently refused any suggestions that she should move out of her home.

THE TRADITIONAL MODEL OF PROFESSIONAL PRACTICE

It is not easy to define precisely what a *professional* is or indeed what *professionalism* is – both concepts are fluid and contested areas (Evetts, 1999, 2012). Traditionally, a professional is someone who is associated with being part of an elite group of experts with claims to specialist knowledge and skills that license their practice. The nature of the work is vocational, and like professional roles such as law and medicine, is valued within society. Professionals exercise their duty in the best interests of their clients and thereby their approach is intentionally altruistic. In that sense professionals may see themselves as the ideal advocates for their clients, being able to define their clients' needs and determine any solutions based on their expertise. Such attributes result in a high degree of professional autonomy and particular trusting relationships with their clients. In healthcare, licensed practitioners are permitted access to the human body in order to undertake intimate or intrusive assessments, clinical examinations and treatments. Thus, professionals have considerable power and higher moral standards are expected of professionals to do what is best for patients; this is enshrined in law as *a duty of care* owed to patients (Dimond, 2015). In the case of Miss Davies (case study), she is owed a duty of care by all three professionals: district nurse, social worker and GP. Therefore, all professionals, and those who are members of recognised professions, share certain characteristics (Box 3.1).

Box 3.1 Characteristics of professions

- A distinct body of specialist knowledge and skills (often rooted in ancient practice or tradition)
- A lengthy and exclusive training leading to registration
- Altruism
- Code of practice
- Duty of care
- Autonomy
- Accountability
- Privileged access to and trusting relationship with clients
- Public trust and good standing
- Higher social status, pay, reward and career structure

Control over who may enter these elite professions is strictly governed, usually through a rigorous selection process. This keeps up demand for such skills by reinforcing their status, value and power (Finlay, 2000a). Professionals can make certain demands, including control over the way they practice, in recognition of their unique skills and status. The process of becoming a professional entails lengthy and rigorous training validated by peers. Historically, those elite professions were male dominated and *patriarchal* in nature. Specialist literature and technical language reinforce 'membership of the club', thus excluding others, particularly their clients. As Williams (2000: 99) noted, professional autonomy 'empowers the strongest at the expense of the weakest'. Professional networks and associations, like membership of Royal Colleges, reinforce entitlement. Professional and statutory regulatory bodies (PSRB) protect the public, policing entry onto and removal from professional registers, for example, the Nursing and Midwifery Council (NMC), the General Medical Council (GMC) and the Health and Care Professions Council (HCPC). The introduction of revalidation and fitness to practice procedures provides additional mechanisms for continuing registration.

ACTIVITY 3.1

Reflection point
Do you consider yourself a professional? What defines you as a professional? How is this different from acting in a professional way?

Many of these features reflect an 'old' model of professional practice associated with what is known as a *medical model of health* (Box 3.2). This model is particularly problematic from a community and public health viewpoint as the focus is on the body, acute illness and the disease process such that social or economic causes of illness are omitted. Concepts within the medical model are informed by and reinforce values, attitudes and practice.

Box 3.2 Features of the medical model of health

Focus on the disease process and cure
Scientific rational approach
Professional as expert
Task focused
Patient as a passive recipient of care
Illness model of health: Little emphasis on prevention or public health

Becoming 'a professional' is a process of acculturation and socialisation where new recruits are exposed to the norms and values that pertain to a particular profession, including language and how to relate to clients. Professional education exposes students to role models or mentors with particular placement experiences that serve to define and reinforce attitudes, values and behaviours as much as the specialist knowledge. This reflects the traditional apprenticeship approach. Training is separate from other professions, and patients do not play an active role in the curriculum, other than permitting students to practice their skills on them. At the end of this acculturation process, there has been a transformation from student to a fledgling practitioner. Benner (1984), cited by Gatley (1992), describes this process in nursing as a continuum 'from novice to expert' whereby experiential learning is central to developing intuitive knowledge and skills. So, while professions share certain common characteristics (Box 3.1), not necessarily all, there remain differences in the way that professionals interact with clients, conceptualise their practice and relate to other professionals.

Training establishes professional identities and it is easiest to make distinctions between or within professions where practice is highly specialised, for example, neurosurgery. Such distinctions may be codified by legislation and regulations, for example, except in an emergency, it is a criminal offence for anyone other than a UK-registered midwife or doctor to attend a woman in childbirth (Dimond, 2015). Such codification has led to the creation of hierarchies even within professional groups and characterising some groups as semi-professions, particularly along gender lines. Boundaries between professionals have emerged such that they jealously guard them in order to protect their roles. This can lead to resistance to change, defensive practice or tribalism (Dalley, 1989; Evetts, 2012). This reflects the traditional view of professions in terms of historical claims to knowledge and expertise and is ultimately an issue of power.

ACTIVITY 3.2

Discussion point

Which professions are legally entitled to prescribe? What are the boundary issues?

You may find Radcliffe (2008) helpful to your discussion.

Differences between professions are frequently reinforced through traditions, training and discourse and to some extent stereotyping (Pietroni, 1991). Theoretical perspectives also underpin this, for example, in social care the concept of anti-oppressive practice (Ward, 2009) is key to explaining social work practice as well as a driver to empower service users. This reflects the *social model of health* (Box 3.3). Doctors are associated with adopting a purely medical model of health while other professional groups across health and social care adopt the social model of health (Brechin et al., 2000) (Box 3.3) that takes in the wider determinants of health and health inequalities (Wilkinson and Pickett, 2010; Marmot, 2010). This is particularly important when taking a public health approach that is population based (Guest et al., 2013). These stereotypes or archetypes are too crude and do not take account of the huge variation across practice areas, different care settings and individual philosophies. In the community, it would be difficult, not to say unethical, for any health or social care practitioner working with service users to ignore wider psychosocial and environmental factors impacting on care (see Chapter 1). For example, in occupational health nursing the work environment is a critical aspect of any care (Black, 2008) and must be balanced with the scientific explanations of occupational exposures to noise, dust or other hazards to health (Aw et al., 2006). However, these concepts and models are useful starting points for challenging assumptions about professions and the extent to which practice is task oriented.

Box 3.3 Features of the social model of health

Health is holistic and not just the absence of disease.
Wider determinants of health are seen as causes of ill-health and health inequalities.
Holistic approach is taken to assessment and sources of evidence.
Service user is expert in their own health.
Emphasis is on health and well-being.
Service user participates in health/community as a full citizen.
Emphasis is on prevention and public health.

ACTIVITY 3.3

Discussion point
List the advantages and disadvantages of having different professionals involved in Miss Davies' care.

Would your list be different if the service user were a child or an employee?

For many years boundaries between professions were fairly rigid and the number of professional groups relatively stable. In primary care, the professional hierarchy was well established (Peckham and Exworthy, 2003), with GPs at the apex. Using prescribing as an example (Activity 3.2), traditionally doctors and dentists were legally empowered to prescribe; in 1992 the Medicines Act (1968) was amended so that all district nurses and health visitors were enabled to prescribe from a community prescribing formulary with training integrated into specialist programmes (Dimond, 2015; NMC, 2006). However, nurse prescribing was hard won; it followed extensive pilots to address the skeptics (Brew, 1997) and was not fully introduced until 1999. This has paved the way for prescribing rights to be extended across nursing and midwifery and to other professional groups such as pharmacists and physiotherapists (Radcliffe, 2008). Interestingly, not all prescribers were granted the same prescribing rights, so new boundaries emerge, and arguably maintain hierarchies (Williams, 2000). There is some contention about whether such developments are *extended roles* or whether this is really *skill substitution*. In the case of nurses they have taken on the work others, namely doctors, no longer wish to do (Williams, 2000); however, increasing the skill mix among the workforce has also been an important mechanism for health service managers to reduce costs (see Chapter 14). In reality, it is a fusion of all these aspects with some degree of compromise between the various vested interests. Boundaries for professional practice are shifting and encompass the legal and policy frameworks within which all practitioners operate (Dimond, 2015; Evetts, 2012).

PRINCIPLES INFORMING PROFESSIONAL PRACTICE

Ethical principles and legal and policy frameworks direct the practice of all professionals. In the community, it is important to understand these principles and be able to apply them in different situations as part of professional decision making. Values encompass personal, societal and professional domains and importantly influence practice. These values are socially constructed and thereby liable to change.

Professionals make decisions with or on behalf of others and need to have clear reasons to justify them. Being accountable is a key element of professional practice and clinical reasoning. Moral reasoning informs decisions, for example, whether or not to treat. A recent feature of professional practice has been the development of *evidence-based practice*, whereby decisions about treatment and care are neither subjective nor capricious. Using research evidence to underpin professional practice has come to be viewed as best practice, being both rigorous and objective following the scientific tradition. The standard by which professionals are judged is in relation to their peers (Dimond, 2015; Greenhalgh, 2006). Steel (2006: 57) makes the point that, 'The development of a more open and evidence-based approach to decision making in healthcare has shown how much personal values influence professional behaviour'. Referring to public health, he warns that science is far from being value free but that it is important to make values clear and decisions explicit (Steel, 2006).

However, the plethora of research published means that professionals need to be able to access, appraise and use research findings to underpin their practice (Greenhalgh, 2006). Given the complexity of research findings, particularly weighted towards quantitative research, this needs to be translated into guidance for practice. Organisations such as the National Institute for Health and Care Excellence (NICE), National Health Service (NHS) Evidence, Health and Social Care Information Centre, King's Fund, professional bodies and peer-reviewed journals often mediate and disseminate guidance. The wholesale adoption of the scientific rational model undermines the 'art' of professional practice, which encompasses tacit knowledge, narrative-based approaches, service user individuality and professional autonomy. Greenhalgh (2006) points out that professionals may be profoundly influenced by their own experiences but this may not always be a good basis for making decisions. It is clearly important to recognise the value of and difficulty in managing both evidence- and narrative-based approaches. For example, an experienced practice nurse may intuitively understand that a woman's reluctance to have cervical screening is due to past sexual violence. A solely evidence-based practice approach may lead to task-focused care to obtain consent for a cervical smear and omit the importance of human interaction and relationships as an integral part of therapeutic care and may transgress patients' values (see Chapter 5).

Decision making is influenced by many factors (Box 3.4) including the context and clinical and ethical aspects (Grundstein-Amado, 1992) sitting within wider health and social care and fiscal policies. Access to high-quality information is required from multiple sources, with interplay between them to draw rational conclusions which can be justified.

Box 3.4 Decision-making factors

- Comprehensive assessment including different stakeholder perspectives
- Wider determinants of health
- Ethical and legal guidance
- Evidence base
- Clinical reasoning
- Options and preferences
- Evaluation
- Accountability
- Safety
- Concordance
- Cost and sustainability

Principles of ethical practice

There is a common set of principles that guides ethical practice in health and social care (Beauchamp and Childress, 2013). Decisions are based not just on clinical evidence but also on a set of moral principles. Health itself is enshrined within human rights values (WHO, 2015). In order to do what is right in the particular circumstances, different stakeholders will have different views which need to be considered when making decisions. In the community, value-based decisions impact not only the service users but also their families and social networks and also their property, for example, the impact of converting a living room into a bedroom. Four ethical principles inform decision making in healthcare practice (Beauchamp and Childress, 2013):

- Respect for autonomy
- Non-maleficence
- Beneficence
- Justice

Respect for autonomy: Individuals have the right to make their own decisions. Professionals must respect the decisions that service users make and ensure their practice is consistent with this (e.g. informed consent). There are exceptional circumstances where individuals are unable to make decisions; professionals must understand the circumstances and legislation that override this self-rule principle.

Non-maleficence: Practitioners should cause no harm, whether intentional or unintentional. Any resulting harm due to a breach in the duty of care owed to that person may be considered negligence, leaving the practitioner open to a charge of professional misconduct and subject to action for compensation through the courts (Dimond, 2015).

Beneficence: It may seem obvious that care offered should be beneficial to service users but this may not always be the case. There may be a clash between the service or policy objectives and the individual, as we saw with the practice nurse. Professionals need to ensure that decisions about care and treatment offered are considered safe and effective (Box 3.4). In the community professionals need to consider the viewpoints, preferences and needs of patients and carers: it must not be assumed that patients' and carers' needs are the same (see Chapter 8).

Justice: Care must be equitable in terms of need and access to resources. In the community this may be a challenge as there will be unequal circumstances and resources affecting quality of care, for example, housing, access to family support or respite. This does not mean that equal time or care has to be allocated among service users but that there should be equitable provision relative to the assessed needs (Thompson et al., 2006). For example, Gerrish's (1999) research showed that there was unequal access to district nursing services for ethnic minority patients because of the way district nursing services were aligned to different GP practices.

Professional practice requires decisions and choices to be made to achieve what is best *and* what is right – though sometimes such choices lead to a moral dilemma. This is where there is conflict between moral principles, in choosing one principle in preference to another (Thompson et al., 2006). In the case of community mental health nursing, where a service user declines treatment but the nurse is aware of the potential harm if the patient does not take his medication, the principle of autonomy conflicts with beneficence, unless the patient is deemed incapable of making such a decision under the Mental Capacity Act (DH, 2005).

Having considered Miss Davies' case regarding her autonomy, she may withhold consent to alternative accommodation or rehabilitation, which she is perfectly entitled to do, providing she is deemed capable of making such decisions. This is at the heart of giving informed consent to treatment. There are four important conditions that need to be in place for informed consent.

ACTIVITY 3.4

Discussion point
Using the four principles of ethical practice above, discuss Miss Davies' case from each person's perspective. What do you think are the key ethical principles here and why? Do you think the district nurse and social worker views will be different? What is guiding their practice?

INFORMED CONSENT

The following conditions need to be present in order for consent to be informed and thereby valid:

1 Sufficient information is made available in order to make a decision, including the potential risks and benefits.
2 The information relevant to the decision must be understood.
3 That information must be used or considered as part of the decision-making process.
4 Consent must be voluntary and without any undue pressure.

In law anyone over 18 years is deemed to be capable of giving consent unless there is evidence to the contrary (Dimond, 2015). In the case of Miss Davies, staff may wish to ensure that she is not only capable of making the decision under the Mental Capacity Act (DH, 2005) but also that there is no undue pressure placed on her to comply with professional advice. Vulnerable people may be susceptible to others' suggestions, feeling they have to comply for fear of losing services or because they wish to be helpful. It may also be the case that older people are used to a paternalistic approach where professionals are seen as expert, not to be challenged, and it is assumed that they always act in the patient's best interest. In Miss Davies' case, both the district nurse and social worker will need to work collaboratively to ensure that she feels supported in whatever decisions she makes and that there are no mixed messages from them.

Children are also vulnerable: those 16 years and over are deemed as having the capacity to give their consent. However, the legal position is different for those under 16 years as children do not have a statutory right to give consent to treatment and Gillick competency must be applied (Dimond, 2015). If the child is mature and is able to understand the nature, purpose and likely effects of any proposed treatment, then valid consent could be given without the involvement of the parents (Dimond, 2015). For example, where a school nurse is asked for contraceptive advice by a young person under the age of 16 years, in making her assessment the nurse would need to satisfy herself not only that the young person understood the significance but also that exceptional circumstances applied (see Dimond, 2015). Assumptions should not be made that informed consent cannot be given purely on the basis of age or condition such as learning disabilities or dementia (see Chapter 16).

PROFESSIONAL VALUES

Alongside these ethical principles, all professions have their own values and concepts that guide and shape practice, providing a means to explore with others the nature of practice and need to be shared (Dominelli, 2009) (Box 3.5). An important aspect of working in the community is the quality of the service user-practitioner relationship, which is key to providing care that is personalised and effective.

Community nurses get to know well service users, families and their circumstances over a period of weeks, months and even years, providing care continuity. Luker's (2002) study on community nurses' construction of quality demonstrates where the 'centrality of knowing the patient and his/her family was an essential antecedent to the provision of high quality palliative care' (Luker, 2002: 775). This value of *knowing the patient* is held in high regard in the community and becomes the crux of person-centred care (The Health Foundation, 2016; NICE, 2015). For example, in Miss Davies' case, the district nurse should seek to establish a relationship stemming from the *first assessment* and subsequent care planning to adopt a collaborative approach. This is where patients are fully engaged in managing their own care, but this is only possible if they feel confident expressing their needs and preferences, resulting in better outcomes (Coulter et al., 2016).

Box 3.5 Common professional values

- Respect and dignity
- Caring
- Empathy
- Autonomy
- Holism
- Confidentiality
- Empowerment
- Partnership
- Equity
- Social justice
- Human rights
- Advocacy

Values need to be shared; at the abstract level they are less problematic but the context in which they apply is where conflict may arise (Dominelli, 2009). Williams' (2000) research showed that despite shared values of caring, compassion and holism between GPs and community nurses, these values were perceived differently by both professional groups, which fuelled communication difficulties. Thompson et al. (2006) state that what appears to be a moral dilemma is more due to inadequate information or a breakdown in communication. Communication is central to all aspects of professional practice and is an area that has warranted numerous policy and practice initiatives to enhance it. For example, the *single assessment process* (SAP) was designed to overcome difficulties in sharing information and duplication for service users (Miller and Cameron, 2011; Worth, 2001). In the case of Miss Davies, a joint assessment ought to result in a comprehensive plan addressing her needs and preferences (see Chapter 7). There is variable support for SAP, which may indicate a failure to understand the values of those who need to use it. Conversely, the learning disabilities *hospital passport* identifies the individual's needs and preferences in advance and crucially is owned by them; it has proven to be an essential document that has saved lives (Skinner, 2011).

PROFESSIONAL CODES OF PRACTICE

These values are expressed in professional *codes of practice*, for example, the NMC (2015) and Health and Care Professions Council (2015a) setting out the ethical standards to which practitioners are held to account, guiding day-to-day practice decisions. Having privileged access to service users, codes are an important way of assuring the public that professionals are regulated so that they can have confidence in them as part of the social contract.

ACTIVITY 3.5

Discussion point

Analyse a professional code of practice from a professional group in relation to the four ethical principles above.

The traditional model pre-dates formal codes of practice; it reflects the utilitarian principle of best interest that bypasses the service user undermining the principle of autonomy. Autonomy is further codified in the Human Rights Act (1998). Conflict may arise between service users' rights and the professionals' duty of care – that is confidentiality, right to privacy or freedom from discrimination (Thompson et al., 2006; O'Keefe et al., 1992).

Box 3.6 Excerpts from HCPC, NMC and GMC codes of practice

HCPC (2016)

1.1 You must treat service users and carers as individuals, respecting their privacy and dignity.

2.2 You must listen to service users and carers and take account of their needs and wishes.

5.1 You must treat information about service users as confidential.

NMC (2015)
1. Treat people as individuals and uphold their dignity.
2. Listen to people and respond to their preferences and concerns.
4. Act in the best interests of people at all times.
5. Respect people's right to privacy and confidentiality.

GMC (2013)
31. You must listen to patients, take account of their views and respond honestly to their questions.
47. You must treat patients as individuals and respect their dignity and privacy.
48. You must treat patients fairly and with respect whatever their life choices and beliefs.
50. You must treat information about patients as confidential. This includes after a patient has died.

While there has been increasing convergence in these codes (Box 3.6), there is a need for a shared code of practice for health and social care professionals based on common ethical principles and values, reflecting a human rights approach. Health and social care professionals are required to keep confidential service users' information, which is reinforced in the respective professional codes of practice (NMC, 2015; HCPC, 2016; GMC, 2013) and legislation (Data Protection Act, 1998). However, failure to share vital information with other professions about service users may not only be inefficient but harmful and in some cases fatal, most notably in child protection (Laming Lord, 2003) and mental health (Cold, 1994). Paradoxically, professionals may use their codes of practice or legislation inappropriately, practising defensively and inhibiting partnership working. Such codes may inadvertently reinforce boundaries and stereotypes between professional groups and represent a conflict of values. Although confidentiality is a common value it does not mean that service users' information can be shared automatically. The Data Protection Act (1998) governs the way in which information is collected, stored and shared (Box 3.7).

Box 3.7 Data protection

Under the Data Protection Act, you must
• Only collect information that you need for a specific purpose
• Keep it secure
• Ensure it is relevant and up to date
• Only hold as much as you need, and only for as long as you need it
• Allow the subject of the information to see it on request

(Information Commissioner's Office (ICO) (n.d.) Health Data Protection – Looking after the information you hold about patients. (Accessed 3 July 2016) https://ico.org.uk/for-organisations/health/.)

Although professionals must understand the law to ensure it is correctly implemented, it is essential that health and social care professionals share information in the best interests of service users. The Caldicott Principles (Dimond, 2015) have been introduced to help practitioners determine what information should be shared and under what circumstances (Box 3.8).

Box 3.8 Caldicott Principles

These good practice principles were updated in 2013 to ensure confidentiality and security of service users' information held by professionals and organisations:

1. Justify the purpose.
2. Don't use personal confidential data unless it is absolutely necessary.
3. Use the minimum necessary personal confidential data.
4. Access to personal confidential data should be on a strict need-to-know basis.
5. Everyone with access to personal confidential data should be aware of their responsibilities.
6. Comply with the law.

(Dimond B, Legal Aspects of Nursing, Pearson Education, Edinburgh, 2015.)

In the case of Miss Davies, the district nurse and social worker may share information through the SAP, and in practice formal agreements are made between organisations with shared service responsibilities. Barriers between organisations and interprofessional working are increasingly being addressed through integrated services (Cameron et al., 2012).

In the community professionals hold a great deal of power over service users due to the invisible nature of the work, staff must be completely trustworthy and uphold codes of practice, to which they are held to account. Staff too may be vulnerable to accusations that may be hard to defend, such as elder abuse or stealing from patients. The expected altruism by professionals working in a service user–centred approach may be countered by how professional power continues to be exercised and maintained beyond direct practice (Box 3.9).

Box 3.9 Critique of professionals

- Are self-interested
- Maintain status quo
- Are incapable of self-regulation
- Retain power
- Block change including policy implementation
- Hide behind rules and regulations or may flout them as a defensive practice

---

Can professionals be trusted?

Trust and professionalism are closely associated (Evetts, 2006a,b). Service users want safe and effective treatment delivered by trusted professionals, but there has been a profound loss of trust in professionals (Evetts, 2006b). Confidence was undermined after a series of scandals where public servants, including health professionals, breached standards (Dimond, 2015). In the community, this was brought to a head by a now seminal case where in 2000 Harold Shipman, a GP in Greater Manchester, was found guilty of murdering 15 patients and forging a will – most of his victims were elderly women living alone, killed by a lethal injection. A subsequent investigation revealed that he had murdered between 215 and 260 patients over a period of 23 years, despite being highly respected by many patients. This rocked the nation's trust in doctors, leading to questioning of the extent of their professional power and that of others. Public confidence has further been shaken by systemic abuse and neglect in hospitals and care homes exposed by the media, leading to public inquiries and calls for radical change to protect the vulnerable (DH, 2012; Francis, 2013). The Francis Inquiry (2013) recommendations led to a change in legislation via the Care Act (2014) providing greater protection from organisations with among others the requirement to disclose failings through a duty of candour (Dimond, 2015). Professionals too are facing greater scrutiny to ensure continuing competence and fitness to practice through more stringent regulation (DH, 2007).

Professional regulatory and statutory bodies such as the NMC, HCPC and GMC have legal powers to regulate their respective professions. They set the standards for education and practice, maintain a register of eligible practitioners, have powers to investigate breaches in professional conduct and revoke the practitioner's licence to practice. Post-Shipman, professional self-regulation has come under greater scrutiny and exposed the lack of transparency, complacency and the reluctance of peers to remove unfit practitioners from the register. This has been addressed through reappraisal of codes, changes to professional education, strengthening the requirements for fitness to practice, including renewal of registration, return to practice and revalidation, and ensuring that more laypeople sit on the professional regulatory boards (King's Fund, 2007).

Traditionally, professionals qualifying were not required to undertake additional training or keep up to date. This does not mean that practitioners did not do this voluntarily and in many cases this was a requirement for specialisation. However health and social care regulators have introduced revalidation requirements and fitness to practice procedures to ensure public protection, which is their central remit (NMC, 2017; HCPC, 2012). For example, all nurses must be able to evidence completion of 450 practice hours over 3 years to be eligible to renew their registration as well declaring themselves fit to do so and need to complete a minimum of 35 hours of continuing professional development activities over a 3-year period (NMC, 2017):

Revalidation
- *is the process that allows you to maintain your registration with the NMC;*
- *demonstrates your continued ability to practice safely and effectively, and*
- *is a continuous process that you will engage with throughout your career.*

Revalidation is the responsibility of nurses and midwives themselves. You are the owner of your own revalidation (NMC, 2017: 6)

Professionals are responsible for maintaining and demonstrating their continuing fitness to practice by submitting evidence to the professional body for scrutiny, usually a portfolio of evidence. Increasingly, self-reported evidence for revalidation is corroborated through peer review exercises and endorsements from employers though service user endorsement is not formally required.

There is now greater convergence across health and social care professions through professional codes of ethics and revalidation of practice (Thistlethwaite, 2007). This reflects a change in language with more active involvement of service users and greater emphasis on teamwork.

The hallmarks of professional practice are summarised in Box 3.10.

Box 3.10 Hallmarks of professional practice

- Critical reflective practice
- Effective communication
- High standards set for safety and effectiveness
- Accountability
- Service users' and carers' participation, feedback and evaluation sought
- Peer review and feedback sought
- Develops others: service users; families; team and students
- Keeps up to date and lifelong learning; can access and use information
- Upholds the code and practices ethically
- Knowledgeable about legal and policy frameworks
- Leadership
- Influences change; research minded
- Develops and maintains networks and partnerships

Service users are generally less reliant on professionals as sole experts or keepers of professional knowledge. Access to the Internet, promotion of self-care and the need to involve service users more means that professionals are less able to hide behind jargon or use terminology that excludes service users. However, for more vulnerable service users this should not be assumed and all patients have a right to be consulted (DH, 2015).

TOWARDS A NEW PARTNERSHIP MODEL OF PROFESSIONAL PRACTICE

Drivers for a new model of professional practice have been gathering momentum and have largely come from outside the professions, reflecting wider societal changes, policy, costs and a recognition of the complexity of health and social care problems. This has also influenced fundamentally professional education with much stronger service user and carer involvement.

The challenge to the old model of professional practice has brought in some radical changes reflecting the shift in societal values that are rights based within a post-modern pluralistic society (DH, 2015).

Although the idea of partnership working with service users has developed over the past 20 years what is new is their role in professional socialisation. The new model of professional practice is one of partnership between service users and professionals and interprofessional working. This is contained within the NMC Standards for pre-registration nurse education (NMC, 2010).

New professionalism?

Although a number of changes have taken place following the reappraisal of professions, professionalism remains a fluid concept and a contested area (Evetts, 2006a, 2012). There is no consensus among researchers about what professionalism is, but the attributes of professional behaviour have been easier to identify (Parker et al., 2006). Parker et al. state that 'the attributes identified as most indicative of professionalism seem to be the subjective, value-laden types such as integrity, regard for the patient and interaction with others' (Parker et al., 2006: 96). The notion that 'good practitioners' know what is quality care is a dated view (Katz et al., 2007). Coulter's (2005) work identifies that patients want professionals who communicate well, keep up to date in clinical knowledge and skills, enable participation in decisions about care and provide emotional support, empathy and respect. Communication skills are inextricably bound up with the quality of the patient's experience (Leatherman and Sutherland, 2007; Freeman and Hughes, 2010).

The balance of power towards service users is changing through a process of deprofessionalisation and patient empowerment (Finlay, 2000b; APPG, 2014); however, many accept that the 'traditional' concept of professionalism is anachronistic and that there has been a paradigm shift to a new norm which is just as problematic to articulate (Davies, 2007; Evetts, 2006a, 2012; Coulter et al., 2016).

Indeed, it is recognised that no single profession is able to meet the health and/or social care needs on their own. In the last half century, myriad new specialties and professions have emerged as healthcare becomes more complex. This has led to greater crossover of traditional roles like prescribing or approved social workers. In many cases this facilitates better access to health and social care services but highlights an increased need for partnership working.

The nature of partnership working

Even if it is agreed that no single profession has all the required knowledge and skills let alone capacity to meet the needs of today's clients, it could be questioned whether these professional differences enhance or complement the assessment of need and planning of care or lead to role conflict and poor teamwork. If there are perceived or actual differences between professional groups, with some seen as more powerful than others, there may be an impact on practice, for example, a GP and a practice nurse, where the GP is also the practice nurse's employer.

Partnership working requires trust and reciprocity (Glendinning et al., 2002) to counter traditional barriers (Hardy et al., cited by Hudson, 2000), avoid blame

> **Box 3.11 Characteristics of effective partnership working**
>
> • Sharing a common vision and goals
> • Planning for the medium term
> • Sharing information
> • Sharing resources
> • Common understanding of need
> • Joint meeting of needs
> • Users experience partnership as coherence in care delivery
> • Equality and trust between partners
> • Common values for social justice
> • Leadership
> • Voluntary

and have clarity about roles and accountability. Interprofessional working in the community (Box 3.11) is essential to avoid gaps and duplication and to focus on agreed outcomes as discussed in Chapter 10.

INFLUENCE OF SERVICE USER INVOLVEMENT ON PROFESSIONAL PRACTICE

Service user involvement is central to health and social care practice whether in direct care, research or education (Cameron et al., 2012; APPG, 2014). This represents a considerable philosophical and practical shift away from seeing the service user as a passive passenger in their journey of care. In refuting the medical model whereby the professionals do not always know best, the emergence of the service user as the expert in their own condition is new (DH, 2006, 2008). Indeed, the notion of being a professional is shifting too, as access to 'elite' information is more readily available and there is greater emphasis on interprofessional working to combat complex health problems. This new paradigm may challenge the traditional hegemony of the medical model of health (Brechin et al., 2000). In addition, service users may now hold special knowledge and experience different from the professionals. Partnership working is a key aspect of this and features strongly in service user involvement.

As professionals have changed so have service users. The move towards health consumerism recasts service users as citizens who must be consulted, offered choice and have a greater say in decisions (Hogg, 1999). By 'reclassifying' health within a wider public health model, the old orthodoxy's power has been challenged, especially in terms of discrimination. This challenge arose from different quarters, reflecting hard-won rights from various groups including women, the disabled and carers. For service users 'having a voice' is not confined to individual care decisions but more fundamentally extends to strategic decisions about the nature and shape of health provision. This involvement extends from policy making and service design to involvement in professional education. Having said this, the reach of professional power in the community for vulnerable and *invisible* people, including carers, has the potential for abuse or disempowerment. Some professionals retain power to control their work, for example, GPs were able to negotiate with the government not to provide *out-of-hours* services (Peckham and Exworthy, 2003), even though improving access to primary care is fundamental.

ROLE OF SERVICE USERS IN PROFESSIONAL EDUCATION

The role of professional education in shaping future practitioners is essential. Changes emphasise the importance of communication and partnership working (HCPC, 2014), recognising that competence alone is not enough to constitute professionalism (Parker et al., 2006). Professionals must balance their technical abilities with those that people value (Leatherman and Sutherland, 2007). These have been codified in the professional standards for education. In this vein, pre-registration nursing has been widely criticised and now an all-graduate qualification has been introduced to redress this imbalance (NMC, 2010). It is an increasing expectation that service users play an active role in all areas of professional education programmes from curriculum design to recruitment of students, teaching and assessment (NMC, 2010).

> An evaluation of service user involvement in health and social care education spanning nursing, social work and allied health professions showed that in contrast to the traditional model service users are now part of the specialisation and acculturation process (Skinner, 2011). Service users and carers then hold a new sort of power, manifested in the power of teaching through stories (Fraser and Greenhalgh, 2001). This brings a direct challenge to professional power as well as a rich reality to education whereby 'knowledge that comes from lived experience be re-valued not necessarily in opposition but alongside more specific professional discourses and bodies of knowledge'. (Brown, in Brechin et al., 2000: 101)

This contrasts with the apprenticeship learning in the traditional model. In the new model of education (and practice) service users participate as experts by experience (Skinner, 2011). Service users in effect now have a quasi-regulatory function locally, by sanctioning aspects of professional education. This could lead to a new form of professional accountability which is shared with or 'controlled' by service users, though professionals decide which service users are involved (Skinner, 2011).

ACTIVITY 3.6

Discussion point

Can you identify service user involvement in your course or practice area? If so, what is its nature?

If you were designing a new service from scratch, how would you go about involving service users? How would you ensure this was 'genuine' and not tokenistic?

There is no *uniform or single set of standards* or benchmarks for service user involvement across the health sector. However, PSRB, including the HCPC and NMC, require assurances about it (HCPC, 2014). Universities determine their own service users' and carers' involvement (SUCI) policy and practice (Skinner, 2011).

Table 3.1 highlights the dichotomy between the old and new models of professional practice, though in reality elements of both models co-exist and different professional groups are at different stages of transition. It may be the case that professionals are regrouping and professional power is still firmly with the professionals, although service users have more rights, powers and resources at their disposal to challenge practice.

Table 3.1 Professional practice: Old and new models

Then – old	Now – new
Patients/individuals	Service users; clients; partners; people/groups/community/ population
Tradition/knowledge handed down/ scientific discovery/experimental treatment	Evidence-based practice; treatment decisions determined externally by peer-reviewed research or regulatory authorities
Apprenticeship model of learning	Service users involved in training and lifelong learning
Expertise rests with professionals	Access to specialist knowledge widely available, e.g. Internet service user as expert
Job for life/way of life/once qualified always qualified	Revalidation – proof of ongoing fitness to practice/maintain competence/ lifelong learning
Clinical autonomy	Patient autonomy – shared decision making with patients and in multidisciplinary teams
Roles distinct and hierarchical boundaries	Role overlap; blurred boundaries; skill mix
Focus on care	Focus on care and experience of care
Focus on skills	Focus on academe; all-graduate profession
Paternalism/professionals define patients' needs	Client-centred care/autonomy/human rights/patient and public involvement
Medical or social models of health	Hybrid holism
Self-regulation; lifelong registration	Lay regulation/regulatory bodies; licence to practice must be reviewed to include proof of fitness to practice, continuing competence, peer review, revalidation
High levels of trust	Less trust and more accountability required
Vocation	Vocation
Best interest; needs determined by professionals	Personal autonomy; rights-based care
Control of resources, e.g. unlimited prescribing	Variable control over resources, direct budgets
Consent	Informed consent
Accountability to peers	Accountability to public and policy makers; codes of practice, duty of candour

CONCLUSION

This chapter highlights a shift in the balance of power towards service users by challenging and redefining what it means to be a health professional in the twenty-first century. Two models of professional practice, old and new, shape relationships between service users and professionals. These models are in a state of flux regarding the conceptualisation of professionalism, role boundaries, core values and power.

Partnership with service users and carers may now play a significant role in the professionalisation of health and social care practitioners. This process not only meets the expected quality and policy agendas to improve fitness to practice but also empowers service users. This is based on mutual respect, trust and reciprocity, which are fundamental to partnership working (Glendinning et al., 2002). Service users and carers are not just being informed about decisions but are key to decision making (Ovretveit, in Brechin et al., 2000).

The professionalisation of health and social care students is being shaped by service user involvement and this may be considered best practice, increasingly reflected in the regulation of professional education (NMC, 2010; HCPC, 2014), although it is too early to judge the extent and permanence of this influence.

Professionals traditionally have wielded considerable power in relation to 'non-professionals' and especially service users. This is viewed as outmoded and undesirable, resulting in a shift in the balance of power towards service users and carers and interprofessional working. This chapter has reviewed the nature of professional practice in relation to two models and the application of ethical principles and values for professional practice within the community. It argues that professional practice has moved from a traditional model of practice towards a more inclusive partnership model involving service users and interprofessional working. The emerging role of service users in the professionalisation process because of their involvement in professional training is explored as part of this new extended partnership model of practice, resulting in a redefinition of what it means to be a health professional in the twenty-first century.

FURTHER RESOURCES

www.cqc.org.uk – Care Quality Commission
www.evidence.nhs.uk – NHS Evidence
www.hscic.gov.uk – Health and Social Care information Centre
www.kingsfund.org.uk – King's Fund
www.nice.org.uk – NICE (National Institute for Health and Care Evidence)
www.wales.nhs.uk/sitesplus/829/opendoc/167542 – Health and Social Care Working
  Together (2010) examples of good practice in Wales

REFERENCES

All Party Parliamentary Group (APPG) (May, 2014) Patient Empowerment: For Better
  Quality, More Sustainable Health Services Globally. A Report by the All Party

Parliamentary Groups on Global Health, HIV/AIDS. Population, Development and Reproductive Health, Global Tuberculosis, and Patient and Public Involvement in Health and Social Care. www.parliament.uk.

Aw TC, Gardiner K and Harrington JM (2006) *Occupational Health Pocket Consultant*, 5th edn. Oxford: Wiley-Blackwell.

Beauchamp TL and Childress JF (2013) *Principles of Biomedical Ethics*, 7th edn. New York, NY: Oxford University Press.

Black C (2008) *Working for a Healthier Tomorrow*. London: The Stationery Office.

Brechin A, Brown H and Eby MA (2000) *Critical Practice in Health and Social Care*, 2nd edn. London: Sage OUP.

Brew M (1997) Nurse prescribing. In Burley S, Mitchell EE, Melling K et al. (eds) *Contemporary Community Nursing*. London: Arnold, pp. 229–43.

Cameron A, Lart L, Bostock L and Coomber C (2012) Factors that promote and hinder joint and integrated working between health and social care services. Social Care Institute for Excellence (SCIE) Research Briefing 41. (Accessed 30 June 2016) http://www.scie.org.uk/publications/briefings/files/briefing41.pdf

Cold J (1994) The Christopher Clunis enquiry. *Psychiatric Bulletin* 18:449–52.

Coulter A (2005) What do patients and the public want from primary care? *British Medical Journal* 351:1199–200.

Coulter A, Kramer G, Warren T and Salisbury C (2016) Building the House of Care for people with long-term conditions: The foundation of the House of Care framework. *British Journal of General Practice* 66:e288–90. doi:10.3399/bjgp16X684745.

Dalley G (1989) Professional ideology or organisational tribalism? The health service–social work divide. In Taylor R and Ford J (eds) *Social Work and Health Care*. Research Highlights in Social Work 19. London: Jessica Kingsley.

Davies C (2007) The promise of 21st century professionalism: Regulatory reform and integrated care. *Journal of Interprofessional Care* 21:233–9.

DH (2005) *Mental Capacity Act*. London: HMSO.

DH (2006) *A Stronger Local Voice: A Framework for Creating a Stronger Local Voice in the Development of Health and Social Care Services*. London: Department of Health.

DH (2007) *Trust, Assurance and Safety: The Regulation of Health Professionals in the 21st Century*. London: TSO.

DH (2008) *Real Involvement Working with People to Improve Health Services Guidance to NHS*. London: TSO.

DH (2012) Transforming Care: A National Response to Winterbourne View Hospital Department of Health Review: Final Report TSO.

DH (2015) The NHS Constitution the NHS belongs to us all England. (Accessed 27 June 2016) https://www.gov.uk/government/uploads/system/uploads/attachment_data/file/480482/NHS_Constitution_WEB.pdf.

Dimond B (2015) *Legal Aspects of Nursing*, 7th edn. Edinburgh: Pearson Education.

Dominelli L (2009). Part 1 Chapter 1. In Adams R, Dominelli L, and Payne M (eds) *Critical Practice in Social Work*, 2nd edn. Basingstoke: Palgrave Macmillan.

Evetts J (1999) Professionalisation and professionalism: Issues for interprofessional care. *Journal of Interprofessional Care* 13:119–28.

Evetts J (2006a) The sociology of professional groups: New directions. *Current Sociology* 54:133–43.

Evetts J (2006b) Trust and professionalism: Challenges and occupational changes. *Current Sociology* 54:515–31.

Evetts, J (2012) *Professionalism: Value and Ideology.* Siociopedia.isa. doi:10.1177/205684601231. (Accessed July 12, 2017) http://www.sagepub.net/isa/resources/pdf/Professionalism.pdf.

Finlay L (2000a) The challenge of professionalism. In Brechin A, Brown H, and Eby MA (eds) *Critical Practice in Health and Social Care.* London: Sage, pp. 74–95.

Finlay L (2000b) Understanding professional development. In Brechin A, Brown H, and Eby MA (eds) *Critical Practice in Health and Social Care.* London: Sage, pp. 48–69.

Francis, R. (2013) Report of the Mid Staffordshire NHS Foundation Trust Public Inquiry Executive summary. (Accessed 26 June 2016) https://www.gov.uk/government/uploads/system/uploads/attachment_data/file/279124/0947.pdf.

Fraser SW and Greenhalgh T (2001) Coping with complexity: Education for capability. *British Medical Journal* 323:799–803.

Freeman G and Hughes J (2010) *Continuity of Care and the Patient Experience An Inquiry into the Quality of General Practice in England Research Report.* London: King's Fund.

Gatley E (1992) From novice to expert: The use of intuitive knowledge as a basis for district nursing. *Nurse Education Today* 12:81–7.

Gerrish K (1999) Inequalities in service provision: An examination of institutional influences on the provision of district nursing care to minority ethnic communities. *Journal of Advanced Nursing* 30:6.

Glendinning C, Powell M and Rummery K (2002) *Partnerships, New Labour and the Governance of Welfare.* Bristol: Policy Press.

GMC (2013) Good medical practice (2013). (Accessed 31 July 2015) http://www.gmc-uk.org/guidance/good_medical_practice.asp.

Great Britain (1998) *Data Protection Act.* London: Stationery Office.

Greenhalgh T (2006) *How to Read a Paper: The Basis of Evidence Medicine*, 3rd edn. Oxford: Blackwell.

Grundstein-Amado R (1992) Differences in ethical decision-making processes among nurses and doctors. *Journal of Advanced Nursing* 17:129–39.

Guest C, Riccardi W, Kawachi I and Laing I (2013) *Oxford Handbook of Public Health Practice*, 3rd edn. Oxford: Oxford University Press.

Health and Care Professions Council (HCPC) (2012) Your guide to our standards of continuing professional development. (Accessed 28 June 2016) http://www.hcpc-uk.org/assets/documents/10003B70Yourguidetoourstandardsofcontinuingprofessionaldevelopment.pdf.

HCPC (2014) Standards of education and training. (Accessed 3 July 2016) http://www.hcpc-uk.org/assets/documents/1000295EStandardsofeducationandtraining-fromSeptember2009.pdf.

HCPC (2016) Standards of conduct, performance and ethics. (Amended 2014). (Accessed 28 June 2016) http://www.hcpc-uk.org/assets/documents/10003B6EStandardsofconduct,performanceandethics.pdf.

Hogg C (1999) *Patients, Power and Politics: From Patients to Citizens.* London: Sage.

Hudson B (2000) Inter-agency collaboration—A sceptical view. In Brechin A, Brown H, and Eby MA (eds) *Critical Practice in Health and Social Care*. London: Sage, pp. 253–74.

Information Commissioner's Office (ICO) (n.d.) Health Data Protection––Looking after the Information you hold about patients. (Accessed 3 July 2016) https://ico.org.uk/for-organisations/health/.

Katz JN, Kessler CL, O'Connell A and Levine SA (2007) Professionalism and evolving concepts of quality. *Society of General Internal Medicine* 22(1):137–9.

King's Fund (2007) *Professional Regulation. King's Fund Briefing*. London: King's Fund.

Laming Lord (2003) *The Victoria Climbié Inquiry Report*. London: Department of Health.

Leatherman S and Sutherland K (2007) *Patient and Public Experience of the NHS*. London: The Health Foundation.

Luker KA (2002) Nurse prescribing from the community: *Nurse's perspective. International Journal of Pharmacy Practice* 10:273–80.

Marmot M (2010) Fair society, healthy lives: A strategic review of health inequalities in England post-2010. (Accessed 14 December 2010) www.marmotreview.org/english-review-of-hi: www.marmotreview.org/AssetLibrary/pdfs/chapters%20of%20fshi/FairSocietyHealthyLivesContents.pdf.

Miller E and Cameron K (2011) Challenges and benefits in implementing shared interagency assessment across the UK: A literature review. *Journal of Interprofessional Care* 25:39–45.

NICE (23 September 2015) Home care: Delivering personal care and practical support to older people living in their own homes NICE guideline. (Accessed July 12, 2017) nice.org.uk/guidance/ng21.

Nursing and Midwifery Council (NMC) (2006) *Standards of Proficiency for Nurse and Midwife Prescribers*. London: NMC. (Accessed 27 June 2016) https://www.nmc.org.uk/globalassets/sitedocuments/standards/nmc-standards-proficiency-nurse-and-midwife-prescribers.pdf.

NMC (2010) Standards for pre-registration nursing education. (Accessed 27 June 2016) https://www.nmc.org.uk/globalassets/sitedocuments/standards/nmc-standards-for-pre-registration-nursing-education.pdf.

NMC (2015) *The Code: Professional Standards of Practice and Behaviour for Nurses and Midwives*. (Accessed 17 June 2016) http://www.nmc.org.uk/globalassets/sitedocuments/nmc-publications/revised-new-nmc-code.pdf

NMC (2017) Revalidation how to revalidate with the NMC requirements for renewing your registration. (Accessed July 12, 2017) https://www.nmc.org.uk/globalassets/sitedocuments/revalidation/how-to-revalidate-booklet.pdf

O'Keefe E, Ottewill R and Wall A (1992) *Community Health Issues in Management*. Sunderland: Business Education.

Parker K, Moyo E, Boyd L et al. (2006) What is professionalism in the applied health sciences? *Journal of Allied Health* 35:2.

Peckham S and Exworthy M (2003) *Primary Care in the UK*. Basingstoke: Palgrave Macmillan.

Pietroni PC (1991) Stereotypes or archetypes? A study of perceptions amongst health care students. *Journal of Social Work Practice* 5:61–9.

Radcliffe V (2008) Non-medical prescribing. In Neno R and Price D (eds) *The Handbook for Advanced Primary Care Nurses*. Maidenhead: Open University Press, pp. 78–88.

Skinner J (2011) VALUE: Valuing Users in Education. An evaluation report. Unpublished.

Steel N (2006) Being explicit about values in public health. In Pencheon D, Guest C, Melzer D, and Muir Gray JA (eds) *Oxford Handbook of Public Health Practice*. Oxford: Oxford University Press, pp. 56–62.

The Health Foundation (2016) Person centred care resource. (Accessed 17 June 2016) http://personcentredcare.health.org.uk/area-of-care/what-is-person-centred-care.

Thistlethwaite J (2007) A commentary from the editorial team. *Journal of Interprofessional Care* 21:2336–9.

Thompson IE, Melia, KM, Boyd KM and Horsbrough D (2006) *Nursing Ethics*, 5th edn. Edinburgh: Churchill Livingstone.

Ward D (2009) Groupwork. In Adams R, Dominelli L, and Payne M (eds) *Critical Practice in Social Work*. Basingstoke: Palgrave Macmillan, pp. 115–24.

Wilkinson R and Pickett K (2010) *The Spirit Level: Why Equality Is Better for Everyone*. London: Penguin.

Williams A (2000) *Nursing, Medicine and Primary Care*. Buckingham: Open University Press.

World Health Organisation (WHO) (December 2015) Health and human rights. Factsheet No. 323. (Accessed 3 July 2016) http://www.who.int/mediacentre/factsheets/fs323/en/.

Worth A (2001) Assessment of the needs of older people by district nurses and social workers: A changing culture? *Journal of Interprofessional Care* 15:257–66.

CHAPTER 4

Managing risk

Jayne Murphy and Debra Smith

LEARNING OUTCOMES

- Explore issues relating to risk assessment of personal safety for nurses working in community settings.
- Explain the importance of preparation needed prior to visiting patients and clients in their homes.
- Critically discuss the implications of risk and use of risk assessment of patients in a community setting.
- Consider the principles of safeguarding individuals in the community.

INTRODUCTION

Working in the community provides many challenges and opportunities. The transition to a non-hospital setting as a student nurse or embarking upon a career as a community staff nurse, requires health professionals to reflect upon their own and others' personal safety, as there will be many situations where the nurse may find themselves working alone. This may include working alone in patients' houses, or working out of hours, weekends and evenings where staff are required to access buildings or other work environments. The importance of appropriate induction and mentorship is crucial to staff who are new to the community setting, to prepare and support them in adapting to this new way of working (Drew, 2011). Working alone enhances the importance of appropriate risk assessment, identification and management in two respects: risk to self and risk to others.

This chapter explores risk from both aspects. The first section of this chapter explores the safety of nurses working in community settings. This includes preparation for home visiting, car safety and the principles of risk management. Risk assessment is fundamental to support the health and safety of both patients and nursing staff (Brennan, 2010), and is part of the clinical governance structure of the organisation. The second part of this chapter focuses upon risk to others, primarily patients and the potential risks to them associated with long-term conditions and living alone. Predictive risk, the use of tools to assess readmission and admission of patients is discussed as well as exploring the care of vulnerable groups, including those with mental health problems, older people, adults and children.

RISK ASSESSMENT IN RELATION TO COMMUNITY NURSES

Personal safety

This section includes the considerations for preparation for home visiting, car safety and organisational support. These issues will be followed by an exploration of the principles of risk management.

Preparation and being streetwise

This includes developing knowledge of the area in which the nurse is to work, developing self-awareness and understanding why and how aggression can escalate.

It is important that the nurse becomes familiar with the geography of the area, whether that is a town, clinic or surgery. This includes becoming familiar with the layout of rooms and buildings and making note of the positions of exits. Finding out what is known about the community is useful and without falling into the trap of stereotyping people, investigate what reputation the area has; for example, finding out about crime rates. Talk to your colleagues about safety. It is strongly recommended that visible security measures, involving personnel and technology, should be evident in health centres and clinics.

ACTIVITY 4.1

Reflection point
You are asked to make a visit to a patient on a local estate which is known to be a very deprived area with a high crime rate. Vandalism, drug use, theft and muggings are increasing. List the precautions that could be taken by the community staff nurse prior to the visit. Reflect upon your own experiences to date.

ACTIVITY 4.2

Review your local policy for lone working, and discuss your findings with an experienced colleague/mentor. Consider whether you will be required to visit out of hours and the local policy to support staff which may involve visiting in pairs. It may also be useful to review the local policy for violence, aggression or harassment.

Before setting out to visit, it is best practice to gather as much information as possible. A survey by the Royal College of Nursing (2007) highlighted that risk assessments are not always considered before first visits and this could potentially put individuals at increased risk. It is important to locate and become familiar with your own organisation's Lone Working Policy.

PREPARATION FOR HOME VISITING

This section will focus on home visits as there are particular features that could, potentially, compromise personal safety.

Bearing the above in mind, first read carefully any records or notes pertaining to the visit. Talk to colleagues who may know the situation and local area and who should make sure that any concerns are shared. Things to think about include does the patient live alone, who else is in the house? Are there any previous issues with violence or aggression? Are there any pets in the house? Look at the location of the visit – think about how you will get there.

Always remember that home visits, however welcome by the patient or client, are an invasion of that individual's space (Table 4.1). It is important to remember that the nurse does not have right of entry into the patient's house. Even when invited, if the patient asks the nurse to leave, and she does not, then the nurse is actually trespassing (QNI, 2013).

The community nurse is a visitor in the patient's home and must wait to be invited in. It is good practice to discourage patients from leaving notes (for example, 'please come round to the back – door open') and hanging keys on strings behind letter boxes. These strategies, obviously, put patients at risk from unscrupulous opportunists and should be discouraged. In addition to these measures, the community nurse should offer personal identification.

Table 4.1 Upon arrival at a patient or client's home

Considerations	Rationale
Remember that you are the visitor.	It is the patient or client's space that you are invading – it is unknown what is or has recently been happening within that person's home.
State clearly who you are and why you have come. Show your identity badge.	Don't assume that the person will recognise a uniform (if one is worn) or will be expecting the visit. It is good practice to encourage patients and clients to ask to see identification. This protects them as well as the professional.
Wait to be invited into the house and ask which room the patient or client would like you to use for your visit.	Being pushy can make people irritated and angry. It may not be convenient for the patient or client to allow you into a particular room. This may be for good reason, e.g. if an unpredictable dog is shut in there!
Note the layout of the house – exits, telephones.	Do this in case a speedy exit is required.
Be careful with people's property – protect their belongings.	Spillages, breakages or rough treatment of belongings will irritate – remember the visitor status.
Be alert – monitor moods and expressions during the visit.	Changes in the demeanour of the patient or client could indicate potential conflict developing.
Be self-aware – monitor the manner in which information is given and care carried out. Do not react to conditions which may seem unacceptable – dirty, smelly environments, for example.	The nurse should not provoke feelings of anger. Remember that this is the patient or client's home.
Trust instinctive feelings. If you feel that leaving quickly is the thing to do – go.	Often assessment of situations takes place on many levels. If uncomfortable feelings are building up do not wait until there is an incident.
If prevented from leaving, try not to panic – see the section relating to interpersonal relationships.	It may be possible for you to de-escalate the situation.

The majority of home visits are very welcome to the patient or client. Relationships between community staff and the people they care for can be very positive and a rewarding aspect of working in primary care. With thought, observation and self-awareness many potential problems may be avoided.

CAR SAFETY

Working in a community setting involves being mobile (Griffith and Tengnah, 2007) and for most community staff, this involves the use of a car.

Some practical measures need to be undertaken relating to car safety (Table 4.2) and areas between car parks and clinic/surgery buildings should be well lit. The nurse should also be aware of the type of car insurance needed when working in the community.

In addition, it is helpful to plan the route to the destination with care. As the geography of the area becomes more familiar, this will become easier. Try not to give the impression that you are unsure of the way. Some police experts are now recommending that car doors are kept locked while driving in more dangerous areas. Good preparation for the journey makes it more likely that the nurse will arrive at the patient's home feeling calm. It is better to avoid road rage – especially if it is your own.

Community nurses should appear purposeful, confident and in control when walking between car and house. Walk towards the curb side of the pavement and away from alleyways and hedges. Footwear should be comfortable and allow for speed, if necessary. It is not a good idea to wear jewellery at work for many reasons. Chains may catch or be pulled; rings and wristwatches are a hazard to patients and clients if physical care is needed. In addition to these (well-known) considerations, jewellery could catch the attention of muggers.

It is important to remember that insurance cover from employers relates to the duration of the shift.

Table 4.2 Car safety

Consideration	Rationale
It makes sense to ensure the vehicle is well maintained.	Not only is it inconvenient, it may be hazardous to break down in a remote place after dark. Well worth the expense of servicing and looking after the car.
Try not to run out of petrol.	The car will not be happy and again this could leave you stranded in remote or unsavoury places.
Park with thought.	Look for safe parking places. In the dark it is helpful to find a street light to park underneath. Try to park near to the destination.
Take out breakdown cover.	At least someone is coming to assist you. Always state that you are alone and make it clear if you are female.
Keep any nursing bags out of view – in addition to any personal valuables.	Some people may believe that nurses carry drugs in their bags – prevent temptation.

ORGANISATIONAL SUPPORT

Organisations that fail to make sure that their employees drive safely may face prosecution. Police may investigate whether basic checks have been made by management (such as whether vehicles have MoT certificates and insurance for business use). There may also be issues around excessive demands being made on staff (Griffith and Tengnah, 2007), such as driving when tired.

Under the 1974 Health and Safety at Work Act and the Management of Health and Safety at Work Regulations (1999), employers have a duty to provide a safe working environment. Along with the responsibilities for employers there are requirements that need to be carried out by employees. First, locate any policies and procedures that exist locally relating to health and safety. Study these carefully and note the reporting arrangements that are laid down for staff to follow.

Nurses must work within the parameters of their Professional Code (NMC, 2015), and this should be enabled by employers.

It is good practice to ensure that your work colleagues are aware of your whereabouts during the day. In addition, contact the work base at the end of the day to let someone know that visits are complete. The team leader or deputy will delegate visits to each member of the staff and will co-ordinate the team. The order in which visits are carried out may not be predictable, but someone will know where each nurse should be visiting on a daily basis.

Most community nurses have the use of a mobile telephone, which can be useful in difficult situations. You need to ensure that your phone has sufficient charge for the day. It may not be possible, however, to access the phone at the very time that you may need it. Mobile phones do not ensure safety, but they help. The use of personal alarms may be useful, to frighten, disorientate and debilitate an attacker. The Suzy Lamplugh Trust (see Further Resources) offers information about personal safety and car travel.

Assessment of risk is a requirement to minimise potential harm and community nurses need to consider safety issues from both practical and professional perspectives.

PRINCIPLES OF RISK MANAGEMENT

Risk management is an analysis of what could potentially harm people, the environment, the organisation and the public, and subsequently assessing measures of prevention (DH, 2007).

These apply to all situations that have potential for risk. It is the case that many interventions carried out by nurses carry risks of harm to patients, the nurse and the general public.

IDENTIFY THE HAZARDS

This includes reports of threats and abuse, not only physical violence, by patients, carers or others. Remember that this could be when the nurse is on or off duty. Incidents include falls, needlestick injuries and stress (Griffith and Tengnah, 2010).

ACTIVITY 4.3

Discussion point

Select one of the identified hazards above. Locate local policies and procedures relating to that hazard and read them. With the chosen topic in mind, work through the stages of risk assessment in Table 4.3 and complete the trust risk assessment documentation if appropriate. Discuss your thoughts with your team leader.

Your discussions may lead you to consider those who may potentially be vulnerable and by working through the following five steps for risk assessment from the National Patient Safety Agency (2007) you can be better prepared for visits.

Table 4.3 Risk identification process

1	Identify the hazard(s) – What can/may go wrong?	Consider things that may have gone wrong in the past, including near-miss incidents.
2	Identify who is at risk – Who might be harmed and how?	Specify who could be harmed by the risk. This could include other members of the nursing team, other professionals and laypeople. Remember that employers have their own duty of care for personal health and safety.
3	Evaluate the risk and decide on precautions.	Assess the seriousness of the situation. Identify what can be done to minimise or eliminate the risk to protect those who could be harmed. Senior nurses will carry out the assessment of the risk with contributing evidence from the team. However, risk assessment is everyone's responsibility in order to identify and report potentially hazardous situations. This may include the use of the organisation's risk matrix.
4	Record the findings and proposed actions.	Decisions taken and workable measures to minimise the risk must be documented. This provides a working plan for staff and managers outlining all of the above in addition to steps that may still need to be taken. Be sure to record events accurately (NMC, 2015). Documentation needs to be comprehensive and accurate, containing a full account of intervention and assessment of the situation (NMC, 2015). Avoid the use of jargon and abbreviations. Incident-reporting systems exist to protect the safety of patients and staff (Armitage, 2005; Evans et al., 2007). Poor communication of risks can result in misunderstanding and failure to pass on vital information to other colleagues.
5	Review and revise the assessment as necessary.	Assessment is a dynamic process. It is important to revisit the document, particularly after incidents are reported. Staff training and communications should also be reviewed. Policies and procedures need to be current, available to those who need them and comprehensive. In order not to compromise patient care, care plans need to be regularly reviewed and updated so that staff are clear what has been found on assessment and what interventions are required.

Patient safety concerns everyone in the National Health Service (NHS), and it is crucial that every member of the staff is aware of these issues. Recent government policy focuses on the delivery of safe, effective, high-quality patient-centred care (DH, 2016a). This can only be achieved if professionals and organisations work within a culture of open information and take responsibility for their contribution to the patients they care for.

ACTIVITY 4.4

Identify whose responsibility it is to review the health and safety policies in your area. Find out where these are kept and how often they are updated. Reflect on your own responsibilities in relation to health and safety. Discuss with your team leader/mentor any education or training that you may need to undertake.

A very useful publication by the National Patient Safety Agency is *Seven Steps to Patient Safety for Primary Care* (2009), a guide to best practices describing key areas of activity that primary care organisations and teams can work through to safeguard their patients (Table 4.4).

Table 4.4 The seven steps to patient safety

Step 1	**Build a safety culture**	Create a culture that is open and fair.
Step 2	**Lead and support your staff**	Establish a clear and strong focus on patient safety throughout your organisation.
Step 3	**Integrate your risk management activity**	Develop systems and processes to manage your risks and identify and assess things that could go wrong.
Step 4	**Promote reporting**	Ensure your staff can easily report incidents locally and nationally.
Step 5	**Involve and communicate with patients and the public**	Develop ways to communicate openly with and listen to patients.
Step 6	**Learn and share safety lessons**	Encourage staff to use root cause analysis to learn how and why incidents happen.
Step 7	**Implement solutions to prevent harm**	Embed lessons through changes to practice, processes.

RISK ASSESSMENT IN RELATION TO PATIENT CARE

Raising concerns

It is the duty of all nurses to raise concerns if they believe that patients in their care are at risk. The Nursing and Midwifery Council (NMC) has produced useful guidance for nurses who are concerned (NMC, 2013). The booklet offers a step-by-step guide to raising and escalating concerns. It recommends following the local 'raising concerns' policy and discussing the issues internally with the respective line manager. These issues may be about the safety and well-being of people in the nurse's care or the environment in which nurses work. To further support individuals to raise concerns, the NMC and General Medical Council (NMC/GMC, 2015) issued a joint statement on the professional 'duty of candour' for their registrants. This requires all health professionals to be open and honest with patients, colleagues, employers and other partner organisations. It suggests that working in a supportive and nurturing environment should support those individuals who wish to raise concerns.

It is therefore evident that organisations must clearly enable nurses to raise concerns, which should then be investigated promptly and thoroughly (RCN, 2015). Further guidance from the RCN explains the process and support mechanisms that are in place for staff.

IDENTIFYING PATIENTS AT RISK OF READMISSION AND ADMISSION

Accident and emergency (A&E) waiting times and NHS winter pressures are reported in the news on a regular basis. Frailty is currently recognised as a long-term condition and is not a consequence of ageing (British Geriatric Society, 2014; NHS England, 2014a). It is apparent that people with long-term conditions, including frailty, are the highest users of acute services but the focus is no longer on admission prevention, instead the focus of healthcare delivery centres on outcomes, on appropriateness of care, on care settings and on improving productivity and delivering better value (see Chapter 12). Leading Change, Adding Value (DH, 2016b) is the follow on from Compassion in Practice (DH, 2012a) and is a framework for all care professionals in all settings, to ensure the best quality of experience and best health and well-being outcomes for patients, using finite resources wisely to get the best value. A variety of initiatives and associated publications across the United Kingdom highlight the need to integrate services to achieve better patient outcomes as well as cost-efficiency savings. Examples of these initiatives include Shifting the Balance of Care (NHS Scotland, 2009), Transforming Your Care (Northern Ireland Health and Social Care Board, 2011), Delivering Local Health Care (NHS Wales, 2013) and the Five Year Forward View (NHS England, 2014b).

Avoidable hospital admissions and prevention of emergency readmissions remain a mainstay of policy discourse and integration of services is geared towards this. Reasons for admission of patients who are deemed at risk of deteriorating health are multi-faceted and often complex. Focus now relies on identifying and minimising these risks and proactively managing patients to avoid incidences of inappropriate admissions. Proactive management involves having appropriate services outside of hospital in order to manage patients and encourage self-management. The ability to predict which patients are at risk of having future unplanned admissions remains key and predictive models are a useful tool to facilitate this. However, according to the Nuffield Trust (Lewis et al., 2011) predictive modelling is a complex area, often surrounded by confusion and there is no specific guidance from the Department of Health (DH) as to which predictive models should be utilised.

There are various different predictive risk models available to the NHS in the United Kingdom and many models differ in the data on which risk is predicted, for instance time period of admission and patient criteria for risk assessment. There are also models that are speciality specific, such as derivatives of the CHADS2 model for atrial fibrillation and stroke risk (Lewis et al., 2011). Some predictive models currently in use in England are the Patients at Risk of Readmission (PARR 30) (Billings et al., 2012) and the Combined Model (Lewis et al., 2011). Scottish Patients at Risk of Readmission (SPARRA) has also been successfully used, in Wales, Prism (Predictive Risk Model) has been utilised (Hutchings et al., 2013) and Northern Ireland have used PARR models (Lupari, 2010). Predictive models identify patients at the highest risk of hospital admission and allow clinicians to engage with high-risk patients to instigate behavioural or treatment changes and introduce preventative measures to reduce risk (Billings et al., 2012). However, few prediction models have been validated and evidence about their effects on patient care is limited (Hutchings et al., 2013). Nonetheless, risk stratification is incorporated in general practitioner (GP) contracts in England (British Medical Association [BMA], 2015) and the importance of admission avoidance remains a significant theme in commissioning services throughout the United Kingdom.

ADULTS AT RISK

Within the community setting, it is difficult to offer any single definition of the term 'vulnerable' and often the concept of vulnerability is open to interpretation by health professionals. In fact, the term 'vulnerable' is now considered as contentious because it is deemed to appear as though the cause of abuse is located with the victim, rather than placing the responsibility on the action or omission on others (Smith et al., 2010). The preferred term currently is 'adults at-risk', although vulnerable is still used. It generally refers to older adults who may be frail due to ill health, physical disability or cognitive impairment, have a learning disability, physical disability or sensory impairment, have a mental health need, a long-term illness, misuses substances or alcohol, is a carer or is unable to demonstrate the capacity to make a decision and is therefore in need of support (Social Care Institute for Excellence, 2015). For the purpose of this chapter, the issues of mental health, falls and safeguarding will be considered in respect of community nurses and their involvement in the care of adults and children at risk.

PEOPLE WITH MENTAL HEALTH ISSUES

Mental illness (discussed in more detail in Chapter 16) is the largest single source of burden of disease in the United Kingdom. It has an impact on every aspect of life, including physical health and risk behaviour (Royal College of Psychiatrists [RCP], 2010). Although mental health issues are not a consequence of ageing, age is a risk factor for developing mental illness and though this includes dementia it is not isolated to dementia alone but also other disorders such as depression, anxiety, schizophrenia, suicidal feelings, personality disorder and substance misuse (Joint Commissioning Panel for Mental Health, 2013). In 2009 in the United Kingdom, mental health problems were present in 40% of older people who attend their GP, in 50% of older adult inpatients in general hospitals, and in 60% of residents in care homes. Just over a quarter of admissions to mental health inpatient services involve people over the age of 65 (Healthcare Commission, 2009). Adults with long-term conditions are more likely to develop mental health problems, such as depression and anxiety (Naylor et al., 2012). They also experience more complications if they develop mental health problems, increasing the cost of care by an average of 45% (NHS England, 2016). The Five Year Forward View For Mental Health (NHS England, 2016) makes 58 recommendations where action is needed to reduce inequalities and to increase access to mental health services in line with accessibility to physical health services.

Physical health is also linked to mental health and poor mental health is associated with other priority public health conditions such as obesity, alcohol misuse and smoking and with diseases such as cancer. Poor physical health also increases the risk of mental illness (RCP, 2010). Action is needed to promote awareness of the importance of mental health and well-being in older age as well as ways to safeguard it (RCP, 2010). The increasing prevalence of multi-morbidity, including co-morbid mental health problems alongside long-term physical health conditions is a central part of the rationale for integrated care, suggested by the King's Fund (Naylor et al., 2016). There is a commitment to value mental health the same way as physical health, enabling people with a mental health condition to get the same access to healthcare services as they would for physical health. This *parity of esteem* was mentioned in 'no health without mental health' (DH, 2011) and has been further reinforced in more recent information from NHS England (2014c). It is recognised that community nurses have an increased role in the care of patients with an established mental health problem or those who may be at risk of isolation, stress and other chronic conditions that may contribute to the development of mental health issues (Haddad, 2010). Community nurses can implement strategies which may include screening, assistance with medication, referral to other specialised mental health services as well as monitoring individuals with established mental health problems (Thompson et al., 2008).

Although the risk of developing dementia increases with age, it is not considered a normal part of ageing. Dementia represents one of the major health and social care challenges facing the United Kingdom, and an ageing population means that dementia will affect an increasing number of people over the coming decades. There are currently 850,000 people in the United Kingdom living with dementia and this figure is set to rise to 2 million by 2051 (Alzheimer's Society, 2015). The term 'dementia' describes a set of symptoms that include loss of memory, mood changes and problems with communicating and reasoning. These symptoms occur when the brain is damaged by certain diseases, such as Alzheimer's disease or a series of small strokes (causing vascular dementia). Rarer causes of dementia include dementia with Lewy bodies and frontotemporal dementia. Dementia is a progressive condition, meaning that people with dementia and their family and carers have to cope with changing abilities over time. These changes include an increasing and fluctuating impairment in the person's capacity to make decisions about major life events and circumstances as well as day-to-day situations (Alzheimer's Society, 2015). Community nurses across the United Kingdom are being asked to carry out cognitive assessments as part of their assessment process and the community nurse's role in identifying people who require investigation in order to discover the causes of cognitive impairment is a crucially important part of improving access to diagnosis and treatment (Nazarko, 2014).

Depression and anxiety are common mental health problems; they are thought to affect about 1 in 10 people in the general population at any time and are the third most common reason for people visiting the GP (Haddad et al., 2011). Available data indicate that fewer than one-third of adults with depression obtain appropriate professional treatment. This is attributed, among other reasons, to the under-recognition of the problem by health professionals (Lazarou et al., 2011). Depression can happen suddenly as a result of physical illness, experiences from childhood, unemployment, bereavement, family problems or other life-changing events. Symptoms include tiredness, sadness that does not go away, loss of confidence, not enjoying things that are usually pleasurable, feeling anxious all the time, sleeping problems, feelings of guilt or worthlessness, appetite changes, thoughts of suicide (Mental Health Foundation, 2006).

Anxiety is one of the most common mental health problems in the United Kingdom and it is increasing. Yet, it remains under-reported, under-diagnosed and under-treated. Experiencing anxiety too much or too often presents the risk of becoming overwhelmed, unable to find balance in life or the ability to relax and recover. Estimates of the number of people who experience anxiety vary because of the different methods for gathering data and the different criteria used in identifying it (Mental Health Foundation, 2014). In order to improve recognition of mental health problems, it is imperative for nurses and especially those working in community settings to appreciate the importance of prompt diagnosis which presumes both an understanding and knowledge of basic aspects of the problem and, an understanding of their role in dealing with depression (Lazarou et al., 2011).

CARING FOR OLDER PEOPLE

Community nursing encompasses caring for people of all ages. However, a large proportion of the community nurses' caseload will involve caring for older people.

This section focuses on living in isolation and will cover falls. There are now more people aged over 65 than aged under 18 in the United Kingdom and the number of older people is set to increase. There are currently 11.4 million people aged over 65 in the United Kingdom and 3 million people are aged over 80. The number of people aged over 65 is set to increase by almost 50% in the next 17 years and one in five people can expect to live to 100 (Age UK, 2016). Increasing age comes with challenges both for the individual and for society. There will be large increases in demand for and costs of health and social care (House of Lords Select Committee, 2013).

Older people are also at risk of isolation for reasons such as bereavement, ill-health, lack of local services or transport and poor physical environment. The number of people living alone also looks set to increase (Age UK, 2014). An evidence review carried out by Age UK (2015a) showed that health conditions or impairments can lead to a curtailment of independence and limit social roles, resulting in feelings of loneliness, just as chronic feelings of loneliness can result in deterioration of health and well-being. Loneliness has also been linked to premature death, cardiovascular disease, lower immunity, increased mental health problems and developing dementia. Despite the recognition that supported self-management can enable older people and their families to live more comfortably with long-term conditions and reduce their risk of developing new ones, they are far less likely to receive such support than younger people in similar situations (Oliver et al., 2014).

Community nurses need to be particularly aware of the needs of older people and to promote self-care initiatives that can encourage and maintain their independence. It is important to know what support there is (both locally and nationally) in terms of health and social care. The range of voluntary services may vary across the United Kingdom, but can still provide valuable advice and resources to individuals and health professionals. Although the provision of advice and information is paramount, it is important to recognise the potential barriers that can exist in the provision of information to these individuals. Some of these barriers include an increasing reliance on the use of the Internet for information and transactions, and the use of language and communication styles. Community nurses need to work closely with these older people to assist them in accessing and understanding information (Hislop, 2010).

FALLS

Falls leading to injury are the leading cause of accident-related mortality in older people. Falls among older people are recognised internationally as a risk to older adults, with the World Health Organization (WHO) producing a global report on falls prevention (WHO, 2007). Guidance, reports and initiatives on falls prevention abound, acknowledging the magnitude of the effects of falls on individuals and society (National Institute for Health and Care Excellence [NICE], 2013, 2015; Age UK, 2013; NHS England, 2015). Falls and fractures, in people aged 65 and over account for over 4 million bed days each year in England alone and the healthcare cost associated with fragility fractures is estimated at £2 billion a year. Falls often lead to reduced functional ability and thus increased dependency on families, carers and services (Royal College of Physicians, 2011).

Falls destroy confidence, increase isolation and reduce independence, with around 1 in 10 older people who fall becoming afraid to leave their homes in case they fall again (Age UK, 2013).

There are many different reasons why people fall and in many cases, it is a combination of risk factors that leads to a fall, such as different medications or medical conditions, poorly fitting footwear or just the physiological conditions associated with ageing, such as natural deterioration in eyesight and muscle strength. A good assessment is essential when it comes to determining the causes of and effective treatment for a fall. A multifactorial risk assessment is paramount and patients should be offered a range of interventions, including medication reviews and home safety assessments (Age UK, 2013). Community nurses may come into contact with individuals who have sustained injuries, or who have lost mobility or have suffered a loss of function and are therefore at high risk of falling. As community nurses are in regular contact with older people, they are in a prime position to make a difference in the prevention and subsequent management of those who are at risk of falling or have actually fallen.

NICE (2015) recommends that older people who have had recurrent falls or who are assessed as being at a high risk of falling should be offered an individualised, multi-factorial risk assessment. Most organisations should have approved documentation for recording the assessment (Robertson et al., 2010). It is acknowledged that this assessment needs to be conducted by an appropriately qualified health professional. Many organisations have introduced a Falls Service to address the needs of this group. Following assessment, if appropriate, the individual may be offered a multi-factorial intervention. The aim of this is to identify and address future risk, as well as promote the individual's independence and improve their overall physical and psychological function. The following components are common to this type of intervention: strength and balance training, home hazard assessment and intervention, vision assessment and medication review (NICE, 2015).

The NHS England Safety Thermometer (ST) introduced in the NHS Operating Framework for 2012/13 (DH, 2012b) announced a new programme to incentivise all providers of NHS care to measure (initially) four common complications (harms): pressure ulcers, falls, catheters and urine infection and venous thromboembolism. The ST has remained for these areas and also covers other areas such as medicines, children and young people, mental health and maternity services (NHS England, 2014d). Data collection for each area is broadly applicable to patients across all healthcare settings, but particularly to older people who, experiencing more healthcare intervention, are at risk of not one but multiple harms. Community nurses and other health professionals working in the community environment have a role in collecting data and monitoring the ST. They should also take the opportunity to routinely ask older patients who they come into contact with about any falls they have had in the past 12 months. This needs to be recorded on appropriate organisational documentation using a recognised assessment tool.

The next activity will enable you to consider the issues in relation to a specific patient.

ACTIVITY 4.5

Reflection point

Discuss predictive risk modelling with a colleague and find out if there is a risk modelling tool that is used locally and how the data gathered impacts service delivery.

Reflect upon an older person you have visited recently. Consider their home environment and identify any hazards that may impact on their health and well-being. Discuss with a colleague ways that you can advise this person to keep himself or herself safe.

With the older population increasing, it is recognised that the consequences of frail individuals falling will pose a greater challenge to both health and social care services. Find out about the falls prevention service in your area. Identify the criteria for referring a client.

SAFEGUARDING ADULTS, CHILDREN AND YOUNG PEOPLE

The Care Act (DH, 2014) sets out a legal framework for how local authorities should protect adults at risk of abuse or neglect, such as implementing preventative measures through a multi-agency approach, enquiring in cases of suspected abuse or neglect, reviewing cases of neglect or abuse, engaging independent advocates where necessary and establishing Adult Safeguarding Boards to share multi-agency safeguarding strategies. It is the responsibility of all health professionals to safeguard against poor practice, harm and abuse of individuals that they care for (DH, 2013). Generally, safeguarding can be defined as 'the function of protecting adults and children from abuse or neglect' (Office of the Public Guardian, 2013). More specifically, child protection can be defined as 'the process of protecting individual children identified as either suffering or likely to suffer significant harm as a result of abuse or neglect' (Department for Children, Schools and Families, 2010).

All adults, children and young people have the right to be protected. It is acknowledged that safeguarding cannot be provided by one single discipline, it requires a multi-agency, collaborative approach. Community nurses are in a unique position to safeguard adults, children and young people as their contact with patients and families allows them to recognise and respond to issues of abuse.

There are many forms of abuse which can be described as a violation of an individual's human and civil rights. Adults at risk (vulnerable adults) are more at risk of abuse if they are isolated, and have limited contact with family and friends; have communication difficulties, are dependent on someone as a carer or if their carer has alcohol or drug addiction issues (DH, 2015a). It is essential therefore that nurses are aware of and can recognise the potential signs of abuse. There are different forms of abuse including, physical, financial, sexual, psychological/emotional, neglect, discriminatory or institutional abuse (Age UK, 2015a). With an ageing population, it is thought that the number of older people at risk of abuse will rise, particularly among those with memory or communication problems (Age UK, 2015b). Similarly, maltreatment of children can manifest in many different ways, including signs of physical, emotional and sexual abuse, neglect and fabricated or induced illness (NICE, 2009). Recent evidence suggests that all four countries in the United Kingdom have seen the number of sexual offences against children increase (Jutte et al., 2015). There are certain factors which may increase the risk for child abuse including living in an environment where domestic violence takes place, having parents with mental health or substance misuse issues, or living in poverty (GMC, 2012). It is important to remember however, that these issues do not necessarily lead to abuse or neglect, as child abuse exists in all areas of society.

In some instances, abuse may result in children being taken into care where a small number of them remain at risk of abuse, neglect or poor standards of care from those who are looking after them (Biehal et al., 2014). In the longer term, when compared with their peers, 'looked after children' generally have poorer outcomes in terms of education and mental health. Many experience poverty, isolation and housing and employment problems in adult life. A child protection issue or concerns regarding the possibility of abuse may arise in a variety of nursing encounters, even when the initial encounter has a completely different focus. It is possible that nurses who are new to the community environment may have received little training and preparation for this element of their role. Furthermore, nurses must recognise the importance of working collaboratively with other health professionals, so that if a nurse suspects that a child is subject to harm or neglect, the nurse has a responsibility to refer their concerns to appropriate personnel (DH, 2015b). This can be a very difficult area of nursing practice which needs to be addressed in a sensitive manner, and with appropriate education and training.

All employers have a duty to ensure that the workforce is competent in the area of adult abuse, child protection and safeguarding. All staff should know what to do if they suspect abuse, or a possible child protection issue and should be able to recognise key indicators that suggest that the individual is a risk of harm or neglect (RCN, 2014; Commissioner for Older people for Northern Ireland, 2014). Often, inter-agency training is delivered, as it is thought to improve collaborative working processes between professionals involved in child protection issues (Charles and Horwath, 2009). The key principles of safeguarding adults include the following:

- Empowerment – Focus on person-led decisions and informed consent
- Prevention – Better to take action before any harm occurs
- Proportionality – The least intrusive response appropriate to the risk presented
- Protection – Support and representation for those in greatest need
- Partnership – Communities working together as they have a role to play in preventing, detecting and reporting neglect and abuse
- Accountability – Accountability and transparency in delivering safeguarding (DH, 2013)

Working Together to Safeguard Children (DH, 2015a) suggests that all training in safeguarding and promoting the welfare of children and young people should be child centred, promote the participation of children and their families in the process, value collaborative working, respect diversity and promote equality (DH, 2015b). Effective communication and partnership working are recognised as key areas in the identification of vulnerable children and protecting them from abuse (Welsh Government, 2014).

To understand and identify significant harm to a child, it is necessary for health professionals to consider

- The nature of harm, in terms of maltreatment or failure to provide adequate care
- The impact on the child's health and development
- The child's development within the context of their family and wider environment
- Any special needs, such as a medical condition, communication impairment or disability, that may affect the child's development and care within the family
- The capacity of parents to meet adequately the child's needs
- The wider and environmental family context (DH, 2003)

Furthermore, it is paramount that the child's needs are put first, and that health professionals ensure that children are listened to and understand the decisions that affect them (Scottish Government, 2014).

Please carry out the next activity to supplement your developing knowledge in this crucial area of practice.

ACTIVITY 4.6

Find out who the lead person is for safeguarding and child protection issues in your organisation. Identify the local policy and guidelines, read them and discuss the referral process with a colleague.

ACTIVITY 4.7

Consider the following case studies and discuss any safeguarding issues or concerns raised with your team leader/mentor:

Jamie is a 3-year-old boy who you meet at the GP practice. He lives with his 20-year-old mother. It is a cold rainy day, but you notice that Jamie only has a thin shirt under his anorak. He is also wearing sandals. On speaking with his mother, she tells you that the staff at the nursery where Jamie attends have spoken to her about his increasingly aggressive behaviour towards some of the other children. Later, when discussing with your colleagues, you discover that Jamie has missed many of his regular, routine health checks, and is not up to date with his vaccinations.

Gladys is 75 years old and lives with her husband George in a bungalow. She has been visited several times by the nursing team over recent months. Gladys was diagnosed with dementia several years ago, and depends upon George for helping with her daily activities. You are visiting Gladys to assess a small laceration which she has sustained to her shin following a fall. During your visit and assessment, you notice that Gladys has some bruises on her upper arms. When talking with Gladys about the bruises she becomes upset and withdrawn. George also appears agitated and anxious.

The above text and activities are designed to assist you in developing your professional practice with at-risk groups. You will need to ensure that this aspect of your work is regularly updated in line with organisational processes and policies.

CONCLUSION

After careful consideration of the issues addressed within this chapter, turn back to the learning outcomes at the beginning and think about each one in turn. Look back and reflect upon the notes made for the first activity at the beginning of this chapter.

If this chapter has raised any concerns for practice, it is important that they are discussed with an experienced community nurse, either informally or through clinical supervision channels. Some useful addresses can be found at the end of this section.

Remember that the majority of staff working in community settings enjoy a close partnership with their patients and clients. The health centre or surgery is at the heart of the local community and relationships may build over a number of years. Visiting patients and clients in their homes is a privilege that greatly enhances the experience of community nursing. Taking practical precautions and taking time to think about the assessment of risk and preparation are crucial elements of nursing in the community.

FURTHER READING

Beckett C (2007) *Child Protection: An Introduction*, 2nd edn. London: Sage.

Corby B (2006) *Child Abuse: Towards a Knowledge Base*, 3rd edn. Berkshire: Open University Press.

Powell C (2007) *Safeguarding Children and Young People. A Guide for Nurses and Midwives*. Berkshire: Open University Press.

Scottish Government (2008) *Getting it Right for Every Child*. Edinburgh: Scottish Government.

FURTHER RESOURCES

www.cqc.org.uk – Care Quality Commission

www.gov.uk – Department of Health

www.hse.gov.uk – Health and Safety Executive

www.suzylamplugh.org – The Suzy Lamplugh Trust

www.nmc-uk.org – Nursing and Midwifery Council

www.npsa.nhs.uk – National Patient Safety Agency

www.rcn.org.uk – The Royal College of Nursing

www.unison.org.uk – Unison

http://www.unitetheunion.org/how-we-help/list-of-sectors/healthsector/healthsectoryourprofession/cphva/ – CPHVA/Unite

www.mind.org.uk – Mind Organization

www.alzheimers.org.uk – Alzheimer's Society

www.mentalhealth.org.uk – Mental Health Foundation

www.wales.gov.uk – Welsh Government

www.gov.ie – Irish Government

www.gov.scot – Scottish Government

REFERENCES

Age UK (2013) *Falls Prevention Exercise—Following the Evidence*. London: Age UK.

Age UK (2014) *Policy Position Paper Loneliness and Isolation (UK)*. London: Age UK.

Age UK (2015a) *Evidence Review: Loneliness in Later Life*. London: Age UK.

Age UK (2015b) *Safeguarding Older People from Abuse and Neglect*. Factsheet 78. London: Age UK.

Age UK (2016) *Later life in the United Kingdom*. Age UK. http://www.ageuk.org.uk/Documents/EN-GB/Factsheets/Later_Life_UK_factsheet.pdf?dtrk=true.

Alzheimer's Society (2015) *Dementia 2015: Aiming higher to transform lives*. London: Alzheimer's Society.

Armitage C (2005) TRAIL: A model to promote active learning from adverse events. *Quality in Primary Care* 13:159–62.

Biehal N, Cusworth L, Wade J and Clarke S. (2014) *Keeping Children Safe: Allegations Concerning the Abuse or Neglect of Children in Care*. London: NSPCC.

Billings J, Blunt I, Steventon A et al. (2012) Development of a predictive model to identify inpatients at risk of re-admission within 30 days of discharge (PARR-30). *British Medical of Journal*. e001667. doi:10.1136/bmjopen-2012-001667

Brennan W (2010) Safer lone working: Assessing the risk to health professionals. *British Journal of Nursing* 19(22):428–30.

British Geriatric Society (2014) *Fit for frailty*. London: British Geriatric Society.

British Medical Association (2015) *General Practice Contract Changes*. http://bma.org.uk/working-for-change/negotiating-for-the-profession/bma-general-practitioners-committee/general-practice-contract.

Charles M and Horwath J (2009) Investing in interagency training to safeguard children: An act of faith or an act of reason? *Children and Society* 23:364–76.

Commissioner for Older people for Northern Ireland (2014) *Protecting our Older People in Northern Ireland. A Call for Adult Safeguarding Legislation*. http://www.copni.org/images/publications/Protecting_Our_Older_People_in_Northern_Ireland_Report_1.pdf. Accessed June 22, 2016.

Department for Children, Schools and Families (2010) *Working Together to Safeguard Children*. London: The Stationery Office.

Department of Health (2003) *Every Child Matters*. London: The Stationery Office.

Department of Health (2007) *Independence, Choice and Risk: A Guide to Best Practice in Supporting Decision Making*. London: The Stationery Office.

Department of Health (2011) *No Health without Mental Health*. London: The Stationery Office.

Department of Health (2012a) *Compassion in Practice*. London: The Stationery Office.

Department of Health (2012b) *Delivering the NHS Safety Thermometer CQUIN 2013/14*. London: The Stationery Office.

Department of Health (2013) *Statement of Government Policy on Adult Safeguarding*. London: The Stationery Office.

Department of Health (2014) *Care Act*. London: The Stationery Office.

Department of Health (2015a) *No Secrets: Guidance on Developing and Implementing Multi-Agency Policies and Procedures to Protect Vulnerable Adults from Abuse*. London: The Stationery Office.

Department of Health (2015b) *Working Together to Safeguard Children*. London: The Stationery Office.

Department of Health (2016a) *The NHS Outcomes Framework 2015/16*. London: The Stationery Office.

Department of Health (2016b) *Leading Change Adding Value*. London: The Stationery Office.

Drew D (2011) Professional identity and the culture of community nursing. *British Journal of Community Nursing* 16(3):126–31.

Evans A, Williams L, Wiltshire M et al. (2007) Incident reporting improves safety: The use of the RAID process for improving incident reporting and learning within primary care. *Quality in Primary Care* 1(5):107–12.

General Medical Council (2012) *Guidance on Protecting Children and Young people*. Manchester: GMC.

Griffith R and Tengnah C (2007) Role of the law in ensuring work related road safety. *British Journal of Community Nursing* 12:574–8.

Griffith R and Tengnah C (2010) Health and safety at work: A guide for district nurses. *British Journal of Community Nursing* 15:77–80.

Haddad M (2010) Caring for patients with long-term conditions and depression. *Nursing Standard* 24:40–9.

Haddad M, Buszewicz M and Murphy B (2011) *Supporting People with Depression and Anxiety: A Guide for Practice Nurses*. London: Mind.

Health and Safety at Work Act (1974) http://www.legislation.gov.uk/ukpga/1974/37/pdfs/ukpga_19740037_en.pdf. Accessed November 10, 2015.

Health and Social Care Board (2011) *Transforming Your Care*. http://www.transformingyourcare.hscni.net/. Accessed June 22, 2016.

Healthcare Commission (2009) *Equality in Later Life: A National Study of Older People's Mental Health Services*. London: Healthcare Commission.

Hislop C (2010) Improving access to information: A key requirement for reducing social exclusion. *Working With Older People* 14:38–43.

House of Lords Select Committee (2013) *Ready for Ageing? Report*. London: The Stationery Office.

Hutchings H, Evans BA, Fitzsimmons D et al. (2013) Predictive risk stratification model: A progressive cluster-randomised trial in chronic conditions management (PRISMATIC) research protocol. *Trials Journal*. 14(301): 1–10. http://www.ncbi.nlm.nih.gov/pmc/articles/PMC3848373/pdf/1745-6215-14-301.pdf.

Joint Commissioning Panel for Mental Health (2013) *Guidance for Commissioners of Older People's Mental Health Services*. www.jcpmh.info. Accessed June 24, 2016.

Jutte S, Bentley H, Tallis D et al. (2015) *How Safe are our Children? The Most Comprehensive Overview of Child Protection in the UK*. London: NSPCC.

Lazarou C, Kouta C, Kapsou M and Kaite C (2011) Overview of depression: Epidemiology and implications for community nursing practice. British Journal of Community Nursing 16(1):41–7.

Lewis G, Curry N and Bardsley M (2011) *Choosing a Predictive Risk Model: A Guide for Commissioners in England*. London: Nuffield Trust.

Lupari M (2010) *PARR in Northern Ireland. Presentation at Nuffield Trust Conference on Predictive Risk 2011*. http://www.nuffieldtrust.org.uk/talks/slideshows/marina-lupari-overview-parr-practicenorthern-ireland. Accessed June 24, 2016.

Mental Health Foundation (2006) *Dealing with Depression*. London: Mental Health Foundation.

Mental Health Foundation (2014) *Living with Anxiety. Understanding the Role and Impact of Anxiety in our Lives*. London: Mental Health Foundation.

National Institute for Health and Care Excellence (2009) *When to Suspect Child Maltreatment*. London: The Stationery Office.

National Institute for Health and Care Excellence (2013) *Falls: Assessment and Prevention of Falls in Older People*. London: NICE.

National Institute for Health and Care Excellence (2015) *Falls in Older People: Assessment after a Fall and Preventing Further Falls*. London: NICE.

National Patient Safety Agency (2007) *Healthcare Risk Assessment Made Easy*. London: NPSA.

National Patient Safety Agency (2009) *Seven Steps for Patient Safety in Primary Care*. London: NPSA.

Naylor C, et al (2012) *Long-Term Conditions and Mental Health: The Cost of Co-morbidities*. London: King's Fund.

Naylor C, et al (2016) *Bringing Together Physical and Mental Health: A New Frontier for Integrated Care*. London: King's Fund.

Nazarko L (2014) Cognitive assessment: A guide for community nurses. *British Journal of Community Nursing* 18(11):550–3.

NHS England (2014a) *Safe, Compassionate Care for Frail Older People using an Integrated Care Pathway*. London: NHS England.

NHS England (2014b) *Five Year Forward View*. London: NHS England.

NHS England (2014c) *NHS England Pledge to Help Patients with Serious Mental Illness*. https://www.england.nhs.uk/2014/01/mental-illness/. Accessed June 24, 2016.

NHS England (2014d) *A Quick Guide to the NHS Safety Thermometer*. http://harmfreecare.org/wp-content/files_mf/NHS-SafetyThermometer_V14.pdf.

NHS England (2015) *Falls Prevention. Reducing Harm Associated with Falls*. http://www.england.nhs.uk/ourwork/patientsafety/falls-prevention/. Accessed June 24, 2016.

NHS England (2016) *The Five Year Forward View for Mental Health*. London: NHS England.

NHS Scotland (2009) *Shifting the Balance of Care*. http://www.shiftingthebalance.scot.nhs.uk/home/. Accessed June 24, 2016.

NHS Wales (2013) *Delivering Local Health Care Accelerating the Pace of Change*. Cardiff: Department for Health and Social Services.

Nursing and Midwifery Council (2013) *Raising Concerns: Guidance for Nurses and Midwives*. London: NMC.

Nursing and Midwifery Council (2015) *The Code: Professional Standards of Practice and Behaviour for Nurses and Midwives*. London: NMC.

Nursing and Midwifery Council/General Medical Council (2015) *Openness and Honesty When Things Go Wrong: The Professional Duty of Candour*. London: NMC/GMC.

Office of the Public Guardian (OPG) (2013) *Safeguarding Policy*. Birmingham: OPG.

Oliver D, Foot C and Humphries R (2014) *Making our Health and Care Systems Fit for an Ageing Population*. London: King's Fund.

Queen's Nursing Institute (2013) *Transition to Community Nursing Practice*. London: QNI.

Robertson K, Logan PA, Conroy S et al. (2010) Thinking falls—Taking action: A guide to action for falls prevention. *British Journal of Community Nursing* 15:406–10.

Royal College of Nursing (2007) *Lone Working Survey*. London: RCN.

Royal College of Nursing (2014) *Safeguarding Children and Young People*. London: RCN.

Royal College of Nursing (2015) *Raising Concerns: A Guide for RCN Members*. London: RCN.

Royal College of Physicians (2011) *Falling Standards, Broken Promises Report of the National Audit of Falls and Bone Health in Older People 2010*. London: RCP.

Royal College of Psychiatrists (2010) *No Health Without Public Mental Health; the Case for Action*. London: RCP.

Scottish Government (2014) *National Guidance for Child Protection in Scotland*. Edinburgh: Scottish Government.

Smith M, et al (2010) Vulnerability: A contentious and fluid term. *Hastings Centre Report* 40(1):5–6.

Social Care Institute for Excellence (2015) *Adult Safeguarding Practice Questions*. London: SCIE.

The Management of Health and Safety at Work Regulations (1999) http://www.legislation.gov.uk/uksi/1999/3242/pdfs/uksi_19993242_en.pdf. Accessed November 10, 2015.

Thompson P, Lang L and Annells M (2008) A systematic review of the effectiveness of in-home community nurse led interventions for the mental health of older persons. *Journal of Clinical Nursing* 17:1419–27.

Welsh Government (2014) *Social Services and Wellbeing Act*. Cardiff: Welsh Government.

World Health Organization (2007) *WHO Global Report on Falls Prevention in Older Age*. Geneva: WHO.

CHAPTER

5

Therapeutic relationships

Jacqueline Corbett, Patricia Wilson and Sue Miller

LEARNING OUTCOMES

- Identify the features and potential benefits of a therapeutic relationship.
- Discuss some of the challenges for community nurses in establishing a therapeutic relationship.
- Critically examine the challenges involved and potential consequences of failing to establish or maintain a therapeutic relationship.
- Analyse the impact of changes in policy on the development of therapeutic relationships.

INTRODUCTION

This chapter focuses upon the relationship that exists between the nurse, the person being cared for and their family. It is recognised that such a relationship should be therapeutic and indeed this is essential to the delivery of effective nursing care. However, it is unwise to assume a therapeutic relationship will automatically occur, as there are many challenges in establishing and maintaining such a relationship in community settings. In this chapter the key features and benefits of a therapeutic relationship will be identified; in addition, some of the challenges of establishing and maintaining that relationship in a community setting will be discussed. This will lead the reader to consider issues of particular relevance to those people receiving his or her community nursing care, to explore some of the consequences of failing to establish and maintain relationships and to identify ways to achieve positive therapeutic relationships. In conclusion, the current and potential changes in healthcare delivery and policy drivers will be reviewed with particular reference to the way these changes might impact on the nurse/person/family relationship.

Varying titles exist for people receiving healthcare in the community often reflecting different community nursing services involved in such care. In this text 'person' is generally used as the preferred term and refers to individuals who may also be identified as patient, client and service user within clinical practice.

THE FEATURES OF A THERAPEUTIC RELATIONSHIP

While there is a lack of clear consensus regarding definition, Pullen and Mathias (2010) describe a therapeutic relationship as one that offers support based on mutual trust, respect, sensitivity to self and others, while nurturing faith and hope and embracing the physical, emotional and spiritual needs of the person. The recognition of the importance of the therapeutic relationship is not a new phenomenon. Peplau's (1952) theory of nursing is based upon the importance of the relationship between the nurse and the individual. She asserts this is pivotal to the way in which all nursing care is delivered. The importance of this relationship has continued to be widely acknowledged. It is recognised as central to advancing the best interest and outcomes for the person and the families (Porr et al., 2012; Canning et al., 2007). However, discussions regarding the quality of relationships inevitably introduce a degree of subjectivity. Furthermore, the inter-subjective qualities involved in therapeutic relationships such as empathy, respect, trust, positive regard, support, communications skills, person- and family-centred care, acceptance, empowerment and so on are not easily measureable (Greenhalgh and Heath, 2010). It is suggested, however, that positive therapeutic relationships can improve communication (Porr et al., 2015; Pinto et al., 2012; Edwards et al., 2006), achieve concordance (Martin et al., 2005), service user satisfaction (NCSBN, 2014), help in professional fulfillment, save time, empower and also reduce risk of litigation (Stewart, 2005). Since a therapeutic relationship is so important, it is essential to consider which key features characterise the relationship. In reviewing various definitions it becomes apparent that important factors include

- Maintaining appropriate boundaries
- Meeting the needs of the person
- Promoting autonomy
- Providing a positive experience for the person and/or family receiving care

Maintaining appropriate boundaries

The Nursing and Midwifery Council (NMC) (2015) highlights the need for clear professional boundaries with people receiving care, including family and carers. This is important whether care is being received at the present time or received in the past, in order to ensure the promotion of professionalism and trust. Boundaries are generally mutually understood and often unspoken physical and emotional limits of a relationship (Farber et al., 1997). However, it is important that the nurse, individual and family are clear regarding their relationship and what is reasonably expected of each party. This will protect all those involved in the relationship.

There is a delicate balance between caring for people and families and becoming over-involved. The process of finding a positive boundary of care, especially nursing in the community, can be challenging to discern as is discussed later in this chapter.

Meeting the needs of the person

The purpose of the relationship between the community nurse and person is to meet the needs of that person. Policy and guidelines support person- and family-centred care (DH, 2015a; Healthcare Improvement Scotland, 2014; NICE, 2012; Davies and Wackerberg, 2012; DHSSPS NI, 2011a). Person- and family-centred healthcare strives to empower individuals and families by providing information and education regarding the person's health condition and encouraging active participation in the decision-making process (Foot et al., 2014). It is therefore important that the needs of the person are discussed at the outset of the relationship in order that mutually identified goals can be set and everyone within the relationship can be clear about their role in achieving these goals. This might include the nurse, the person receiving care, carers, family members or friends, other health and social care professionals or relevant agencies. Discussion will require expert communication skills on the part of the nurse in order that a relationship of trust can develop. Although the relationship exists to meet the needs of the person, it is likely that the nurse will experience satisfaction in helping to ensure the needs are met. This is entirely appropriate. However, it is important that nurses do not allow their personal needs for positive self-esteem, control and belonging to undermine the professional relationship (Milton, 2008). This requires enhanced self-awareness, engagement in reflective inquiry and critical-thinking skills (Waugh et al., 2014). It may also require a willingness to seek support from others (Foster and Hawkins, 2005).

Promoting autonomy

Autonomy is derived from the Greek *autos-nomos* meaning self-determination or self-rule. While the original meaning of autonomy relates to 'self-rule', it can also refer to liberty of thought, freedom of choice, freedom of action, self-determination and freedom from coercion (Dworkin, 1988). Therefore, it is about self-governance, the ability to make choices and decisions about things that will affect oneself (Ellis, 2015). This further supports the need for excellent communication skills on the part of the nurse in order to assist the person and to understand the person's perspective and situation. There is general acknowledgement regarding the therapeutic value of empathically understanding the person (Clarke, 2010). Empathic understanding is deemed to facilitate autonomy and so empathy is explored later in this chapter. Within a relationship that promotes autonomy the person receiving care can contribute to the achievement of personal goals and move towards independence.

Providing a positive experience for the person

The experience of participating in a therapeutic relationship will be positive for all, given needs will be met in a way that is most appropriate for the person and their family. Truly therapeutic relationships can be remembered and valued for a long time. They empower the person, the family and the nurse, they facilitate trust, respect, autonomy, and encourage self-awareness for the nurse and person alike. A positive experience for the person is supported by the National Institute for Health and Care Excellence (NICE, 2011) in the publication of 'The quality standard for the service user experience in adult mental health services' and NICE (2012) in 'The quality standard for the patient experience in adult NHS services'. Person-centred care is supported by organisations like the Picker Institute (www.pickereurope.org); it monitors patients' experience of care and highlights deficiencies. Community nurses providing care need to be mindful with regard to the key determinants of a good experience and be proactive in seeking and acting on individual feedback (Spencer and Puntoni, 2015).

These features are evident in guidance provided by the NMC (2015) which highlights the importance of relationships prioritising people and promoting professionalism and trust.

ACTIVITY 5.1

Reflection point

Is there potential to improve your approach towards therapeutic relationships? Think about entering a person's home and establishing a therapeutic relationship. Ask yourself to what extent am I able to connect emotionally and show unconditional regard? Do my therapeutic relationships allow any 'hidden agenda' to surface and be addressed? To what extent do I acknowledge the need for that person's autonomy and accept their perspective as legitimate in the communication? If I score poorly on these do I need additional support? Discuss your ideas with your mentor/preceptor. Questions are adapted from Greenhalgh and Heath (2010).

CHALLENGES OF DEVELOPING THERAPEUTIC RELATIONSHIPS IN COMMUNITY SETTINGS

Having considered the features of a professional relationship, some of the challenges of achieving such a relationship in the community setting will be discussed. Professional relationships with people are influenced by a number of factors that are illustrated in Figure 5.1.

Location of care

The delivery of care within the home can provide a feeling of security for the person and his or her carers as they are on familiar territory. This can make it easier to develop a positive relationship, such that they are able to share their concerns and worries. It is also probable that individuals and carers will be able to learn new skills more readily as they are likely to feel more relaxed within their 'normal' environment.

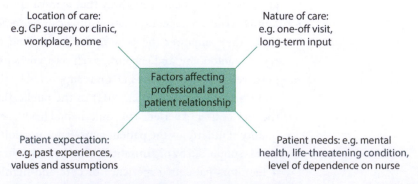

Figure 5.1 Factors affecting the therapeutic relationship.

Example 5.1

Consider Mrs Patel whose 2-year-old son has recently been in hospital as a result of an asthma attack. Mrs Patel speaks some English but found the experience of her son being in hospital very stressful. When the health visitor made a visit to the home Mrs Patel was unsure how to use the prescribed medication, particularly the spacer device to administer the inhalers. Teaching within Mrs Patel's home is likely to be more successful as she will be more relaxed and it will be possible for the health visitor to reinforce any aspects of the care at a later date if this is necessary.

However, caring in the home environment can leave the nurse feeling vulnerable. The Queen's Nursing Institute (QNI, 2015) highlights some of the challenges facing community nurses, in particular if they first move from hospital-based jobs to work in the community. Despite the use of mobile phones and pagers it is more difficult to seek the advice of a colleague, and help may not be instantly at hand. A nurse who feels vulnerable and isolated will find it more difficult to inspire confidence.

Working in the relative isolation of the home can provide challenges to nurses in maintaining standards of care. If the relationship is not 'therapeutic' it can be difficult for the nurse to identify this himself or herself, particularly if the situation has developed over time. The support and guidance of colleagues is essential, as is the willingness of the nurse to be open to that support. It is important that peers recognise unhealthy situations that colleagues are involved in (Halter et al., 2007). However, it can be difficult to express concerns with colleagues and so a shared culture of open discussion where the person is the priority as directed by Francis (2013) is essential.

Furthermore, the QNI provides a useful online resource, 'Transition to Community Nursing Practice', which offers practical support and guidance for community nurses to address personal challenges and identify sources of support which can reduce feeling of isolation. The resource can be found at www.qni.org.

Care given by the nurse within the person's workplace will also be different from the more traditional hospital setting. The occupational health nurse addresses the health and well-being of the working population in their place of work (Thornbury, 2013). They are often the first point of contact for individuals with health-related problems. Moreover, the occupational health nurse holds a unique public health role towards the improvement of health, social well-being and towards improving the quality of working lives in the workplace (RCN, 2015a).

Example 5.2

Although work-related mental ill health is being increasingly recognised as a legitimate occupational health issue (TUC, 2015) many employees will still consider it detrimental for their career prospects to report mental health needs to their occupational health nurse. The challenge for the nurse within this context is to promote trust with the employees in order to facilitate a therapeutic relationship.

Developing therapeutic relationships can also be affected by a clinic or surgery setting, where the person may gain the impression of busy workloads inhibiting the time they spend with the nurse. Paterson (2001) identified lack of time as a major inhibitor in developing participatory relationships. More recently Ball et al. (2013), in a survey of district and community nurses identified 13% of respondents cited 'lack of patient contact time' as a significant frustration affecting quality of care. Similarly, the King's Fund (2016) highlights research indicating activity amongst district nurses has increased significantly both in terms of people seen and complexity of care provided. While the community nurse is likely to be as busy if not more so, when undertaking home visits, there may be fewer distractions than in a busy clinic. However, it can be argued that even the briefest episode of caregiving presents the community nurse with an opportunity to capitalise on time (Chan et al., 2013) and with purposeful focused communication enhance the therapeutic relationship.

Example 5.3

Consider the scenario of the new mother trying to explain her depression to the health visitor and how much harder this might be in a busy baby clinic rather than in the privacy of her own home. In other cases the relative anonymity that the surgery or clinic provides may be of benefit in facilitating the development of a therapeutic relationship. Clearly, as a community nurse it is important to recognise the impact that the working environment has upon relationships with people, carers, family and colleagues. It is a key element of care influencing communication together with the quality and safety of healthcare provided (Godsell et al., 2013). Initial assessments are often the first point of contact between community nurse and the person receiving care; the nurse must develop skills to enable a conducive environment, in order to establish the start of a therapeutic relationship (Hagerty and Patusky, 2003).

ACTIVITY 5.2

Reflection point
Do you wear a uniform when working in the community? What are the advantages and disadvantages of wearing a uniform? If you had a choice, would you wear a uniform?

Working in the community many nurses find not wearing a uniform removes an unnecessary barrier and makes the development of a therapeutic relationship an easier task. It does however require skills on the part of the nurse to gain access to the a person's home, gain the trust and explain the nursing role since a symbol, which for many carries some degree of status, has been lost (Shaw and Timmons, 2010).

For those community nurses who do wear a uniform other challenges arise. Wearing of a uniform can enable almost instant entry to some homes, but may present a barrier to acceptance by some people. This may be especially apparent with children who have perhaps learnt to associate uniforms with pain and discomfort. In these situations it will take time to address prior conceptions before a therapeutic relationship can be established.

If nurses do not wear a recognised uniform it is particularly important to consider the appropriateness of the clothing that is worn. Entering a home inappropriately dressed may cause offence and prevent establishment of a relationship. Perhaps this might require the nurse to cover her arms and legs if visiting Asian families, or maybe to remove shoes prior to entering some homes. In order to meet the needs of individual families the nurse must enquire about family preferences and be willing to adapt behaviours to respect values different from her own in order to facilitate positive relationships.

A final point about dress code: whether wearing uniform or not it is essential to carry identification at all times in order to protect the well-being of people living in the community.

ACTIVITY 5.3

Nature of care
Discussion point
Have you cared for someone over a long period of time? How did your relationship with that person develop? Did you find yourself becoming 'closer' to the individual? How did this make you feel? Discuss this with your mentor/preceptor.

A key element in the nature of the therapeutic relationship is the duration of the relationship. Morse (1991) describes three appropriate relationships. First, she describes the one-off clinical encounter that, for example, a practice nurse may have with a person seeking healthcare in a travel clinic. There are also encounters that last longer but focus on a specific need, such as maintenance of hormone replacement therapy. Both of these relationships are mutual and appropriate to certain situations, but Morse argues that within a much longer-term nurse-person relationship, there should be a different focus, with the development of what she terms a connected relationship. Morse suggests that the key characteristic of a connected relationship is that the nurse views a person as a person first rather than a patient, client or service user, and so on.

Example 5.4

A district nurse has been visiting an elderly lady for several years. The visits now may often include a chat over a cup of tea about how the grandchildren are progressing or other issues in the person's life that the nurse has developed a wealth of knowledge on over the years. Although it may be a venous ulcer that initiated the referral to the district nurse, the connected relationship that has developed with time allows the nurse to deal with other issues that may be far more important to the person, such as feelings of loneliness. During the chat, a skilled nurse will be able to assess for signs of depression or other psychosocial needs that are common for people experiencing long-term conditions. Although for many families and professionals this can only be positive, there is a potential to step over the professional boundary and it is essential to maintain the appropriate balance within the therapeutic relationship. The consequences of not maintaining the balance will be returned to later in the chapter.

ACTIVITY 5.4

Reflection point
Have you ever cared for someone who did not follow the recommended treatment programme? Why do you think that they did not adhere to the treatment regimen? How did it make you feel?

In the home environment individuals and carers could be perceived to have greater control within the relationship. Should a person decide not to concur with recommended treatment, this may not be immediately evident as the nurse is generally spending only a short period of time within the home environment. If unbeknown to the nurse, lack of adherence to treatments takes place, the therapeutic relationship may be threatened. However, the focus for the community nurse needs to be towards concordance and facilitation of person/family centred care. At times challenging, this is about ensuring a partnership approach with people and families. This approach can facilitate decisions that reflect the person's needs and preferences and ensure individuals have the education and support required to make such decisions and participate in their care (IOM, 2001). It is less about fitting people into predetermined services and more about empowering people to work towards outcomes that matter to themselves (King's Fund, 2015a; Healthcare Improvement Scotland, 2014; WG, 2014; The Health Foundation, 2014; DHSSPS NI, 2010). Therefore, within a therapeutic relationship a person receiving care is comfortable enough to tell the nurse of his or her intentions. This might allow treatment to be modified to the extent that the person feels able to follow the regimen, but even if this is not the case at least the community nurse is aware of the true situation and can modify the nursing care accordingly.

Example 5.5

Consider the following scenario and your responses.

Rosie is 14 years old and has been diagnosed as having type 1 diabetes for 6 months. She has been asked to record her blood glucose levels once daily, varying the time of day she takes the readings, but she finds this requirement tiresome and does not do it. Prior to the community children's nurse's visit she wonders what to do – should she make up some values to keep the nurse happy or should she tell the truth? Hopefully if Rosie and the community nurse have a good relationship Rosie can be truthful and they can work together on what can reasonably be expected. A study by Schaeuble et al. (2010) found teenagers felt it took time to develop trust in healthcare providers, with respect from the provider being a paramount issue. Some of the adolescents in the study stated that they withheld information out of fear of a provider's reactions; however, they still wanted to know the consequences of refusing or delaying treatment. Concordance describes a partnership approach to treatments and care; it recognises the importance of individuals being able to make their own decisions about lifestyle and whether or not to adhere to advice from health professionals (DH, 2015b). Therefore, concordance returns us to the theme of person-centred care and decision making. The subject is visited again in the next and last sections of this chapter.

Expectations

Expectations of the nurse and community nursing service may also impact on the therapeutic relationship. Over the past 25 years, there has been a rapid rise in consumerism resulting in the NHS becoming more business-like with a rise in expectation and subject to similar consumer drivers identified in other parts of society (Sturgeon, 2014). Recent health policy emphasises person-centred choice and involvement in care (Foot et al., 2014). Many people have clear ideas on the service they expect from community nurses, with a consequential detrimental effect on the therapeutic relationship when these expectations either are not met or are unrealistic. However, despite trends in healthy ageing and participation in healthcare (Healthcare Commission, 2006), many older adults were brought up in a society where medicine was seen to have all the answers and the public was expected to be the passive recipient of care (Coulter, 1999). There is some evidence that some people do not wish to be an active partner in the therapeutic relationship (Davis et al., 2007), and some may prefer a more paternalistic model of care (Roberts, 2001).

The community nurse may find a challenge in helping some people to develop the confidence and ability to self-care, and so the therapeutic relationship will be focused on trust and the facilitation of realistic independence. Self-care is key policy strategy for the NHS across all countries in the United Kingdom (Drakeford, 2013; DHSSPS NI, 2012; DH, 2009; Scottish Government, 2008). Skills for Health (2015) set out some key principles to support self-care; it involves creating environments in which people who need care and support are perceived as active and equal partners, rather than passive recipients. It includes self-management, which means people drawing on their strengths and abilities to manage or minimise limitations imposed by a condition, as well as what they can do to feel happy and fulfilled (Skills for Health, 2015). Furthermore, it is suggested by Drakeford (2013) that self-care links closely to person-centred care, person experience, co-production and improving quality. Therefore, the nurse 'doing for' the individual rather than enabling them to self-care contradicts current perspectives on best practice (Wilson et al., 2007).

Needs

The main purpose of the nursing or health-visiting intervention may also have a significant impact on the therapeutic relationship. The patient within the relationship may have significant physical and emotional needs such as in palliative care. The relationship developed within these cases may be based on intensive input by the nurse (Dunne et al., 2005). In contrast, the practice nurse or occupational health nurse may see a patient for health screening with less obvious health needs as the focus of the intervention.

The substantial shift of care from hospitals to the community for those with mental health needs (Malone et al., 2007) has resulted in a rapidly developing role for community nurses in supporting this patient group. With approximately one in six people at any one time experiencing mental illness in the United Kingdom and one in four of people experiencing problems some time in their life (DH, 2011) the role for community nurses supporting people living in the community is constantly evolving. Recent mental health frameworks and guidance (DH, 2012; Scottish Government, 2012; DHSSPH NI, 2011b; WG, 2010) are firmly underpinned with focus on the patient. However, empowering people with mental health needs and implementing empowerment initiatives is often challenging. The World Health Organization (WHO, 2010) suggests it requires the person, service and societal levels to be aligned for this to happen and for stigma, discrimination and marginalisation to be prevented. Therefore, the therapeutic relationship with this group is essential in empowering people to actively participate in decisions about their care. Peplau's (1952) developmental model is often used as the framework for developing a therapeutic relationship (Merritt and Procter, 2010), with the assessment (or orientation) phase focusing on the development of mutual trust and regard, as well as data gathering. Developing a therapeutic interpersonal relationship is the foundation stone of quality nursing care (McKenna and Cutcliffe, 2008), and the community nurse may take on a number of roles to facilitate this, including that of counsellor, resource, teacher, coach, leader or surrogate. All nurses working in the community develop knowledge of local resources and other agencies and facilitating individuals and families to access these may be the key component within this relationship.

It should also be acknowledged that the therapeutic relationship in the community setting is not only formed between nurse and the person, but will often encompass a family carer. Carers UK (2014) suggest that there are 1.4 million people providing care round the clock in the United Kingdom and approximately six and half million people providing some level of care supporting friends and family with various conditions and disabilities. The law relating to carers differs across the four countries of the United Kingdom. The Care Act (2014) in England, the Social Services and Well-being (Wales) Act 2014, Carers (Scotland) Bill (2014) and Carers and Direct Payments Act (Northern Ireland) 2002 have provided carers the legal right to needs assessment and support. The law across the United Kingdom requires local authorities assess carers' need for support wherever they appear to have such needs. For the community nurse this reinforces that an individual therapeutic relationship must also be developed with the family carer, but this poses a number of challenges.

Caring is associated with increased risk of mental health problems (Stansfield, 2014). It is important for community nurses to recognise the potential need for interventions and be familiar with local services available to reduce the stress of caring. Unfortunately some family carers will be unknown to the community nurse (Simon and Kendrick, 2001). The more a family carer does for a person, the less intervention there will be from the community nurse (Gerrish, 2008). Consequently, the family carers most likely to benefit from a therapeutic relationship are less likely to be visited by the community nurse. This highlights the need for the community nurse to identify carers and liaise with other health professionals, social services and other agencies accordingly. Furthermore, there are often misguided assumptions by many professionals that family carers should undertake the caring role and that the role is taken on very willingly (Procter et al., 2001). All too frequently, community nurses first meet a family carer when there is a crisis and the physical input and support are limited to when the crisis is over or the person has been admitted to hospital. The therapeutic relationship with family carers should ideally be long term, with the nurse aiming to provide information and acting as a resource (Seddon and Robinson, 2001) and responding to the role the carer is happy to undertake. Twigg and Atkin (1994) describe three different responses by individuals to the informal caring role (Table 5.1).

It is important for the community nurse to recognise the carer's response to their situation and not take the carer for granted as a readily available resource (Manthorpe et al., 2003).

Table 5.1 Responses to the caring role (adapted from Twigg and Atkin: 1994)

Response to the caring role	Features of response
Engulfment mode	Cannot articulate needs as a carer
	No other occupation
	Generally female spouse
	Total sense of responsibility and duty
Balancing/boundary setting mode	Have a clear picture of themselves as carers (e.g. how they save nation money)
	Generally male
	Often adopt language of an occupation – treat role as a job
	May emotionally detach themselves from recipient
Symbiotic mode	Positive gain by caring
	Does not want role taken away

Example 5.6

Imagine the case of Lily, a 75-year-old mother caring for her son Ted, who has Down's syndrome. She is devoted to her son and has no other life than caring for him. The general practitioner has referred Ted for a wound assessment, but when the nurse arrives it is apparent that Lily is exhausted by her role. The challenge for the nurse is to establish a relationship which enables Lily to acknowledge her individual needs and helps her to accept help without feelings of guilt. This may involve developing a long-term relationship and not simply the organising of respite, which many informal carers do not want (Stockwell-Smith et al., 2010).

Another frequently met scenario is that of the husband caring for his wife. He has every detail organised and is business-like in his approach to the community nurse. Again, this may hide a number of physical and emotional needs for which the community nurse must develop a therapeutic relationship in order to enable him to express these. The needs of family carers should be recognised, and the community nurse must develop a relationship and provide interventions appropriate to both the person and the carer as individuals. You can explore carers in greater detail in Chapter 8.

WHEN THE BALANCE IS NOT MAINTAINED: FAILURES IN THERAPEUTIC RELATIONSHIPS

ACTIVITY 5.5

Discussion point

How do you define friendships? What are the potential dangers in becoming friends with people and families that you are caring for in the community? What dangers exist in discussing personal issues and treating as your friend someone who is receiving care from your community nursing service? In keeping secrets with the person? In believing you are the only member of staff that can provide the correct level of care for that person? In meeting outside the work environment as friends? In speaking in a derogatory way regarding other members of staff or the work setting? In showing favouritism? What can you do if someone that you are providing care for wants to develop a friendship with you? Discuss your ideas with a professional colleague. (Questions are adapted from NCSBN, 2014.)

In reality it is hard to learn about boundaries unless one is involved in setting them, and extending beyond the therapeutic boundary may only be apparent once it has been breached. It may be that it is in the interests of an individual and his or her carer to encourage the professional to develop a relationship of friendship since this has the potential to 'normalise' the situation, as it is 'normal' to have friends who visit. This is perhaps more likely to occur if nurses do not wear uniforms. Families may be keen that friendships do develop since a friend is likely to respond to requests for help, perhaps more swiftly than a detached professional. Therefore, nurses must consider their actions carefully in case actions are misinterpreted, as perhaps was the case when Ann attended John's party.

Example 5.7

Consider the case of Ann, who is John's community children's nurse. Ann has cared for John, aged 5, for the last 2 years and supported Gill, his single mother, through some difficult times while John has received treatment for acute lymphoblastic leukaemia. During Ann's recent visit to the home, Gill and John invite her to John's sixth birthday party the following weekend. Ann considers this briefly and agrees to come. At the end of the party, Gill asks Ann if she would be willing to babysit for John, as 'she's the only person she feels she can trust to care for John'. What should Ann do now? It would appear the edges of the professional boundary have become significantly blurred such that Gill feels it is appropriate to ask Ann to babysit.

Hylton Rushton et al. (1996) describe over-involvement as a lack of separation between the nurse's own feelings and those of the person receiving care. Typically the nurse may spend off-duty time with the client, appear territorial over the care or treat certain clients with favouritism (Parkes and Jukes, 2008). The consequences for the person may result in an over-dependence on that particular nurse and a lack of support in reaching therapeutic goals (Moyle, 2003). For the community nurse, the implications can involve significant stress, eventual compassion fatigue and burnout especially where clients are experiencing trauma, pain and suffering (Gandi et al., 2011). The NMC (2015) directs nurses to stay objective and have clear professional boundaries always with people (including those cared for in the past), their families and carers. Of course, the balance in the therapeutic relationship may be tipped the other way. The detached, cold nurse who seems indifferent to a person's emotional needs may be familiar to the reader. The results of under-involvement are a lack of understanding by the nurse of the person's perspective, conflict and standardised rather than contextually dependent care (Milton, 2008). The overwhelming feelings that a nurse may have for a person's situation can lead to dissociation by the nurse within the therapeutic relationship (Crowe, 2000). The consequence of under-involvement is that the nurse can have a lack of insight into the other person's perspective and be unable to facilitate a person in meeting therapeutic goals.

Mackintosh (2006) suggests that it is the inter-personal aspects of the caring relationship that nurses value most highly. Ensuring therapeutic relationships is viewed as having an important place (Brunero et al., 2009). To establish the goal empathy is often regarded as one of the most desirable qualities for a nurse. It is described as the process of understanding a person 'as if' you were that person (Drydon and Mytton, 1999). Definitions also stress empathy as the ability to perceive the meaning and feelings of another and to communicate those feelings to the other person (La Monica, 1981; Wiseman, 1996: Stein-Parbury, 2005). It is often viewed as having two parts; cognitive and affective (Verducci, 2000; Hojat et al., 2002). The cognitive domain involves understanding of the other's inner experience and feelings with an ability to view the world from the other's perspective. The affective domain involves entering or joining in the emotional experience of the other. It may be difficult for nurses acting in the affective domain as they are at risk of losing objectivity and becoming overwhelmed by the emotions of others (Brunero et al., 2009).

Empathy is also seen as a crucial part of emotional intelligence and highlights the importance of having emotionally skilled community nurses. Gandi et al. (2011) argues that nurses' empathy for and connection with people demonstrate core professional values which are often seen as essential but as a consequence attract certain factors capable of inducing stress. It is suggested that when caring for those experiencing trauma, pain and suffering, nurses can be affected resulting in compassion fatigue. Therefore, behaviour can reveal a central theme of the 'negative effects' of overly identifying with those receiving care, and as mentioned, this can result in unintentional vicarious experience of the other person's pain and anxiety (Abendroth and Flannery, 2006). Community nurses need to strive towards being skilled and competent nurses who are also emotionally skilled, able to understand the benefits and dangers of empathy and also able to recognise indifference among others within teams. Empathy and empathic listening skills have the potential to enable community nurses to deliver dignified and compassionate care while building therapeutic relationships. However, knowledge and understanding regarding the benefits of cognitive empathy and empathic concern, and an appreciation of the danger of excessive affective empathy and emotional contagion are required.

Viktor Frankl, post holocaust, powerfully describes the choice that humans have in taking time to respond and choose an attitude in a particular set of circumstances (Frankl, 2006). It is important for community nurses to take time. Taking time during the therapeutic relationship can be facilitated with clinical supervision as part of continuing professional development. Clinical supervision can offer a valuable opportunity to explore self and promote emotional skill and empathy in community nursing practice in order to enhance the therapeutic relationship.

ACTIVITY 5.6

Reflection point
Think of a likeable person with whose care you have recently been involved. Reflect on the following: What were the characteristics of the individual and their care that made it a positive experience for you? If other colleagues were involved, do you think they felt the same way? Was the care you gave the person affected by these feelings? Are there any consequences for yourself, the person and other people on your caseload?

Maintaining a therapeutic relationship is particularly challenging within the community because of the commonly intense nature of care, duration of contact and the non-clinical environment. Reflection with colleagues and clinical supervision become invaluable tools to facilitate the nurse in developing appropriate relationships with people.

INFLUENCE OF THE CURRENT AND FUTURE CONTEXT ON THERAPEUTIC RELATIONSHIPS

Long-term care interventions within the community setting will continue to increase with an ageing population (King's Fund, 2015b) and this chapter has already explored the impact of duration of care on the therapeutic relationship. One response by policy makers to the rise in long-term conditions is the facilitation of individuals to self-manage their own conditions.

There are a number of well-established self-management programmes that aim to empower people to improve their health. The Expert Patient Programme (DH, 2001) is based on the Stanford model of self-management education and is widely delivered by publically funded healthcare organisations in the United Kingdom, the United States and Australia (Greenhalgh, 2009). A generic approach, this chronic disease self-management programme, consists of six weekly, lay tutored sessions fostering self-management skills via participative techniques such as modelling and action planning (Griffiths et al., 2007).

Therapeutic relationships in the current climate must be based on an acknowledgement that the person may have considerable expertise in their own condition, exceeding the nurse's. There can be little doubt that a therapeutic relationship needs to take into account the knowledge that both nurse and person bring. The Expert Patient Programme is one example of a policy that is based on personal responsibility and a partnership approach with people (Wilson, 2001). There has been an acknowledgement that healthcare professionals need appropriate training and support in order to develop partnership approaches (Health Foundation, 2008). The partnership approach is based on the principle of concordance (Horne et al., 2005) where the person's views are considered of equal importance and central to decision making.

Chapter 12 offers opportunity to explore in greater depth the care and management of people experiencing long-term health conditions.

ACTIVITY 5.7

Discussion point
A child has severe eczema that has not responded well to normal treatments. The parents insist on trying a homeopathic remedy recommended to them by a self-help group. How would you feel about this? What issues would you need to take account of? What are the implications for the therapeutic relationship?

Community nurses are required to demonstrate evidence-based practice (Woodward, 2001) and the challenge of today's therapeutic relationship is to balance this with informed choice (Wilson, 2002; RCN, 2015b). There is a balance to be maintained between the rights of the child (dependent on their age and understanding) and the rights of the parents in decision making, against the risks of significant harm that might result from the treatment. The parents in the above scenario should be advised to ensure the advice regarding the complementary treatment comes from a registered practitioner. Community nurses need to assess their own knowledge base regarding complementary therapy and seek specialist advice if necessary. Within a therapeutic relationship the nurse will be aiming to facilitate an atmosphere where the parents feel able to be honest about the treatments the child is currently receiving, and should be able to direct children and their families to sources of appropriate information.

A final feature of the current context of care that may have an effect on the therapeutic relationship is the fragmentation of care. It can be seen that the failure to deliver public service integration has resulted in dissatisfaction by service users who can at times experience services that appear confusing, fragmented and inflexible (Scottish Government, 2015; Wales Audit Office, 2014; DH, 2013). Despite the move towards integrated care, within the United Kingdom there is generally a division of health and social care (Wilson et al., 2009), this means that people within the community sometimes have to deal with a vast array of professionals, which can be an inhibitor in the development of a therapeutic relationship (Hyde and Cotter, 2001). The picture in Northern Ireland is different. Since 1973 Northern Ireland has had an integrated structure of health and social services. Nevertheless, ultimately strong leadership and clear vision by stakeholders throughout the United Kingdom are required to ensure a seamless service (Ham et al., 2013). The QNI (2013) also highlights the importance of a model for community nursing services facilitating strong leadership that promotes seamless and effective joined up care across professions and agencies. The community nurse has a role to be mindful of the risk of fragmentation and to strive towards improved integrated working, liaison and positive communication with relevant health professionals and agencies in order to build the potential for strong therapeutic relationships with service users. See Chapter 15 for more discussion on leadership.

CONCLUSION

In this chapter features and benefits of a therapeutic relationship have been identified, leading to an exploration of some of the challenges community nurses face in establishing therapeutic relationships. In future community healthcare provision, challenges will be shaped by an increasingly multicultural, ageing and informed population. The growing provision of healthcare in the community only serves to reinforce the need to establish appropriate relationships with people receiving healthcare in the community, their families and other carers. Current government policy emphasises partnership in care at all levels; the challenge for the community nurse is to develop this opportunity in everyday working practice.

FURTHER READING

Norcross JC and Wampold BE (2011) Evidence-based therapy relationships: Research conclusions and clinical practices *Psychotherapy* 48(1):98–102

Smith P (1992) *The Emotional Labour of Nursing.* Basingstoke: Macmillan.

Theodosius C (2008) *Emotional Labour in Health Care: The Unmanaged Heart of Nursing.* Abingdon: Routledge.

REFERENCES

Abendroth M and Flannery J (2006) Predicting the risk of compassion fatigue. *Journal of Hospice and Palliative Nursing* 8:346–56.

Brunero S, Lamont TS and Coates M (2009) A review of empathy in education in nursing *Nursing Inquiry* 17(1):65–74.

Ball J, Philippou J, Pike G and Sethi J (2013) *Survey of District and Community Nurses in 2013 Report to the Royal College of Nursing.* London: King's College London. (Accessed 18 November 2015) https://www.kcl.ac.uk/nursing/research/nnru/publications/Reports/DN-community-RCN-survey-report---UPDATED-27-05-14.pdf.

Canning D, Rosenberg JP and Yates P (2007) Therapeutic relationships in specialist palliative care nursing practice *International Journal of Palliative Nursing* 13(5):222–23.

Carers and Direct Payments Act (2002). (Accessed 30 July 2015) http://www.legislation.gov.uk/nia/2002/6/contents.

Carers Scotland Bill (2014) (Accessed 30 July 2015) http://www.scottish.parliament.uk/ResearchBriefingsAndFactsheets/S4/SB_15-24_Carers_Scotland_Bill.pdf.

Carers UK (2014) *Facts about Carers.* London: Carers UK.

Chan EA, Jones A and Wong K (2013) The relationships between communication, care and time are intertwined: A narrative inquiry exploring the impact of time on registered nurses' work. *Journal of Advanced Nursing* 69(9):2020–29. doi: 10.1111/jan.12064

Clarke AJ (2010) Empathy: An integral model of the counseling process *Journal of Counselling and Development* 88:348–355.

Coulter A (1999) Paternalism or partnership? *British Medical Journal* 319:719–20.

Crowe M (2000) The nurse–patient relationship: A consideration of its discursive context. *Journal of Advanced Nursing* 31:962–7.

Davies J and Wackerberg N (2012) *Person Driven Care A study of The Esther Network in Sweden and the lessons that can be applied to enable NHS Wales to become a patient-centred healthcare system* Cardiff: 1000 Lives Public Health Wales

Davis RE, Jacklin R, Sevdalis N and Vincent C (2007) Patient involvement in patient safety: What factors influence patient participation and engagement? *Health Expectations* 10:259–67.

DH (2001) *The Expert Patient—A New Approach to Chronic Disease Management for the 21st Century.* London: Stationery Office.

DH (2009) *Your Health, Your Way—A Guide to Long-Term Conditions and Self-Care* London: Department of Health.

DH (2011) *No Health without Mental Health; A Cross-Government Mental Health Outcomes Strategy for People of all Ages.* London: Department of Health.

DH (2012) *No Health without Mental Health: Implementation Framework.* London: Department of Health.

DH (2013) *Integrated Care: Our Shared Commitment.* London: Department of Health.

DH (2015a) 2010 to 2015 *Government Policy: Compassionate Care in the NHS.* London: Department of Health.

DH (2015b) *Concordance and Partnership in Taking Medicines* Department of Health at (Accessed 26 November 2015) http://webarchive.nationalarchives.gov.uk/+/www.dh.gov.uk/en/publicationsandstatistics/publications/publicationspolicyandguidance/browsable/DH_5354368.

DHSSPS NI (2010) *A Partnership for Care: Northern Ireland Strategy for Nursing and Midwifery.* Belfast: Department of Health Social Services and Public Safety

DHSSPS NI (2012) Living with Long Term Conditions; a policy framework. (Accessed 16 November 2015) http://www.dhsspsni.gov.uk/living-longterm-conditions.pdf.

DHSSPS NI (2011a) *Transforming your Care available.* Department of Health Social Services and Public Safety Northern Ireland. (Accessed 31 July 2015) http://www.dhsspsni.gov.uk/transforming-your-care-review-of-hsc-ni-final-report.pdf.

DHSSPS NI (2011b) *Service Framework for Mental Health and Wellbeing.* Belfast: Department of Health, Social Services and Public Safety.

Drakeford M (2013) *Everyone has a roleo to play in Self Care.* (Accessed 16 November 2015) http://gov.wales/newsroom/healthandsocialcare/2013/131120selfcare/?lang=en.

Drydon W and Mytton J (1999) *Four Approaches to Counselling and Psychotherapy.* London: Routledge.

Dunne K, Sullivan K and Kernohan G (2005) Palliative care for patients with cancer: District nurses' experiences. *Journal of Advanced Nursing* 50:372–80.

Dworkin G (1988) *The Theory and Practice of Autonomy.* Cambridge: Cambridge University Press.

Edwards N, Peterson WE and Davies BL (2006) Evaluation of a multiple component intervention to support the implementation of a 'Therapeutic Relationships' best practice guideline on nurses' communication skills. *Patient Education and Counseling* 63:3–11.

Ellis P (2015) *Understanding Ethics for Nursing Students.* London: Sage.

Farber N, Novak D and O'Brien M (1997) Love, boundaries, and the physician-patient relationship. *Arch Int Med* 157:2291–94.

Foot C, Gilburt H, Dunn P et al. (2014) *People in Control of their Own Health and Care.* London: King's Fund.

Foster T and Hawkins J (2005) Nurse–patient relationship. The therapeutic relationship: Dead or merely impeded by technology? *British Journal of Nursing* 14:698–702.

Francis R (2013) *The Mid Staffordshire_NHS Foundation Trust Public Inquiry.* London: Stationary Office.

Frankl V (2006) *Man's Search for Meaning.* Boston, MA: Beacon Press Books.

Gandi J, Wai P, Karick H and Dagona Z (2011) The role of stress and level of burnout in job performance among nurses. *Mental Health in Family Medicine* 8:181–94.

Gerrish K (2008) Caring for the carers: The characteristics of district nursing support for family carers. *Primary Health Care Research and Development* 9:14–21.

Godsell M, Shaban RZ and Gamble J (2013) 'Recognizing rapport' health professionals lived experience of caring for patients under transmission-based precautions in an Australian health care setting. *American Journal of Infection Control* 41:971–5.

Greenhalgh T (2009) Chronic illness: Beyond the expert patient. *British Medical Journal* 338 7695:629–31.

Greenhalgh T and Heath I (2010) *Measuring Quality in the Therapeutic Relationship: An Inquiry into the Quality of General Practice in England*. London: King's Fund.

Griffiths C, Foster G, Ramsay J et al. (2007) How effective are expert patient (lay led) education programmes for chronic disease? *British Medical Journal* 334:1254–56.

Hagerty BM and Patusky KL (2003) Reconceptualizing the nurse–patient relationship. *Journal of Nursing Scholarship* 35:145–50.

Halter M, Brown H and Stone J (2007) *Sexual Boundary Violations by Health Professionals—An Overview of the Published Empirical Literature*. London: The Council for Healthcare Regulatory Excellence.

Ham C, Heenan D, Longley M and Steele DR (2013) *Integrated Care in Northern Ireland, Scotland and Wales; Lessons for England*. London: King's Fund.

Healthcare Improvment Scotland (2014) *Person Centred Health and Care Collaborative Health Inequalities Impact Assessment—Final Report*. NHS Scotland. (Accessed: 31 July 2015) http://www.healthcareimprovementscotland.org/our_work/person-centred_care/person-centred_collaborative.aspx.

Health Foundation (2008) *Co-creating Health*. London: The Health Foundation.

Healthcare Commission (2006) *Living Well in Later Life: A Review of Progress Against the National Service Framework for Older People*. London: Healthcare Commission.

Hojat M, Gonnella J, Nasca, T et al. (2002) Physician empathy: Definition components, measurement, and relationship to gender and speciality. *American Journal of Psychiatry* 159:1563–9.

Horne R, Cribb A and Kellar I (2005) *Report for the National Co-ordinating Centre for NHS Service Delivery and Organisations R&D (NCCSDO)*. London: Centre for Health Care Research.

Hyde V and Cotter C (2001) The development of community nursing in the light of the NHS plan. In Hyde V (ed) *Community Nursing and Health Care. Insights and Innovations*. London: Arnold, pp. 230–44.

Hylton Rushton C, Armstrong L and McEnhill M (1996) Establishing therapeutic boundaries as patient advocates. *Pediatric Nursing* 22:185–9.

IOM (2001) *Crossing the Quality Chasm* Institute of Medicine. (Accessed 16 November 2015) https://iom.nationalacademies.org/~/media/Files/Report%20Files/2001/Crossing-the-Quality-Chasm/Quality%20Chasm%202001%20%20report%20brief.pdf.

King's Fund (2015a) *Patient and Family Centred Care Toolkit*. King's Fund. http://www.kingsfund.org.uk/projects/pfcc%20. (Accessed 13 July 2017)

King's Fund (2015b) *Long-term conditions and multi-morbidity*. http://www.kingsfund.org.uk/time-to-think-differently/trends/disease-and-disability/long-term-conditions-multi-morbidity. (Accessed July 2017)

King's Fund (2016) Understanding quality in district nursing services, learning from patients carers and staff (Accessed July 2016) https://www.kingsfund.org.uk/sites/files/kf/field/field_publication_file/quality_district_nursing_aug_2016.pdf

LaMonica E (1981) Construct validity of an empathy instrument. *Research in Nursing and Health* 4:389–400.

Mackintosh C (2006) Protecting the self: A descriptive qualitative exploration of how registered nurses cope with working in surgical areas. *International Journal of Nursing Studies* 42:179–186.

Malone D, Marriott S, Newton-Howes G et al. (2007) Community mental health teams (CMHTs) for people with severe mental illnesses and disordered personality. *Cochrane Database of Systematic Reviews* 3:CD000270.

Manthorpe J, Iliffe S and Eden A (2003): Testing Twigg and Aitkin's typology of caring: A study of primary care professionals' perceptions of dementia care using a modified focus group method. *Health and Social Care in the Community* 11:477–85.

Martin LR, Williams SL, Haskard KB and DiMatteo MR (2005) The challenge of patient adherence. *Therapeutics and Clinical Risk Management* 1(3):189–99.

McKenna H and Cutcliffe J (2008) *Nursing Models, Theories and Practice*. Chichester: Blackwell Publishing.

Merritt MK and Procter NG (2010) Conceptualising the functional role of mental health consultation-liaison nurse in multi-morbidity, using Peplau's nursing theory. *Contemporary Nurse* 34:140–8.

Milton C L (2008) Boundaries: Ethical implications for what it means to be therapeutic in the nurse–person relationship. *Nursing Science Quarterly* 21:18–21.

Morse J M (1991) Negotiating commitment and involvement in the nurse–patient relationship. *Journal of Advanced Nursing* 16:455–68.

Moyle W (2003) Nurse–patient relationship: A dichotomy of expectations. *Journal of Mental Health Nursing* 12:103–9.

NCSBN (2014) *A Nurse's guide to professional boundaries* National Council of State Boards of Nuring. (Accessed: 31 July 2015) https://www.ncsbn.org/ProfessionalBoundaries_Complete.pdf .

NICE (2011) *Quality Standard for Service User Experience in Adult Mental Health* London: NICE.

NICE (2012) *Quality Standard for Patient Experience in Adult NHS Services*. London: NICE. http://www.nice.org.uk/guidance/qs15/chapter/introduction-and-overview#/overview (Accessed July 2017)

NMC (2015) *The Code: Professional Standards of Practice and Behaviour for Nurses and Midwives*. London: NMC.

Parkes N and Jukes M (2008) Professional boundaries in a person-centred paradigm. *British Journal of Nursing* 17:1358–64.

Paterson B (2001) Myth of empowerment in chronic illness. *Journal of Advanced Nursing* 34:574–81.

Peplau HE (1952) *Interpersonal Relations in Nursing*. New York, NY: Putnam's Sons.

Pinto RZ, Ferreira ML, Oliveira VC, et al. (2012) Patient-centred communication is associated with positive therapeutic alliance: A systematic review *Journal of Physiotherapy* 58:77–87.

Porr C, Drummond J and Olson K (2012) Establishing therapeutic relationships with vulnerable and potentially stigmatized clients *Qualitative Health Research* 22(3):384–396.

Pullen RL and Mathias T (2010) Fostering therapeutic nurse relationships. *Nursing Made Incredibly Easy* 8(3):4. (Accessed 24 July 2015) http://journals.lww.com/nursingmadeincrediblyeasy/Fulltext/2010/05000/Fostering_therapeutic_nurse_patient_relationships.1.aspx.

Queen's Nursing Institute (QNI) (2013) *Report on District Nurse Education in England, Wales and Northern Ireland 2012/13*. London: Queen's Nursing Institute.

Queen's Nursing Institute (QNI) (2015) *Transition to Community Nursing Practice.* (Accessed 16 November 2015) http://www.qni.org.uk/for_nurses/transition_to_community.

RCN (2015a) *Public health—Topics: Occupational health nursing.* (Accessed 18 November 2015). http://www.rcn.org.uk/development/practice/public_health/topics/occupational-health-nursing.

RCN (2015b) *Quality and Saftery Bulletin.* (Accessed 29 November 2015) https://www.rcn.org.uk/development/practice/clinical_governance/quality_and_safety_e-bulletin.

Roberts K (2001) Across the health–social care divide: Elderly people as active users of health care and social care. *Health and Social Care in the Community* 9:100–7.

Schaeuble K, Haglund K and Vukovich M (2010) Adolescents' preferences for primary provider interactions. *Pediatric Nursing* 15:202–10.

Scottish Government (2008) *Gaun Yersel! The Self Management Strategy for Long Term Conditions in Scotland.* Glasgow: Scottish Government.

Scottish Government (2012) *Mental Health Strategy for Scotland 2012-2015.* Glasgow: Scottish Government.

Scottish Government (2015) *Integration of Health and Social Care.* (Accessed 19 November 2015) http://www.gov.scot/Topics/Health/Policy/Adult-Health-SocialCare-Integration.

Seddon D and Robinson CA (2001) Carers of older people with dementia: Assessment and the Carers Act. *Health and Social Care in the Community* 9:151–8.

Shaw K and Timmons S (2010) Exploring how nursing uniforms influence self image and professional identity. *Nursing Times* 106, www.nursingtimes.net/nursing-practice-clinical-research/acute-care/exploring-how-nursing-uniforms-influence-self-image-and-professional-identity/5012623.article. (accessed July 2017)

Simon C and Kendrick T (2001) Informal carers—The role of general practitioners and district nurses. *British Journal of General Practice* 51:655–7.

Skills for Health (2015) *Common Core Principles to Support Self-Care.* Bristol: Skills for Care. (Accessed 28 November 2015) http://www.skillsforcare.org.uk/Document-library/Skills/Self-care/Commoncoreprinciples.pdf.

Social Services and Well-being (Wales) Act (2014) (Accessed 31 July 2015) http://www.legislation.gov.uk/anaw/2014/4/pdfs/anaw_20140004_en.pdf.

Spencer M and Puntoni S (2015) *Improving Healthcare White Paper Series Listneing and Hearing to Improve the Experience of Care Understanding What it Feels Like to use Services in NHS Wales.* Cardiff: Public Health Wales 1000 Lives.

Stansfield S, Smuk M, Onwumere J, et al. (2014) Stresses and common mental health disorders in informal carers—An analysis of the English adult psychiatric morbidity survey 2007 *Social Science and Medicine* 120:190–198.

Stein-Parbury J (2005) *Patient and Person,* 3rd edn. Sydney: Elsevier.

Stewart M (2005) Reflections on the doctor-patient relationship: From evidence and experience. *British Journal of General Practice* 55(519):793–801.

Stockwell-Smith G, Kellet U and Moyle W (2010) Why carers of frail older people are not using available respite services: An Australian study *Journal of Clinical Nursing* 19(13–14):2057–64.

Sturgeon D (2014) The business of the NHS: The rise and rise of consumer culture and commodification in the provision of healthcare services. *Critical Social Policy* 34(3):405–16. ISSN 0261-0183

The Care Act (2014) (Accessed 31 July 2015) http://www.legislation.gov.uk/ukpga/2014/23/contents/enacted.

The Health Foundation (2014) *Person-Centred Care Made Simple; What Everyone Should Know About Person-Centred Care.* London: The Health Foundation.

Thornbury G (ed) (2013) *Association of Occupational Health Nursing, Contemporary Occupational Health Nursing, A Guide for Practitioners.* London: Routledge.

Trades Union Congress (TUC) (2015) *Good Practice in Work Place Mental Health; Report of the TUC Seminar February 2015.* London: TUC. (Accessed 1 September 2015) https://www.tuc.org.uk/sites/default/files/GoodPracticeMentalHealth_0.pdf.

Twigg J and Atkin K (1994) *Carers Perceived.* Buckingham: Open University Press.

Verducci S (2000) A conceptual history of empathy and a question it raises for moral education. *Educational Theory.* 50(1):63–79.

Wales Audit Office (2014) *The Management of Chronic Conditions in Wales—An Update.* Cardiff: Wales Audit Office.

Waugh A, McNay L, Dewar B and McCraig M (2014) Supporting the development of interpersonal skills in nursing, in an undergraduate mental health curriculum: Reaching the parts other strategies do not reach through action learning *Nurse Education Today* 34:1232–1237.

WG (2010) *The Mental Health (Wales) Measure.* Cardiff: Welsh Government.

WG (2014) *Prudent Health Care.* Cardiff: Welsh Government. (Accessed 31 July 2015). http://gov.wales/topics/health/nhswales/prudent-healthcare/?lang=en.

Wilson PM (2001) A policy analysis of the expert patient in the United Kingdom: Self-care as an expression of pastoral power? *Health and Social Care in the Community* 9:134–42.

Wilson PM (2002) The expert patient: Issues and implications for community nurses. *British Journal of Community Nursing* 7:514–19.

Wilson PM, Bunn F and Morgan J (2009) A mapping of the evidence on integrated long term condition services. *British Journal of Community Nursing* 14:202–6.

Wilson PM, Kendall S and Brooks F (2007) The expert patients programme: A paradox of patient empowerment and medical dominance. *Health and Social Care in the Community* 15:426–38.

Wiseman T (1996) Concept analysis of empathy *Journal of Advanced Nursing* 23(6): 1162–67.

Woodward V (2001) Evidence-based practice, clinical governance and community nurses. In Hyde V (ed.) *Community Nursing and Health Care. Insights and Innovations.* London: Arnold, pp. 206–29.

World Health Organization (2010) *User Empowerment in Mental Health—A Statement by the WHO Refional Office in Europe.* Copenhagen: WHO

Care across the lifespan

Helen McVeigh

Helen McVeigh

> **LEARNING OUTCOMES**
>
> • Compare and contrast the different theories of growth and development.
> • Evaluate the issues that influence caring for clients across the lifespan.
> • Critically analyse how an understanding of a lifespan approach can enhance the quality of care provision.

INTRODUCTION

This chapter explores the concept of a lifespan approach to healthcare. It is an approach that is able to reflect on and adapt to changes in demographics, society and the expectations of individuals within the community. The health of an individual is influenced by a complex interaction of a range of factors including physiological, psychological, social, cultural and environmental issues. A sound understanding of the factors that influence growth and development across the lifespan can enable the community nurse to adopt a truly holistic approach in the assessment, planning, implementation and analysis of healthcare interventions; however, it is recognised that health professionals may have distinct roles in the community, often focused on specific stages of the lifespan (e.g. Health Visitor – child health 0–5 years). The importance of developing a broad viewpoint and an awareness of all aspects of the lifespan continuum should underpin effective care provision.

THEORIES OF GROWTH AND DEVELOPMENT

There are many theories which explore the concept of human growth and development; however, it is beyond the scope of this chapter to consider them all. A basic understanding of these theories will enable the health professional to understand the individual, their illness and their reaction to illness.

Growth can be defined as an increase in physical size and maturity, whereas development describes an increase in functional ability; however, this is a fairly simplistic approach and a lifespan perspective recognises that changes in physical, cognitive and social domains are all influential (Boyd and Bee, 2015; Cameron, 2006). Aspects of growth and development can be related to all stages of the lifespan, although it is suggested that growth and development apply to the period from conception to young adulthood whereas the notion of ageing is more readily applicable from middle age onwards (Taylor et al., 2003).

It is useful to consider some of the theories which underpin growth and development and a lifespan approach. These theories can be grouped into several different categories and classified according to the following broad headings: biomedical, psychodynamic, cognitive, behavioural, humanist and sociocultural (see Box 6.1).

Box 6.1 Theories of growth and development

Biomedical – Focus is on the change in body mechanics
Psychodynamic – Focus is on development of personality traits and psychological challenges at different ages
Cognitive – Focus is on the advancement and development of thinking
Behavioural – Describes the development of human behaviour and behavioural learning changes
Humanist – Describes the influence of human experiences such as love and attachment on personality development
Sociocultural – Describes how culture and society influence behaviour.

Although exploration of the various theories can provide key information on the different life stages, it is important to recognise that a lifespan approach adopts an eclectic approach which successfully combines aspects of all of these elements (Boyd and Bee, 2015).

Utilising a lifespan approach

The changes in physiology, psychology and behaviour that occur normally at different stages of the lifespan and how these are influenced by their interaction with other factors including life experience, social norms, culture, health status and the environment are explored in this chapter through the use of a multigenerational case history (Figure 6.1). Aspects of need and healthcare at various life stages are considered and related to the different theoretical approaches. A wide range of healthcare professionals will input into this family's life history along their lifespan. Whichever professional you are, an understanding of the roles of others and how they may meet the needs of the clients is important, along with a holistic approach to healthcare reflecting not only knowledge of the individual but some understanding of how this is influenced by their environment, society and the relationships they are in. How life is lived will influence health and most health outcomes are related to the choices made by the individual at each stage of the lifespan (Barry and Yuill, 2012; Leifer and Hartshorn, 2004). For example, the elderly patient with chronic obstructive pulmonary disease (COPD) may well regret choices made as a teenager to adopt an unhealthy lifestyle and to smoke. Some understanding of why we behave in specific ways at certain life stages may help us in effectively targeting lifestyle choice and in providing health promotion and healthcare effectively tailored to meet the needs of our client group. We also need to remember that most individuals do not exist in isolation and healthcare needs will frequently impact on families and carers. The challenge for the community nurse is to recognise these influences and offer sensitive healthcare that reaches the client and their family/carers.

BIOMEDICAL INFLUENCES

Historically, the biomedical approach has directed the organisation and provision of healthcare and remains the dominant model in Western culture (Naidoo and Wills, 2015; Taylor and Field, 2007). The biomedical approach ignores social and environmental factors and taken in isolation is essentially a reductionist method focusing on body mechanics, which assumes that the mind and body can be treated separately and that they can be repaired (Naidoo and Wills, 2015; Nettleton, 2013). The emphasis is on what causes illness and how it should be treated, with responsibility for treatment seen as principally resting with the medical profession (Ogden, 2012). Nurse education is underpinned by a sound understanding of human anatomy and physiology, and it is essential that nurses are able to recognise normal physiology and changes to this in order to provide safe and effective care (NMC, 2015). This knowledge should include knowing not only how the different organs and systems of the body work, but also how they grow and develop. An understanding of growth norms is useful when monitoring child health and in health surveillance. If we consider Samuel, who is rather small for his age, knowing there is an adolescent growth spurt which differs between the sexes, and that the male spurt although greater in intensity is usually on average 2 years behind that of females (Boyd and Bee, 2015) can enable us to determine whether this is normal variance or not. Tools such as human growth curve charts, which record the growth of an individual from 0–18 years, allow us to monitor and interpret recorded results.

A sound understanding of physiological changes and the normal patterns of ageing may aid us in the diagnosis and treatment of disease. An awareness of biomedical aspects such as genetic programming, wear and tear theory (cells having a specified life cycle), cell programming (cells divide until they are no longer able to), immune theory (immune response diminishing with age) (Aldwin and Gilmer, 2013; Grossman and Lange, 2006) and how the body handles significant changes, for example, drug administration, bacterial or viral invasion, is fundamental to effective healthcare. Recognition that homeostasis (the ability of body systems to maintain equilibrium) may be impaired in the very young or elderly patient is essential knowledge for effective care provision. For example, individuals with the influenza virus are more likely to be seriously ill and at increased risk of mortality if they are at each end of the lifespan. Biologically this correlates with human development and physiology, lung function continues to increase and develop from birth until adulthood (around age 20 years) staying stable on average for around 15 years and then it begins to decline (Farley et al., 2011).

Knowledge of the stages of wound healing and the normal progression of wound healing should underpin nursing care for Margaret and Samuel. Samuel as a young

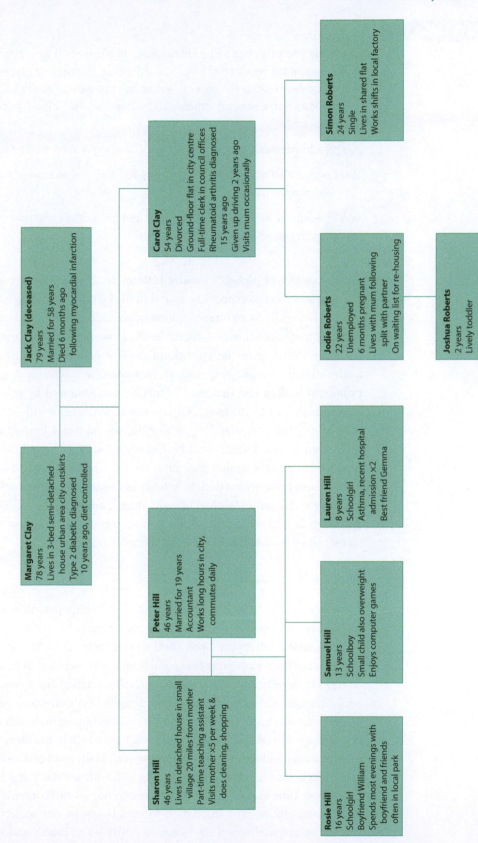

Figure 6.1 Case history genealogy.

ACTIVITY 6.1

Reflection point

Recently, Margaret has had a fall resulting in a pre-tibial laceration to her lower leg which required the community nurse to visit and assess. Margaret has been self-treating for several weeks but the wound is not healing and the community nurse notes it appears to be infected. Her blood glucose levels are also elevated.

Using a biomedical approach, what is influencing wound healing for Margaret?

Samuel has also lacerated his leg playing football and Sharon has taken him to the surgeon for advice.

What advice would you give to Samuel and his mother and how might that differ from the advice given to Margaret?

healthy child will probably require little more than one or two simple dressing changes as we would expect his wound to heal within 4–7 days. Advice to Samuel and Sharon would focus on recognition of possible infection and risk management (playing football) while the wound heals. However, for Margaret decreased cell turnover, thinning of the epithelium, loss of collagen within the dermis and a diminished immune response, factors consistent with ageing, will result in prolonged healing and this may be further compromised by other physiological factors such as her diabetes. Advice and management will be more complex; establishing her understanding of why the wound is not healing and how this is influenced by her diabetes will be essential. Using a biomedical focus to guide practice can give the community nurse an indication of what to expect as the body ages, although patterns of decline will not necessarily follow a predictable sequence and may vary from individual to individual (Farley et al., 2011; Cameron, 2006). Although crucial to care provision it is important to recognise that biomedical factors will be overlaid by psychosocial influences.

PSYCHOSOCIAL INFLUENCES

Sociology can be defined as the study of social relationships; holistic healthcare recognises that people's lives and behaviour cannot be divorced from the social contexts in which they participate (Beckett and Taylor, 2013; Taylor and Field, 2007). Psychosocial theory attempts to explain human development in terms of individual changes in cognitive function, behaviour, roles, relationships, coping abilities and social change, and as such it provides insight into individual personalities and attitudes across the lifespan. Psychosocial factors impact on health across all stages of the lifespan in relation to onset of illness, health beliefs, health behaviour, health-seeking advice and adaptation to, progress of and outcomes of illness (Ogden, 2012). Life expectations and our understanding of health are not static but develop and evolve over time and are frequently linked to our socio-economic circumstances. Health inequalities exist in relation to social class in our society, influenced by wealth, income and access to resources. Attitudes to health and illness may also be shaped by generational features related to the era an individual was born into and the social norms and expectations they have been exposed to (Barry and Yuill, 2012). For example, attitudes to smoking in the last century have impacted on lung cancer incidence and may influence attitudes to smoking cessation advice.

The concept of health

The concept of health is important and it is essential to consider the individual's subjective interpretation of the meaning of health and illness. Health may be viewed negatively

• The absence of disease or illness
  or positively

• A state of complete physical, mental and social well-being, not merely the absence of disease or infirmity (WHO, 1946)

The concept of health is explored in more detail in Chapter 2.

ACTIVITY 6.2

Reflection point

What is your interpretation of health?

Consider how an individuals' notion of health may change across the lifespan.

How might Carol define being healthy? How would this differ from Simon's definition?

The way in which we define health will impact on our life choices and subsequent behaviour. Simon's definition may reflect strength and fitness, whereas Carol may focus on the ability to cope with life and the demands of work. Health perception will vary across the lifespan and genders. Nettleton (2013) suggests that for young men it may equal strength and physical condition, whereas for young women it may equal vitality, energy and an ability to cope. As we age, the emphasis shifts from notions of mental and physical well-being and the ability to do things well in middle age, to wisdom, contentment, happiness and resilient ageing in late adulthood (Hicks and Conner, 2014; Alder et al., 2004). Perceptions will be influenced by physiological, social and environmental factors. For example, a working individual or young mother may consider that she has no time to be ill and Carol's perception will be influenced by her rheumatoid arthritis. It is important to recognise that views on 'what is health' are varied and those of our patients may well be different from our personal perspectives.

Health promotion

The promotion of health is an essential role for every community nurse, and strategies to support healthy behaviour and lifestyle are at the heart of improving the quality of life for individuals (Cox and Hill, 2010; Leifer and Hartshorn, 2004). Statistics on mortality indicate that up to 50 percent of deaths from the 10 leading causes of death in the United Kingdom can be attributed to health-related behaviour (Ogden, 2012).

The process of promoting health involves enabling individuals to take control of their own health and is focused on a proactive preventative approach. Individuals are encouraged to take responsibility and to be more knowledgeable about the behavioural and social factors that influence health although it is important to recognise that wider social and structural influences may be outside of their control (Nettleton, 2013; Thornton, 2012). Current health policy supports patient empowerment and personal responsibility (Scottish Government, 2016; Welsh Government, 2015; DH Northern Ireland, 2014; NHS England, 2014; Scottish Government, 2013a; DH 2010a,b). The community nurse needs to develop a reflective approach that combines knowledge of health promotion strategies with an understanding of lifespan influences. For example, the teaching style and strategy we might adopt for an adolescent may well be very different to that which would be effective for an older person, where a paternalistic approach of 'doctor knows best' may be expected. Objective analysis also suggests that there may be a tendency for health promotion to be targeted at those in younger age groups (Taylor et al., 2003). However, it is important to remember that opportunities exist across the whole lifespan and that the effectiveness of any health message is reliant on how well it reaches the target audience. The Family Planning Association campaign 'Middle-age Spread' to encourage increased responsibility in the over-50s in relation to risky sexual behaviour in response to increasing incidence of sexually transmitted infection (STI) in older adults demonstrates the importance of differing approaches (FPA, 2010). Health promotion should be aimed at enabling the individual to make an informed choice while recognising the uniqueness of the lived experience of health, illness and their health beliefs.

Children and families

Aspects of growth and development in childhood are rooted in the context of family life. The fundamental structure of the family in the United Kingdom has evolved from origins of the extended family group all living under one roof to more nuclear families living separately, divided by greater geographical mobility, and increasingly diverse family groupings, which include more single parents, remarriages and working families, which may well impact on child development. The family construct can be considered to have a growth and development lifespan originating in marriage/living together through having children, child rearing, separation and ageing family responsibilities (Boyd and Bee, 2015; Leifer and Hartshorn, 2004). A sound understanding of the concept of family and its construct enables planning of individualised care for family members.

The basis of effectively meeting the needs of children is underpinned by an understanding of child development milestones (Sharma et al., 2014). Insight into emotional and behavioural development can enable us to respond effectively to children and family groups. At 2 years old, Joshua is developing social interaction and language skills (he has a vocabulary of around 100 words) and is mastering an element of self-control (he is toilet trained and dry through the day). However, the arrival of a new sibling may provoke regression as he struggles to adjust to the change in relationship with his mother. A sensitive approach and allowing him to participate in caring for the new baby may help with the process of adjustment. Support from the Health Visitor including statutory developmental checks and advice on access to local educational and day care facilities can provide support and reassurance for Jodie and optimise Joshua's socio-emotional development and well-being (NHS Scotland, 2016; NICE, 2014a; DH, 2009a)

It is important to recognise that children cannot be cared for in isolation from their families who will have an established health belief system (Naidoo and Wills, 2015; Smith and McSherry, 2004). Attitudes underpinning health belief are very hard to change, so the community nurse needs to understand what contributes to family decision making about health. The Health Belief Model (Becker, 1974) highlights the purpose of beliefs in decision making. The model suggests that behaviour change is underpinned by a cost–benefit analysis and evaluation of its feasibility (Naidoo and Wills, 2015).

ACTIVITY 6.3

Reflection point

Lauren has asthma; recently her symptoms have been much worse and she has had two severe attacks requiring overnight hospitalisation.

Since the death of her father Sharon has visited her mother most days after work and Lauren has spent time with her best friend Gemma after school. Gemma has a pet cat; previous allergy testing revealed that Lauren is allergic to cat fur.

Using the Health Belief Model and a lifespan approach, consider how Sharon and Gemma will respond.

Sharon's concern about the increased risk to Lauren of further asthma attacks through spending time at her friend's house may be tempered by the needs of her elderly mother, work commitments and the tearful remonstrations of her daughter. Lauren's response is less rational and she is less likely to comprehend the consequences of continuing with the current arrangement. Understanding of chronic illness is dependent in some degree on the age of the child. A child aged 4–7 may perceive causality of asthma as related to magic or naughtiness; by ages of 7–11 they may have developed some understanding of allergies; while the older child will start to comprehend relationships (Alder, 2013). Lauren is likely to have an understanding of the cause of her asthma but may not be able to relate this to cause-and-effect principles and coping mechanisms (Leifer and Hartshorn, 2004). As a community nurse supporting Sharon and Lauren, a holistic approach to care encompasses not only the needs of the individual but the family as well. Care delivery should recognise that the family has complex needs while encouraging both Lauren and her family to take an active role in healthcare decisions.

Adolescents

Adolescence is a time of significant changes marking the transition between childhood and adulthood. The characteristic physical changes of puberty are heightened by corresponding psychosocial development. In Western society factors such as earlier onset of the menarche and increasing time in formal education have

ACTIVITY 6.4

> **Reflection point**
>
> Rosie is not getting on very well with her parents and is frequently argumentative and confrontational. She has started going out in the evenings, often coming home late. Rosie has a boyfriend and a large circle of friends. There is very little to do in the village and they spend most of their evenings at the local park. She is very close to her cousin Jodie and confides in her that she is worried that she might be pregnant as she has been sleeping with her boyfriend.
>
> Jodie has gone with Rosie to see the practice nurse. The pregnancy test is negative.
>
> Consider the type of approach you might adopt in giving advice and support to Rosie.

widened the gap between physical maturity and adulthood (Alder, 2013). There is increased emphasis on social conflicts and personal dilemmas during this time as the individual endeavours to identify their role within society (Erikson, 1980). This challenges and changes relationships between parents and peers, and there is often increased conflict in families as the individual experiments with a variety of roles and styles. Disputes are frequently related to differences of opinions around rights and responsibilities (Boyd and Bee, 2015; Alder et al., 2004). In our case history Rosie is frustrated by the attitude of her parents who consider her old enough to babysit for her younger siblings but not old enough for a sexual relationship, whereas from Peter and Sharon's perspective, Rosie wants sexual freedom without the responsibility of the potential consequences. The challenge of achieving a sense of self and independence may impact on healthcare, which may be particularly relevant for adolescents with a long-term condition. Peer pressure and the need for self-identity may mean that social logic replaces that of medical logic (Nettleton, 2013).

It is important to take an approach which establishes a level of trust with Rosie. Rosie may be worried about the community nurse sharing information with her parents; therefore, an honest approach is important. It is important to take adolescents' psychosocial and cultural experiences and expectations into account (Briggs, 2010). Although Rosie's pregnancy test was negative, she needs advice on sexual health in the future as adolescents are likely to have a greater sense of invulnerability in relation to risk taking and are also influenced by peer group norms and pressures (Beckett and Taylor, 2013; Ogden, 2012). The community nurse needs to adopt a non-judgmental, approachable and friendly attitude in providing advice and support. The emphasis should be on helping her to enjoy her teenage years while minimising the risk of unwanted/unplanned pregnancy, STIs, HIV, cancer of the cervix and female infertility (NICE, 2014b; DH, 2013; Briggs, 2010). Providing health advice for adolescents can be challenging and requires an approach in which establishing trust and offering sound advice and respecting them as individuals are key.

Adulthood

Early adulthood is generally defined as being between the ages of 20 and 40. The body has reached physical maturity and expectations are to be in good health and at the peak of physical strength, endurance and energy. The focus at this time is on forming relationships, finding love and is typically the period in which long-term relationships are established. Work, career choices, security and satisfaction are important values. Intellectual growth is a feature and individuals learn how to evaluate opposing views and assess practicality alongside creative and social concerns (Leifer and Hartshorn, 2004). For the healthcare professional, this may be an important time to highlight risk factors and establish preventative goals as personal concerns for health and well-being may be of low priority.

ACTIVITY 6.5

Reflection point

Simon confides in his sister that he is worried about his health. He no longer enjoys going out with his friends and has increasingly lost interest in taking part in any activities outside of work. He confesses that he has not been sleeping and that this is impacting on his ability to cope and make decisions at work. His poor performance has been noted at work and his employer has asked him to see the occupational health nurse. He tells his sister he cannot afford to be sick and cannot see what the nurse will be able to do to help; he's just a bit low and feels he just needs to 'snap out of it'.

What psychosocial factors may be influencing Simon's reluctance to access a healthcare professional?

Simon is probably aware that he has a mental rather than a physical health problem. His reticence to see the nurse may be influenced by a variety of psychosocial factors. Gender-related expectations of manliness combined with Western cultural influence which places an emphasis on self-reliance may cause him to feel guilty about his lack of ability to cope and therefore to fail to seek help (Barry and Yuill, 2012; Hammen and Watkins, 2013). The impact of stigma associated with mental health may also be a factor, although current healthcare approaches are working hard to change this negative view (TNS BRMB, 2014). Myths and unhelpful media portrayal, such as characterisation of villains as having mental imbalance, continue to reinforce negative stereotypical views (Barry and Yuill, 2012). Simon may well be worried about the impact any diagnosis of mental ill health such as depression may have on his personal, social and work relationships. It is important that the nurse recognises how factors such as stigma and attempts to fit in with social expectations of normality may influence his access to healthcare, management of his ill health and concordance with prescribed treatment.

Middle age and the world of work

Middle age is considered to be the period between 40 and 60 years of age. Physical growth and development has been replaced by aspects of ageing. The challenges of this period are often associated with work and maintaining roots within the community. Erikson (1980) noted that middle age is defined as a time of conflict between contribution to the family or community (generativity) and concern for self (stagnation). The consequences of ageing may be an emerging worry. Alder et al. (2004) highlight the concept of 'the mid-life crisis' as a period of uncertainty and change that may be perceived as a last opportunity to achieve some of life's goals. Middle age may also be a time of re-evaluation and self-reflection, a time to focus on health behaviour and lifestyle choices. Opportunities exist for the community nurse to effectively manage risky behaviours. Changing demographics along with increases in the age of retirement indicate that in the future older people will account for an increased proportion of the working age population (NICE, 2015; ONS, 2013). Therefore, opportunities to promote health and well-being in the work environment and to support individuals in changing lifestyle behaviours which aims for healthier ageing are set to become increasingly important. Occupational health and general practice nurses are in an ideal position to effectively target these individuals.

It may be appropriate to identify how Sharon and Peter view their health and their ability to control it. Health promotion and changing behaviour may be easier if individuals have an internal locus of control where they feel they have some say

ACTIVITY 6.6

Reflection point

Sharon and Peter are rather overweight. They both enjoy a glass of wine in the evenings, often eating late when Peter returns from work.

They feel that their busy lives do not allow them time to take regular exercise.

Consider how psychosocial factors will influence effective health promotion for Sharon and Peter.

in their future health rather than an external locus of control where individuals feel that their health is governed from the outside and would therefore not take responsibility for making changes to improve well-being (Naidoo and Wills, 2015). Decisions to change lifestyle may be based on weighing up any benefit against disadvantage highlighted in the Health Belief model (Becker, 1974). Concern for family (generativity) can be a positive influence; Samuel is an overweight teenager and an increased knowledge that childhood obesity will tend to carry over into adulthood (Larkin, 2009) may support behaviour changes. Research highlights the positive association of parental attitude to food, diet and eating behaviour on the dietary behaviour of their children (Ogden, 2012). Exercise advice can be promoted not only to prevent declining health but as an opportunity for a family social activity. The value of implementing a health-promoting social activity with additional social benefits can act as a useful motivator for ongoing behaviour change (Ogden, 2012). Activities such as organised bike riding, for example, 'Big Bike Events' (Sky Ride, 2016), illustrate this approach. For the community nurse, an understanding of social, cultural and environmental factors at this point in the family's lifespan is essential, and the emphasis should be on shared decision making.

An individual may be challenged by long-term illness at any age, although the likelihood will increase with age. Long-term illness can confront our sense of self and reminds us that normal functioning is often central to social relationships and activities (Nettleton, 2013). The impact of long-term illness on life is twofold: its consequence, that is, its effects, on the practical aspects of life (work and play), and its meaning as significant to our sense of self (Bury, 1991).

ACTIVITY 6.7

Reflection point

Carol has rheumatoid arthritis. Recently, her symptoms have become much worse and she finds sitting for long periods very difficult. Although her employers have been very supportive Carol is finding it increasingly difficult to manage at work. She is frequently tired in the evenings and is finding it quite stressful living with her daughter and a lively 2 year old. Consider the consequence and meaning of long-term illness for Carol.

It is important to recognise that expected norms across the lifespan may be challenged and changed by long-term illness. Carol's disability has resulted in her developing a set of coping mechanisms; however, recent exacerbation of symptoms has created new problems for her. The biomedical approach would emphasise the importance of maintaining mobility and minimising resultant disability, the focus being on the individual's limitations and incapacity. However, her ability to cope is influenced by several psychosocial factors:

- Social imagery associated with rheumatoid arthritis; limited mobility, severe disability and wheelchair use
- Individual sense of self
- Reaction of others

The social model argues that attitudes and physical restrictions are often imposed by society and as a consequence opportunities and functional capability are decreased (Larkin, 2009). For Carol, increasing difficulties at work have resulted in the realisation that she is less able to function in what might be termed socially accepted normality and that her increasing disability generates barriers in employment. Her capacity to cope may also be influenced by her mental health (many patients who suffer from a long-term condition may also suffer from depression) (Boyd and Bee, 2015), her health beliefs, and her perceived ability to overcome her disability, which may have been exacerbated by the demands of having her daughter and grandson living with her. For the community nurse, supporting an individual with a long-term condition it is important to recognise that there is no timetable of events as to how a condition may progress (Barry and Yuill, 2012) and that the individual is constantly responding to emergent changes and resultant adaptation to their own normality. The ability to cope has to be revised on all aspects of life, their understanding of self, relationships (family, work and social), the impact of treatment regimes, the demands of compliance and their engagement with healthcare professionals (Barry and Yuill, 2012). A collaborative approach which focuses on promoting equality and empowerment with sensitivity and compassion is essential.

Ageing

Knowledge and understanding of the ageing process and the meaning of being old are essential for effective individualised care of clients in the community. Old age is often considered to begin at 65, but increasing life expectancy means we now have subgroups of young old, old and the very old (over 85 years) (Erber, 2013). Trends show there are fewer younger people and more older people in the United Kingdom with increasing numbers of those living to be very old (Clarke, 2013). By 2051 estimates indicate that 1:4 people will be over the age of 65 and 1:15 will be over 85 (HSCIC, 2014). Our understanding of ageing is influenced by the concept of ageism, stereotypical ideas, social norms and expectations. We live in an ageist society, where physical change such as greying hair and loss of skin elasticity is viewed negatively, particularly in relation to women (Clarke and Korotchenko, 2010; Alder et al., 2004), whereas in men it may suggest increasing maturity and competence (Alder, 2013). Ageism may influence the provision of healthcare, while the National Health Service (NHS) Constitution (NHS, 2013) and Equality Act (DH, 2010c) protect the rights of the individual against ageist practices and indirect ageism, for example, negative assumptions that the health of the older person is less significant than the younger still exist (Narayanasamy and Narayanasamy, 2012). Popular stereotypes of ageing portray individuals as demented and in poor health and are synonymous with decline, dependency and vulnerability (Barry and Yuill, 2012). Many elderly individuals may hold stereotypical ideas of themselves; therefore, respect for individuality is vital (Taylor et al., 2003). Some individuals may retain a view of the inner self which is younger than their body as a means of negating ageist expectations and preserving a sense of dignity (Boyd and Bee, 2015; Alder et al., 2004).

As we age we carry an increasing wealth of health experiences with us, shaped by the cultural and social norms of the world we live in. Successful ageing may be marked by an ability to look back on life with a sense of fulfilment and wholeness, or the extent to which an individual is able to remain socially engaged (Beckett and Taylor, 2013; Antai-Otong, 2007). Erikson (1980) noted that individuals who could reflect on life with a sense of satisfaction achieved a sense of integrity rather than despair. Meaning in life is closely related to health and declining health often equates to a sense of loss (Grossman and Lange, 2006). Feeling old may relate to feelings of fear, helplessness, feeling different from peers and losing a sense of control over one's life (Nilsson et al., 2000). Physical changes may restrict the capability for social involvement while factors such as changing role and status in the community or decline in mental ability will impact on the individual's experience of ageing. Economic aspects will also impact on the ageing process as opportunities for positive approaches to fulfilment in ageing may be linked to financial standing and deprivation (Barry and Yuill, 2012).

Positive ageing is dependent on a complex interaction of physical and psychosocial factors. However for individuals who have a long-term condition(s) and/or declining health ageing may be associated with increasing vulnerability and frailty. Frailty is not a diagnosis but can be classed as a long-term condition, it refers to a state related to ageing in which body systems lose their built-in reserves and fail to integrate adequate responses in response to changes in health or stress, and as a result the individual becomes increasingly vulnerable (Harrison et al., 2015; NHS England, 2014; Cornwell, 2012). Frailty presents unique challenges to healthcare professionals and its management requires knowledge, skill, empathy and compassion. A positive climate for care can be achieved through advance care planning and integrated approaches on a multi-disciplinary level (Cornwell, 2012). Preventative approaches to care which employ supportive and educative practices for individuals in managing, recognising and understanding their condition can aid independent living and reduce levels of risk and episodes of crisis management.

ACTIVITY 6.8

Reflection point

On her visits to Margaret, the community nurse has noted that the house is rather untidy and that Margaret often looks unkempt and appears very uninterested. Carol is also concerned about her mother; she tells the nurse that prior to Jack's death her mother had enjoyed an active social life, as both her parents had been keen members of the local bowls club.

Critically consider how an understanding of ageing can influence the quality of care for Margaret.

Social aspects of ageing may be characterised by patterns of adjustment that result in a process of disengagement in which the older person gradually withdraws from society. Social practices in retirement and cultural norms and values may mean that the older person becomes excluded from a variety of social settings and relationships; this may also be influenced by poverty and social class (Barry and Yuill, 2012). Old age is also a time of increased losses and a period when the individual is less able to cope with crises and loss (Walsh, 2009; Nilsson et al., 2000). Margaret is clearly struggling to maintain her emotions in the face of bereavement, which has also affected her role and social status within the community. She appears to have lost the social contact and network of support she had with Jack, and without an active social network she may be at increased risk of developing mental health problems (Walsh, 2009). Strategies to enable Margaret to move through this period of loss and bereavement may include replacing the losses in some way with different roles or people (Wadensten, 2006).

Dementia is a major cause of disability and an increasing challenge for healthcare in older age. Dementia is a known risk factor which contributes to frailty (Cornwell, 2012). Approximately 850,000 people in the United Kingdom have dementia, it affects 1:20 of those aged over 65 and 1:6 over 80 and two-thirds will be women (Alzheimer's Society, 2015). The financial costs are estimated at £26 billion p.a., with family carers saving the United Kingdom around £11 billion p.a. (Alzheimer's Society, 2015). The management of dementia is explored in more detail in the chapter on mental health.

Reflection point

As time progresses, Margaret continues to struggle to manage at home. Carol confides in you that her mother seems to be becoming very forgetful and frequently repeats elements of conversations. She has not been eating properly and has been forgetting to take her medication. You talk to Margaret about how she feels and she admits she is a 'bit forgetful at times and her memory is not what it used to be'. She says Carol thinks I am going 'daft'. However she agrees to a consultation with the GP. Several weeks later, Carol asks to meet with you at her mothers. She informs you that investigations following a period of assessment have confirmed that Margaret has early indications of Alzheimer's disease. Carol is worried about her mothers' safety and how she will cope with caring for her.

Consider how you might support Carol in coming to terms with her mother's diagnosis.

How might your understanding of a lifespan approach influence care for Margaret?

Margaret will be feeling vulnerable as she is aware that her cognitive function is changing and she is losing a sense of self and control. She is also probably acutely aware of the changes in how people react to her and this is impacting on her ability to maintain relationships and socialise. The way in which we present ourselves as a social being is underpinned by our ability to communicate effectively through conversation (Barry and Yuill, 2012) and for Margaret this is becoming increasingly challenging.

The impact of diagnosis is frightening for Margaret and devastating for Carol. The issue of stigma and negative responses to diagnosis on both personal and social levels alongside concerns about the likely progress of the disease, are all important factors to consider in supporting both Carol and Margaret. Raising awareness and understanding, providing support and enabling the individual to live well with dementia, supported by competent healthcare professionals are all key elements of current policy (DH, 2009b, 2015; Scottish Government, 2013b; DH Northern Ireland, 2011; Welsh Government, 2011). Carol will need advice and support on how to cope with the cognitive and behavioural changes her mother is experiencing. Identifying strategies to manage cognitive symptoms such as memory books and reminiscence techniques may be useful. Recognising that behavioural symptoms may be as a result of attempts to communicate and often reflect unmet needs may also be valuable (Sandilyan and Dening, 2015). For the nurse an understanding of Margaret's life history, personality and her personal reality may be important to maintaining her safety and maximising her quality of life. A multi-professional approach is essential; Margaret would be entitled to an assessment of need for social care and support that places her well-being at its core (DH, 2014). The impact of additional caring responsibilities may result in stress for Carol, she would be entitled to a carer's assessment and would need advice and support on how and where to access both financial and social help. The challenge for the healthcare professional is to provide safe patient- and family-centred care that will enable the individual to live well with dementia and to remain independent for as long as possible.

Communication skills

How well we communicate with patients can influence the quality of the relationship we develop with them. Person-centred communication which takes account of patient perspectives, expectations, feelings, needs and wants and has an understanding of the uniqueness of that individual is essential. Taking a lifespan approach to communication will enable us to utilise the most effective methods of communication with each client group. Communication with children requires concurrent dialogue with the family, and using a partnership approach will enhance empowerment and the effectiveness of healthcare interventions (Glasper, 2015). How we explain illness to a young child needs to be thought through in light of their cognitive abilities; for example, Piaget noted that before the age of 7 years the child has an inability to distinguish between cause and effect (Beckett and Taylor, 2013). Communication with adolescents needs an engaging non-judgemental approach initiated through open dialogue. Good communication strategies will be based on a sound understanding of their needs and some insight into adolescent culture (Briggs, 2010). The types of resources used will be an important consideration in reaching certain groups; examples such as the successful YouTube video highlighting teenage pregnancy demonstrate effective communication with their target group (NHS Leicester City, 2009). The use of media as a method of communication when used appropriately can be a powerful tool in shaping the norms, expectations and patterns of behaviour of individuals, families and communities (Livazovic, 2014).

The ability to communicate effectively is an important aspect of healthy ageing. Older people may be hampered by age-related changes, such as hearing loss and decreased vision, which influence how they perceive and control external cues (Tolson and Wilson, 2012). Barriers to communication with older adults include ageism, hurried approaches, lack of respect and a lack of appreciation for the individual's life experience (Antai-Otong, 2007). Inter-generational communication may be influenced by nurse assumptions and maintaining a professional, respectful approach which avoids overly familiar terms such as 'sweetie' and 'love' is of paramount importance (Knifton, 2009). Older people may need longer to retrieve learned material from their memory store and story-telling may be a valuable means of effective communication (Tolson and Wilson, 2012); therefore, strategies that allow greater time for assessment may be useful.

The opportunity to utilise effective communication skills with patients at whatever point in the lifespan is key to effective healthcare delivery. The quality of face-to-face interaction may become increasingly important as healthcare interventions become progressively driven by technology (McCabe and Timmins, 2012). Developing a therapeutic relationship can be enhanced by recognising the psychosocial and age-related factors that influence methods of communication.

The challenges of developing effective communication are explored in more detail in chapters on the therapeutic relationship and eHealth.

Gender issues

Gender issues influence health across the lifespan. Life expectancy is greater for women than men in the United Kingdom by an average of 3.8 years (ONS, 2014). Biomedical factors indicate that males may be inherently more vulnerable and are less likely to survive the first year of life (Taylor and Field, 2007). However, it is the interaction between biological and social factors that is significant in relation to health. Boys are more likely to die from accidents or have an accidental injury; gender roles increase the health risk for males as boys are encouraged to be more active (White, 2013). Female longevity may be linked to more positive health behaviours; for example, women are more likely to consume a healthy diet, although conversely more likely to develop an eating disorder (Taylor and Field, 2007). Male behaviour may be influenced by expectations and pressures of contemporary society to demonstrate masculinity (Barry and Yuill, 2012). Into adulthood, male probability of early death is increased by risk-taking behaviour such as dangerous sports, fast driving, hazardous consumption of alcohol and illicit drug use (White, 2013). However, we should remember that this is not necessarily a static picture. Evidence shows there is a narrowing of the gap in life expectancy, which may in part be explained by increasing risk-taking behaviours in females (e.g. smoking and alcohol consumption) (ONS, 2009, 2016).

The Equality Act (DH, 2010c) supports gender-sensitive healthcare. The community nurse needs to recognise that men and women may access services and present symptoms differently, and this may impact on the accessibility of services. The likelihood of seeing a GP varies with age and gender; females and older individuals are more likely to access these services. Men are less likely to attend for screening, preventative health checks and issues such as mental health and obesity (White, 2013). Women are more likely to recognise symptoms of illness and seek help earlier (Taylor and Field, 2007). Women are also more likely to ask questions, be given information and be involved in shared decision making than men (Antai-Otong, 2007). Although we could argue that female participation and uptake of services may be related in some part to need, that is, reproductive years and increased morbidity in later life, this cannot be entirely explained by these factors, and issues such as masculinity and gender roles may be relevant (White, 2013). Evidence would indicate that men may delay seeking help as a result of stoicism, ideals of being strong and being able to endure pain (Barry and Yuill, 2012). Access to services may also be linked to social factors such as employment. Peter's busy schedule means he is less likely to seek advice if he cannot attend in the evening, whereas Simon's choice may be guided by the impact on his salary.

Issues of sexual orientation may also influence access to healthcare. This may be of particular relevance in adolescence when individuals may be developing an awareness of their sexual identity as lesbian, gay, bisexual or transgender

(Boyd and Bee, 2015). Evidence suggests that sexual minorities have a greater tendency to exhibit health risk factors (e.g. smoking, alcohol consumption), have an increased incidence of mental health problems and that they may have reduced access to healthcare (Hsieh and Ruther, 2016; Beckett and Taylor, 2013). The experience of an individual may be influenced by inequalities in service provision, perceived discrimination and poorly informed healthcare practitioners (Aleshire, 2016; McCann and Sharek, 2016). It is important that assumption-free, non-judgmental attitudes are embedded within the provision of culturally sensitive healthcare.

Understanding how age, gender and gender identity and expression may influence uptake and accessibility is important in the planning and delivery of services to effectively meet the needs of the local community.

CONCLUSION

This chapter has explored a lifespan approach to healthcare. Multi-dimensional views that take account of not only the biological and psychological but increasingly the social, cultural and environmental aspects of health and illness are essential. Age, gender and individual perceptions of health will all influence individual needs, assessment and care provision. It is important to recognise that each person is part of a family system, and that the healthcare needs of the individual may well impact on the family. Proactive person-centred approaches and developing positive health should underpin holistic healthcare provision. Understanding how aspects of the lifespan relate to the physical, psychological, social, environmental and spiritual elements of an individual's life can positively influence care provision and the quality of life for clients, their families and carers.

FURTHER READING

There is a vast amount of literature relating to the theories of growth and development and the application of these concepts to healthcare and your interest may well be guided by your professional role and client group focus. The following texts take a broad view.

Boyd D and Bee H (2015) *Lifespan Development*, 7th edn. Harlow: Pearson Education.
Beckett C and Taylor H (2013) *Human Growth and Development*. London: Sage.
Crain W (2014) *Theories of Development: Concepts and Applications*, 6th edn. Harlow: Pearson Education Ltd.

REFERENCES

Alder B (2013) *Psychology of Health Applications of Psychology for Health Professionals*, 2nd edn. Hove: Taylor-Francis, pp. 75–93, 143–64.
Alder B, Porter M, Abraham C and van Teijlingen E (2004) *Psychology and Sociology Applied to Medicine*, 2nd edn. Edinburgh: Churchill Livingstone, pp. 8–45, 112–13.
Aldwin C and Gilmer D (2013) *Health, Illness, and Optimal Aging: Biological and Psychosocial Perspectives*, 2nd edn. New York, NY: Springer Publishing Company, pp. 38–46.
Aleshire M (2016) Sexual orientation, gender identity and gender expression: What are they? *The Journal for Nurse Practitioners* 12(7):329–30.

Alzheimer's Society (2015) Statistics. http://www.alzheimers.org.uk/. Accessed July 28, 2016.

Antai-Otong D (2007) *Nurse–Client Communication: A Life Span Approach*. Burlington, MA: Jones & Bartlett, pp. 20–97.

Barry A and Yuill C (2012) *Understanding the Sociology of Health*, 3rd edn. London: Sage Publications, pp. 129–63, 206–21.

Becker M (1974) *The Health Belief Model and Personal Health Behaviour*. Thorofare, NJ: Slack.

Beckett C and Taylor H (2013) *Human Growth and Development*. London: Sage, pp. 1–17, 61–73, 92–109, 178–89.

Boyd D and Bee H (2015) *Lifespan Development*, 7th edn. Harlow: Pearson Education, pp. 26–65, 218–21, 288–93, 334, 454–79.

Briggs P (2010) Strategies for discussing sex with teenagers. *Practice Nursing* 21:71–4.

Bury M (1991) The sociology of chronic illness: A review of research and prospects. *Sociology of Health and Illness* 13:451–68.

Cameron N (2006) *Human Growth and Development*. San Diego, CA: Elsevier, pp. 1–20.

Clarke A (2013) *The Sociology of Healthcare*. London: Routledge, pp. 194–226.

Clarke L and Korotchenko A (2010) Shades of grey: To dye or not to dye one's hair in later life. *Ageing and Society* 30(6):1011–26.

Cornwell J (2012) *The Care of Frail Older People with Complex Needs: Time for a Revolution*. King's Fund, pp. 1–9. https://www.king'sfund.org.uk/sites/files/kf/field/field_publication_file/the-care-of-frail-older-people-with-complex-needs-mar-2012.pdf. Accessed June 21, 2017.

Cox CL and Hill MC (2010) *Professional Issues in Primary Care Nursing*. Chichester: Wiley Blackwell, pp. 78–94.

DH (2009a) *Healthy Child Programme: The 2 Year Review*. London: DH.

DH (2009b) *Living Well with Dementia: A National Dementia Strategy*. London: DH.

DH (2010a) *Equity and Excellence Liberating the NHS*. London: DH.

DH (2010b) *Healthy Lives, Healthy People: Our Strategy for Public Health in England*. London: DH.

DH (2010c) *Equality Act*. London: DH.

DH (2013) *A Framework for Sexual Health Improvement in England*. London: DH.

DH (2014) *Care Act*. London: DH.

Department of Health (DH) (2015) *Prime Minister's Challenge on Dementia 2020*. London: DH.

DH Northern Ireland (2011) Improving dementia services in Northern Ireland—A regional strategy. https://www.health-ni.gov.uk/publications/improving-dementia-services-northern-ireland-regional-strategy. Accessed July 28, 2016.

Department of Health (DH) Northern Ireland (2014) Making life better: A whole system strategic framework for public health 2103-23. https://www.health-ni.gov.uk/sites/default/files/publications/dhssps/making-life-better-strategic-framework-2013-2023_0.pdf. Accessed July 28, 2016.

Erber J (2013) *Aging and Older Adulthood*, 3rd edn. Chichester: Wiley-Blackwell, pp. 8–14.

Erikson EH (1980) *Identity and the Life Cycle*. New York, NY: Norton and Company, pp. 94–107.

Family Planning Association (FPA) (2010) Sexual health week 2010: The middle-age spread. www.fpa.org.uk/home. Accessed July 28, 2016.

Farley A, McLafferty E and Hendry C (2011) *The Physiological Effects of Ageing: Implications for Nursing Practice*. Oxford: Wiley-Blackwell, pp. 1–6, 67–91.

Glasper E (2015) *Children and Young People's Nursing at a Glance*. Oxford: Wiley Blackwell, pp. 54–85.

Grossman S and Lange J (2006) Theories of aging as basis for assessment. *Medsurg Nursing* 15:77–83.

Hammen C and Watkins E (2013) *Depression*, 2nd edn. Hove: Psychology Press.

Harrison J, Clegg A, Conroy S and Young J (2015) Managing frailty as a long term condition. *Age and Ageing* 44:732–45.

Hicks M and Conner N (2014) Resilient ageing a concept analysis. *Journal of Advanced Nursing* 70(4):744–55.

HSCIC (2014) Focus on the Health and Care of Older People. Health and Social Care Information Centre, pp. 1–49. http://content.digital.nhs.uk/catalogue/PUB14369/focu-on-hac-op-dat-qual-note.pdf. Accessed June 21, 2017.

Hsieh N and Ruther M (2016) Sexual minority health and risk factors: Intersection effects of gender, race and sexual identity. *American Journal of Preventative Medicine* 50(6):746–55.

Knifton C (2009) Dementia. In McVeigh H (ed) *Fundamental Aspects of Long Term Conditions*. London: Quay Books, pp. 153–76.

Larkin M (2009) *Vulnerable Groups in Health and Social Care*. London: Sage, pp. 29–46, 71–86.

Leifer G and Hartshorn H (2004) *Growth and Development across the Lifespan*. St Louis, MO: Saunders, pp. 50–65.

Livazovic G (2014) The role of media in adolescent social relationships. In Runcan G and Rata G (eds) *Applied Social Psychology*. Cambridge: Cambridge Scholars Publishing, pp. 69–88.

McCabe C and Timmins F (2012) Communicating care. In McSherry W, McSherry R and Watson R (eds) *Care in Nursing: Principles, Value, and Skills*. Oxford: Oxford University Press, pp. 137–49.

McCann E and Sharek D (2016) Mental health needs of people who identify as transgender: A review of the literature. *Archives of Psychiatric Nursing* 30:280–85.

Naidoo J and Wills J (2015) *Health Studies: An Introduction*, 3rd edn. London: Palgrave, pp. 35–63, 135–6.

Narayanasamy A and Narananasamy G (2012) Diversity in Caring. In McSherry W, McSherry R and Watson R (eds) *Care in Nursing: Principles, Value, and Skills*. Oxford: Oxford University Press, pp. 61–69.

NICE (2014a) Health visiting. https://www.nice.org.uk/guidance/lgb22/resources/health-visiting-60521203534021. Accessed July 28, 2016.

NICE (2014b) Contraceptive services for under 25's. https://www.nice.org.uk/guidance/PH51/chapter/1-Recommendations#recommendation-3-providing-contraceptive-services-for-young-people. Accessed July 28, 2016.

National Institute for Health and Care Excellence (NICE) (2015) Workplace health and management practices. https://www.nice.org.uk/guidance/ng13/resources/workplace-health-management-practices-1837269751237. Accessed July 28, 2016.

Nettleton S (2013) *The Sociology of Health and Illness*, 3rd edn. Cambridge: Polity Press, pp. 3–75.

NHS (2013) NHS Constitution for England 2013. Department of Health, pp. 1–16.

NHS England (2014) Safe compassionate care for frail older people using an integrated care pathway. https://www.england.nhs.uk/wp-content/uploads/2014/02/safe-comp-care.pdf. Accessed July 28, 2016.

NHS Leicester City (2009) Leicester teenage pregnancy and partnership. (Accessed 18 May 2009) www.youtube.com. Accessed July 28, 2016.

NHS Scotland (2016) Child health surveillance programme pre-school. http://www.isdscotland.org/Health-Topics/Child-Health/Child-Health-Programme/_docs/CHSP-PS-Clinical-Guidelines-140316.pdf.

Nilsson M, Sarvimaki A and Ekman SL (2000) Feeling old: Being in a phase of transition in later life. Nursing Inquiry 7:41–9.

NMC (2015) *The Code: Professional Standards of Practice and Behavior for Nurses and Midwives*. London: NMC, Standard 13.1.

ONS (2009) Alcohol-related deaths 2007. *Health Statistics Quarterly* 41:4.

ONS (2013) Statistical bulletin: National population projections 2012 UK. http://webarchive.nationalarchives.gov.uk/20140616025728/http://www.ons.gov.uk/ons/dcp171778_334975.pdf. Accessed July 28, 2016.

Office for National Statistics (ONS) (2014) *Statistical Bulletin: National Life Tables, United Kingdom*. Newport: ONS, pp. 1–15.

Office for National Statistics (ONS) (2016) Alcohol related deaths in the United Kingdom registered 2014. https://www.ons.gov.uk/peoplepopulationandcommunity/healthandsocialcare/causesofdeath/bulletins/alcoholrelateddeathsintheunitedkingdom/registeredin2014.

Ogden J (2012) *Health Psychology: A Textbook*. Maidenhead: Open University Press, pp. 35–181.

Sandilyan MB and Dening T (2015) Diagnosis of dementia. *Nursing Standard* 29(41):42–51.

Scottish Government (2013a) Route map to the 2020 vision for health and social care. http://www.gov.scot/Topics/Health/Policy/Quality-Strategy/routemap2020vision.

Scottish Government (2013b) Scotland's National dementia strategy. http://www.gov.scot/Topics/Health/Services/Mental-Health/Dementia/DementiaStrategy1316.

Scottish Government (2016) A national clinical stategy for Scotland. http://www.gov.scot/Publications/2016/02/8699. Accessed July 28, 2016.

Sharma A, Cockerill H, Okawa N and Sheridan M (2014) *Mary Sheridan's from Birth to Five Years: Children's Developmental Progress*, 4th edn. Abingdon: Routledge, pp. 85–92.

Sky Ride (2016) Big bike events. http://www.goskyride.com/. Accessed July 28, 2016.

Smith J and McSherry W (2004) Spirituality and child development: A concept analysis. *Journal of Advanced Nursing* 45:307–15.

Taylor S and Field D (2007) *Sociology of Health and Illness*, 4th edn. Oxford: Blackwell, pp. 3–44, 93–112.

Taylor R, Smith B and van Teijlingen E (ed) (2003) *Health and Illness in the Community*. Oxford: OUP, pp. 105–85.

Thornton S (2012) Caring for communities. In McSherry W, McSherry R and Watson R. *Care in Nursing: Principles, Value, and Skills*. Oxford: Oxford University Press, pp. 81–91

TNS BRMB (2014) Attitudes to Mental Illness 2013 Research Report. https://www.time-to-change.org.uk/sites/default/files/121168_Attitudes_to_mental_illness_2013_report.pdf.

Tolson C and Wilson D (2012) Communication. In Reed J, Clarke L and Macfarlane A. *Nursing Older Adults*. Maidenhead: Open University Press, pp. 158–74.

Wadensten B (2006) An analysis of psychosocial theories of ageing and their relevance to practical gerontological nursing in Sweden. *Scandinavian Journal Caring* 20:347–54.

Walsh L (2009) *Depression Across the Lifespan*. Oxford: Wiley Blackwell, pp. 106–10.

Welsh Government (2015) Prudent health care and patient activation. http://gov.wales/topics/health/nhswales/planned/?lang=en. Accessed July 28, 2016.

Welsh Government (2011) National dementia vision for wales. http://gov.wales/docs/dhss/publications/110302dementiaen.pdf.

White A (2013) Raising awareness of men's risk of premature death. *Nursing Standard* 25(50):35–41.

World Health Organization (WHO) (1946) *Constitution*. Geneva: WHO.

CHAPTER 7

Community nursing assessment

Helen Gough

LEARNING OUTCOMES

- Explore the meaning of assessment.
- Explore the concept of need.
- Discuss assessment frameworks.
- Analyse conceptual aspects of assessments.
- Critically reflect on decision making.

INTRODUCTION

The aim of this chapter is to examine community nursing assessment by defining terminology and identifying what constitutes a holistic assessment. The concept of need and its relationship to assessment will be explored along with existing assessment frameworks and models that have been developed to meet the wide range of assessment perspectives that exists within a community setting. Decision making and its essential alignment with community nursing assessment will then be discussed, with opportunities to guide reflection on current practice.

EXPLORING THE MEANING OF ASSESSMENT

Assessment is a core skill for nurses, as any subsequent care depends on the accuracy of the assessment. This means that any mistakes in this process will inevitably lead to flawed care. Developmental changes to UK health policy, which include improving the health of the population and providing healthcare locally, placed the community nursing workforce at the forefront of early developments (Scottish Executive, 2005; Department of Health [DH], 2006). This emphasis on convenient access to care closer to and within the patient's home continued to gain momentum and identified the need for flexible and adaptable community nurses (Scottish Government, 2007; DH, 2008). More recent developments in relation in UK health policy have driven the integration of health and social care for adults which stresses the importance of seamless care (Scottish Government, 2015; NHS England and Local Government Association, 2013). Indeed health and social services are experiencing a rapid period of transition in order to respond to the needs of the aging population and are engaged in strategic change within professional practice (UK Parliament, 2013; Scottish Parliament, 2013). This means community nurses remain in a unique position to reflect on existing assessment practices and review these for suitability and/or adaptation to meet the changing political and professional agenda. The Nursing and Midwifery Council (NMC) Code (2015) reinforces the need for effective practice, and this suggests that current community nursing assessment practice is worthy of exploration as it provides nurses with an opportunity to reflect on their current assessment skills and knowledge and to identify ways to improve their practice. A starting point is examining what we actually mean by assessment.

DEFINING ASSESSMENT

It is perhaps somewhat surprising that concise contemporary definitions of nursing assessment can be challenging to find in current literature. Seminal nursing theorists Roper et al. (1990) were quite specific in relation to patient assessment, highlighting that it included collecting information about the patient, identifying the problems and then determining the priorities. Although this first appears as a superficial approach, far more detail is then provided and it is clear that assessment is an ongoing activity that gathers biographical and health data before considering assessment of the patient's activities of living (Roper et al., 1990). In contrast, a patient-centred definition of assessment was provided by Worth in 2001 that highlighted the ways in which the needs and requirements of the person drove the subsequent planned care and services. While this approach emphasises patient need, the need was usually determined by the professional, therefore diminishing the opportunity for a partnership approach. In a succinct definition, Kenny (2009: 386) explains assessment as, 'an ongoing process of data collection to determine the client's strengths and health concerns'. This definition suggests the person is at the centre of care and a partnership approach is assumed, making the patient visible.

Making the patient visible is reflected by the Royal College of Nursing (2014) where assessment guidance includes seeking patient's views, expectations and preferences. More recently, the NMC too have articulated patient involvement in care in the 2015 Code, using a key theme of 'prioritising people' to underpin the guidance and promote a partnership approach to assessment. This places the patient at the centre of care. Therefore it is perhaps misguided to suggest that historically nurses have not been involving people in their care when it may simply be due to a lack of an authentic description in the literature.

PATIENT-CENTRED CARE

The idea of patients being at the centre of their care was established in the Patients' Charter in 1991, and introduced the concept of the named nurse (King's Fund, 2009).

Box 7.1 Principles of patient-centred care

Consideration of

- The patient's needs and beliefs
- The patient as an individual
- The patient's view in decision making
- The patient's fears and concerns
- The patient's family, carers and friends

Principles of patient-centred care are detailed in Box 7.1, and it is clear that these key areas represent an approach to practice, as opposed to a definitive framework.

Furthermore, the principles of patient-centred care link to holistic assessment, recognising need and shared decision making. Support for this patient-centred approach is augmented in practice by the growing understanding of the term concordance and the resulting 'informed partnership agreement which is negotiated between the professional and the patient' (Beckwith and Franklin, 2007). This partnership agreement was explained in more detail by the Department of Health (DH) (2007) originally in relation to prescribing, and differentiates between concordance and compliance in relation to medicines management by stating:

> Concordance describes a partnership approach to medicine prescribing and taking. It is different from 'compliance', which describes the patient's medicine taking in relation to the prescriber's instructions. Concordance recognises that people make their own decisions about whether or not to take a prescribed treatment and acknowledges that a well-informed patient may decide to decline treatment after learning about the relative benefits and risks. It is this approach to shared decision making and information exchange where the patient shares their knowledge of their illness and the clinician shares evidence based information that highlights an authentic partnership approach. (Foot et al., 2014)

In an alternative stance where the focus is on the practitioner within the assessment process, Muncey (2002) suggests that the assessment activity undertaken by the expert nurse is 'invisible'. Muncey (2002) explains that this is because assessment is a cognitive process which is then only articulated, and therefore 'visible', once documented in written form. Only then can the visual representation of the assessment findings and their priority be identified.

Regardless of visibility, this partnership or sharing of power between patient and professional is a cornerstone of person-centred care, a term promoted in the literature by McCormack and McCance (2010) that has since been embraced by a range of organisations including The Health Foundation (2014). The Health Foundation (2014: 4) describes person-centredness as a situation where there is 'recognition of the active roles that individuals can play as partners in their health and health care'. Notwithstanding, person-centred care can introduce complex challenges for community nurses as sharing evidenced-based information to enable authentic, shared decision making can be time consuming. At a time where resources are constrained and community nurses need to justify the time spent in patients' homes, the concern is that achieving genuine holistic person-centred care could be compromised.

ACTIVITY 7.1

Defining terms: Holism

From your own perspective note the key components of holism. Now link these ideas to community nursing assessment and write a short definition of 'holistic nursing care'. Continue reading through the chapter and then review your definition against those drawn from the literature in the following section.

HOLISM

Although holism is a term used frequently within nursing literature in relation to health assessment (Roper et al., 1990; Aggleton and Chalmers, 2000; Fox, 2003; Royal College of Nursing 2006; Beckwith and Franklin, 2007), a more detailed analysis of the term is often absent. According to Dossey and Guzzetta (2005: 8), holistic nursing consultants in the United States, 'Holistic nursing is the most complete way to conceptualise and practice professional nursing'. The bio-psycho-social-spiritual concept that Dossey and Guzzetta (2005: 8) describe for patient care necessary to achieve the best results closely resembles the approach supported by Cornforth (2013), Gough (2008), Freeman (2005) and Haworth and Dluhy (2001). This concept embraces physical, psychological, social, environmental, spiritual and cultural factors that make up an individual as a whole (Haworth and Dluhy, 2001; Freeman, 2005; Gough, 2008). This is a sound perspective for community nurses to start from, as it reflects a social model of health and places the patient in a community setting. This approach links to Kennedy's (2004) earlier work, which looked at community nursing assessment and reinforced the wider aspects of care that included psychosocial and spiritual features and the impact these factors have on a person's health and well-being. This focuses on the interaction and relationship between all those involved in care, and not only aligns with a patient-centred approach but also advocates a holistic approach (McCormack and McCance, 2010). Therefore, holistic assessment involves gathering information from a person using a partnership approach in relation to their physical, psychological, social, environmental, spiritual and cultural well-being. Although the Family Health System (FHS) described by Anderson and Tomlinson (1992) and Anderson (2000) has much earlier roots, it also embraces a holistic approach for assessment and care delivery for families, centering on significant areas of concern intimated by the family. This suggests that the emphasis to develop more partnership approaches in relation to nursing assessment is not new but better articulated in family assessment literature. Given this focus on partnership approaches to assessment practice, it is reassuring to discover that compatible assessment perspectives from the disciplines of community and family nursing co-exist. Despite this alignment, it is worthwhile taking time to explore the background to nursing models, as these models were the earliest frameworks that introduced a systematic approach to nursing assessment.

NURSING MODELS

Nursing models were introduced into the UK nurse education and practice in the 1980s. Designed to inform assessment by collating appropriate data (Aggleton and Chalmers, 2000), they were developed to guide nurses to deliver practice in a less chaotic and more organised fashion. Roper et al. (1990) model for nursing is perhaps the most well known in the United Kingdom, which is no surprise as the authors are British. Although the five components of the model include the activities of living and influencing factors, the lifespan, dependence–independence continuum and individuality in living (Roper et al., 1990), it is almost always the activities of living that are evident in assessment frameworks within practice. Unfortunately, if the whole model is not used, the activities of living become a checklist and as a result the information gathered can often become superficial and lack crucial detail. It is perhaps no surprise that current literature which promotes the use of nursing models in contemporary community nursing practice is scarce, and this may reveal a lack of interest from educators and practitioners alike. Not surprisingly, when models of nursing, such as Orem's self-care model and Roy's adaptation model (Aggleton and Chalmers, 2000), are explored for clarity and understanding it becomes evident that the terminology implemented is not always user friendly and the language used is somewhat complicated. Furthermore, Whetsell et al. (2011) and Kenny (2009) suggest that a wide, advanced-level knowledge base is required in order to interpret and apply nursing models in practice, and perhaps it is this difficulty in application combined with a complicated language that has contributed to their decline. Notwithstanding it is likely that a search for the perfect assessment tool for community nursing is not realistic; however, there are various diverse theories and concepts available in the literature to assist nurses to develop holistic approaches for their area of practice.

DISCUSSION OF ASSESSMENT FRAMEWORKS

A starting point for analysis of existing frameworks is consideration of those currently in place that guide community nursing assessment.

ACTIVITY 7.2

Reflection point

Reflect on the way in which you currently assess a patient/client in practice including the assessment framework or model that guides you. Consider the age and context of the framework/model that you currently use and judge the following:

1. It is fit for purpose?

2. *You may wish to consider its strengths and limitations (is it simply a tick list,* electronic or otherwise?) and its ease of completion along with any gaps you identify. Gaps in assessment frameworks often result in the practitioner having to key in additional information.

3. Does it have an evidence base?

4. *Can you clearly identify the literature or research that underpins the tool?*

If you are using a Trust/National Health Service (NHS) assessment framework then you still need to question the evidence base and identify the literature or research that underpins the tool.

It may be that you are unsure what assessment framework is available to you in practice: this is an important discovery. Practitioners can find themselves using the documentation that their employing organisation provides them with and mistakenly believe this to be an assessment tool. Of course in some cases, a validated assessment tool will be incorporated into the documentation, and as practitioners you should be able to identify this clearly. In an article on patient documentation by Irving et al. (2006), there is an assumption made that nursing records mirror the assessment made.

The problem with this is that although the nurse enters the findings from the assessment into the nursing record, there is no guarantee that the documentation is in fact an assessment tool. This is then problematic if it is the documentation that drives the assessment because the focus may not be holistic or, even worse, crucial information shared by the person may be missed. Furthermore, if the tool only allows the nurse to document 'tasks' or tick boxes, then the ethos of holistic assessment and responding to need, which are the key elements of community nursing practice, are lost.

EXPLORING THE CONCEPT OF NEED

A key aspect of health assessment links to the concept of need, and it would be difficult to undertake holistic assessment without consideration of need. Health needs can relate to different levels depending on the context, for example, helping patients to identify their own health needs takes a different approach from identifying broad health needs within a local community (Coles and Porter, 2008). Seminal work by Bradshaw in 1972 identified a taxonomy of need from a sociological perspective that helps to explain individual need, and this is outlined in Box 7.2.

> **Box 7.2 Bradshaw's taxonomy of need**
>
> *Normative need* is explained as the need that the health/social care professional identifies. Although professionals are educated to recognise need, it has to be acknowledged that various professionals may identify different needs from each other. Furthermore, health needs can change over time.
>
> *Felt need* is described as a need identified by the patient or carer. Although the patient or carer will be able to identify some of their own needs, they may not have a grasp of all that they require.
>
> *Expressed* need is the articulation of a felt need by the patient or carer.
>
> *Comparative need* is when in certain areas the patients or carers are not receiving the same standard of care that is available elsewhere.

Although this does provide a theoretical perspective of need that can be practically applied by community nurses, it is worth pointing out that there is no acknowledgement within the taxonomy of any associated resources, including availability of services. This means that although needs in relation to individuals or families may be identified, an issue arises when the resources are limited and these needs cannot be met. In reality, this means that although assessment identifies healthcare needs in partnership with an individual, for example, referral to an additional service, third sector organisation or a nursery placement, any treatment or service provision will need to be justified economically. Furthermore, if the need cannot be met because there is no transport to the service or the nursery has no spaces, then alternatives have to be considered. Working within these constraints can be very challenging for the community nursing team and can result in frustration and concerns when trying to deliver evidence-based practice. As determining need along with being aware of local available resources is part of the assessment process, then analyzing current conceptual aspects of assessment is the next logical step.

ANALYZING CONCEPTUAL ASPECTS OF ASSESSMENT

Rushworth (2009) and Wilson and Giddens (2012) state that individual health assessment is undertaken by taking a health history and conducting a physical examination, and this is then followed by a diagnosis and treatment plan. Bickley and Szilagyi (2016) support this approach and explain comprehensive assessment in relation to a health history and complete physical examination, which includes family, personal and social history as part of the seven components required. Therefore, the focus of the consultation is usually around the presenting complaint and has a strong physical component. Even though this type of consultation clearly has a place in community nursing, for example, in long-term condition management and prescribing, the emphasis can appear medicalised with less focus on the person. However, this is tempered by the position statement on advanced level nursing (DH, 2010) where the emphasis is clearly around the significance of advanced health needs assessment for nurses working at this level.

In contrast, Wright and Leahey (2013) look at family assessment and include physical or spiritual suffering, illness, relationship issues or family crisis as indications for a family assessment. Although a health history described by Bickley and Szilagyi (2016), and Wilson and Giddens (2012) is suitable for the context of individual patients presenting with a physical complaint or illness, this is clearly a different context from that of a family with health needs in the community setting that Wright and Leahey (2013) are alluding to. This highlights the complex nature and diversity of community nursing assessment, as it is often the client group along with the community nursing service involved that dictate the form of assessment. Indeed new community nursing roles have been developed in order to meet the evolving needs of patients in the community and the resultant service developments.

ADOPTING NEW ROLES

The context of health assessment, however, can subtly change its focus directly due to nurses adopting new roles in practice. This can be seen when the term 'patient consultation' is introduced into contemporary nursing along with details of consultation models which have found their way into nursing literature (Hastings, 2006; Young et al., 2009; Harper and Ajao, 2010; Young and Duggan, 2010). The aforementioned authors analysed the history-taking process in relation to a patient consultation, and it is clear that this reflects advanced skills in comparison to assessment of need by current community nurses. Among other things, these skills include *clarifying the complaint* and *identifying any red flags* (Young et al., 2009; Young and Duggan, 2010), and for those with a prescribing background these terms in relation to risk assessment will no doubt be familiar. Although current consultation models clearly have an assessment component drawn from nursing, along with recognition of interpersonal skills, this does introduce advanced clinical proficiencies that nurses moving into these roles need to develop and maintain (Young et al., 2009), while simultaneously continuing to advocate person-centred care. Advanced physical examination and interpretation of diagnostic tests are developing skills for nurses particularly within the home setting, and this highlights the continued development of advanced level of assessment, although this advanced stage of nursing is linked to a level of expertise well beyond initial registration and would be undertaken only by those practitioners who had additional education and expertise.

Retrieving guidance in the form of a model or framework that assists the practitioner to undertake a holistic assessment however is not straightforward. Some years ago, in an attempt to provide novice prescribers with guidance for assessment, Gough (2008) developed a holistic assessment model based on relevant theoretical perspectives. Although a limitation of this holistic framework is that it has not been formally validated to determine its inter-rater reliability, the content can guide practitioners and help them evaluate the assessment and consultation models that they currently use. Developing an assessment tool for a group of patients is not a new phenomenon, although failure to disseminate it through nursing literature perhaps is.

The holistic assessment tool created by Gough (2008), which can be viewed in Box 7.3, was developed with a prescribing focus in mind. That said, the tool is arguably useful for guiding community nurses to engage in a partnership approach when assessing people who have an identified health need within a community setting. Drawing on the dimensions of health (adapted from Aggleton and Homans, 1987; Ewles and Simnett, 1999), the Determinants of Health (Dahlgren and Whitehead, 1991; Bickley and Szilagyi, 2016) physical examination and history taking along with the prescribing pyramid (National Prescribing Centre [NPC], 1999), which includes the Mnemonic WWHAM used in pharmacies for advising about over-the-counter treatments (Box 7.4), a flexible assessment tool emerged. The tool provides guidance for community nurses to undertake a holistic assessment and although every aspect may not be assessed at the first visit, the assessment tool allows community nurses to respond to the needs determined by both the patient and nurse thus implementing a partnership approach.

While the flexibility of the assessment tool developed by Gough (2008) promotes the identification of priorities and provides an opportunity to include additional information at a later date, it can only be used to guide or prompt practitioners. This is because Trusts and NHS organisations have their own discrete documentation which is increasingly electronic, that must be completed. Developments in relation to mobile technology have promoted agile working across the United Kingdom and as a result electronic assessment forms are frequently used. While some of these electronic forms may sustain the tick box approach, the holistic tool detailed below can act as a prompt to enhance a holistic approach that involves the patient in an authentic partnership.

Box 7.3 Holistic assessment tool for community practitioner nurse prescribers (Gough, 2008)

Name and address
DOB
Occupation

(hazards, working conditions, risks)

Reason for assessment/presenting complaint

Physical health

Onset, duration and severity of condition

Previous history of complaint, treatment and results

Previous medical history

Family history

Current health status and appearance

Medication

Prescription-only medication (POM), pharmacy medication (P), general sales
list (GSL) and other

Herbal/homeopathic

Known allergies (drugs and substances)

Alcohol history (can include family if client a child)

Smoking history (can include family if client a child)

Diet and fluids

Mobility (aids and adaptations)

Dexterity (aids and adaptations)

Visual acuity (aids and adaptations)

Additional physical findings specific to complaint (e.g. bowel habit, oral
hygiene, broken skin)

Clinical findings (if examination required)

Additional specific assessment tool required (pain, wound, depression,
nutritional assessment tool)

Emotional and psychological health

Emotional effects of condition

Cognitive (ability, disability, memory)

Mental health (anxiety, worry, confusion, depression, dementia)

Social/environmental health

Home occupants

Dependents

Carers (statutory and voluntary)

Living conditions (housing, access, safety)

Financial (needs, allowances, exemptions)

Local amenities (shops, transport, sanitation)

Sexual health

Impact of condition on sexuality and sexual health

Spiritual health

Impact of condition on religion, beliefs, faith and culture

Additional information

Box 7.4 Mnemonic WWHAM

W Who is it for?

W What are the symptoms?

H How long have the symptoms been present?
A Any action taken so far?
M Any other medication?

(NPC, 1991)

ACTIVITY 7.3

Reflection point

Holistic assessment tools must often be supplemented by additional specific assessment tools, for example, for pain assessment, for assessment of postnatal depression, nutrition or assessing spiritual needs. Now consider any additional specific areas of assessment (pain, wound, memory, mental state, nutrition, etc.) that you might want to undertake with people whom you work with in the community. What evidence-based tools or frameworks are available to you in your area? What educational preparation and practice supports do you apply in the clinical setting and how do you support learners to engage with these within the local setting? Now identify any additional assessment tools that you are currently unfamiliar with and the ways in which you could access continued professional development (CPD) to develop your skills.

Not surprisingly, assessment practice does not stand independently and decision making is a close relation that needs to be embraced in tandem alongside it. Decision making is part of the crucial cognitive process when assessment is being undertaken and ties together the evidence base that should underpin community nursing assessment practice.

CRITICAL REFLECTION ON DECISION MAKING

It is clear therefore that assessment cannot exist in a vacuum without decision-making processes with which to move the episode of care along.

ACTIVITY 7.4

Reflection point

Reflect on your current practice and determine what currently guides your decision making. If you are unable to answer this then please do not panic as help is at hand in the following section.

If you can identify a guide to your decision-making practice, now consider whether it has an evidence base.

Can you clearly identify the literature or research that underpins this guide?

If not then this is something that you can investigate within your local Trust/ NHS organisation.

Sometimes it can be difficult to actually unpick what we mean when thinking about what guides decision making, but what is clear is that for community nurses, nursing care must be evidence based and not as a result of a whim or, worse, a comment like 'we always do it like this here'. As accountable practitioners our decisions are rightly scrutinised and never more so than when a critical incident has taken place. Therefore, a robust rationale needs to be provided for our actions and decisions (NMC, 2015) and having a guide to support and understand our decision making with an opportunity to reflect with afterwards, helps us to learn from experience.

CONTEXT OF DECISION MAKING

As already mentioned, within community nursing there is a wide variety of contexts of practice in relation to the patient group and the discipline involved, for example, young children and the potential input from health visitors/public health nurses or community children's nurses, those with mental health conditions and likely input from community mental health nurses and finally unwell older adults receiving care from district nurses and practice nurses. These contexts are important as they determine the skills and knowledge required to deliver care and are highlighted specifically in relation to decision making and healthcare by Croskerry (2009). Croskerry (2009) highlights two main systems of decision making. The first is *system one*, the intuitive route, which relies on a reflexive approach that expends little effort and does not depend on evidence to underpin the decision. Although this will be familiar to community nurses, the problem is that it can be unreliable and errors are frequent, so relying on this approach is unlikely to provide quality patient care and in the extreme could be fatal. Errors in decision making are explained as slips, lapses and mistakes. Pearson (2013) has an alternative view of intuition and suggests that it is based on pattern recognition drawn from experience in clinical practice and is in fact a cognitive skill. However, Pearson (2013) does agree with Crosskerry that intuition should be used along with evidence-based practice. The scientific approach then described by Pearson (2013) that involves hypothesis and cue acquisition or gathering of objective and subjective data aligns to Crosskerry's system two. Furthermore, mistakes take place when the practitioner's thinking is faulty; for example, the diagnosis of a red painful wound as infected when it is actually inflamed.

System two described by Croskerry (2009) is the analytical route, which relies on a rule-based approach that requires significant effort and has a scientific base. The problem with this analytical approach is that although it is a more reliable system of decision making, there is an associated cost and time issue that cannot be ignored. Therefore, a balance or blend between both systems needs to be considered. This is supported by Person (2009), who argues that a combination of intuition and scientific evidence-based approaches can be used successfully to achieve effective outcomes. The following case study illustrates this from a community nursing practice perspective.

CASE STUDY

Mrs Grant is aged 84 years and is unknown to you. She has requested that you visit as she would like some help and advice in relation to a problem with constipation.

Intuitive approach – Fast, reflexive with minimal effort
Your experience with patients in this age group links constipation to medication side effects, reduced fibre in the diet along with a lack of fluids and low mobility. This intuitive approach relies on the context to guide the

decision and in this case it's the gender, age and assumed co-morbidity of the patient.

Analytical approach – Slower, deliberate with considerable effort

Your experience with patients in this age group links constipation to medication side effects, reduced fibre in the diet along with a lack of fluids and low mobility. However, you are aware that a change in bowel habit and any bleeding could indicate bowel disease or cancer. This knowledge combined with the use of the Bristol Stool Chart and a history of the complaint will identify a normal bowel pattern and stool consistency.

It is not Mrs Grant who has constipation as you first thought, and it turns out that Mrs Grant would like some help and advice about her husband as she is his main carer. Mr Grant has multiple sclerosis and poor mobility, and he has had several recent falls. As a result he has stopped the osmotic laxative he had been taking for several months as his bowel movements are loose and he needs to rush to the toilet fairly frequently. He has been soiling underwear and sheets, which has been upsetting for them both, and now his normal bowel pattern has ceased. Mr Grant now feels very uncomfortable and nauseous. This analytical approach extracts any irrelevant information (in this case the patient with constipation is not Mrs Grant), does not focus on the specific context and uses guidelines to support clinical practice. While repeated specific experiences may convert analytical decisions into intuitive ones, a raised awareness of the context of situations, although helping us to make sense of the situation, can also provide a distraction from the reality and lead us to assumptions that are not accurate. Earlier work by Croskerry (2002) in relation to pattern recognition explains a situation whereby a patient presenting with particular visual aspects of a complaint and their appearance can trigger a bias in the decision making. Furthermore, any subsequent data gathered from the patient can be used to confirm the initial diagnosis, even when it is not accurate. For example, a patient presenting with a painful mouth with evidence of an ulcer and white plaques on their tongue who confirms that they have just completed a course of antibiotics may result in a bias towards oral thrush when the ulcer may actually be the beginnings of oral cancer. Although this article by Croskerry (2002) is aimed at medics and in particular those who work in emergency medicine, it can illustrate how a failed approach to decision making can occur, a fundamental message that community nurses need to be aware of.

CONCLUSION

So it would seem that in order to deliver effective care to patients in the community, assessment needs to be placed under scrutiny. Determining existing assessment strategies and underpinning theory that supports assessment in practice is a starting point. Holistic assessment in community nursing practice involves a person-centred partnership approach where information is gathered in relation to the individual's physical, psychological, social, environmental, spiritual and cultural well-being using recognised evidence-based frameworks. Family and carers are included in the assessment where appropriate, and, depending on the needs prioritised, the focus of the assessment can move along a spectrum from concentrating on a physical assessment utilising advanced clinical skills with one individual, to focusing on a broad family assessment. It is this flexible approach practiced by a body of community nurses that is a real strength. Undertaking robust evidence-based assessments that have clinical decision making embedded in the process, evidences accountability and the essential underpinning knowledge and skills in relation to delivering patient care using shared decision making. This continued approach will facilitate community nurses to deliver the high-quality care that most patients expect and deserve. By revisiting theories of assessment, including assessment tools and decision-making frameworks, current and future community nurses will be able to provide a clear rationale for their practice and take responsibility for implementing any improvements within their own clinical area.

REFERENCES

Aggleton P and Chalmers H (2000) *Nursing Models and Nursing Practice*, 2nd edn. London: Macmillan Press Limited.

Aggleton P and Homans H (1987) *Educating about AIDs*. Bristol: NHS Training Authority. Cited in Naidoo J and Wills J (2000) *Health Promotion: Foundations for Practice*, 2nd edn. Edinburgh: Harcourt Publishers.

Anderson KH (2000) The family health system approach to family systems nursing. *Journal of Family Nursing* 6:103–19.

Anderson KH and Tomlinson PS (1992) The Family Health System as an emerging paradigmatic view for nursing. Journal of Nursing Scholarship 24:57–63.

Beckwith S and Franklin P (2007) *Oxford Handbook of Nurse Prescribing*. Oxford: Oxford University Press.

Bickley LS and Szilagyi PG (2016) *Bate's Guide to Physical Examination and History Taking*, 12th edn. Philadelphia, PA: Lippincott Williams & Wilkins

Bradshaw J (1972) The concept of social need. *New Society* March:640–3.

Coles L and Porter E (2008) *Public Health Skills: A Practical Guide for Nurses and Public Health Practitioners*. Oxford: Blackwell Publishing.

Cornforth A (2013) Holistic Wound assessment in primary care. *British Journal of Community Nursing* 18:12- S28.

Croskerry P (2002) Achieving quality in clinical decision making; cognitive strategies and detection of bias. *Academic Emergency Medicine* 9:1184–204.

Croskerry P (2009) Context is everything or How could I have been that stupid? Healthcare Quarterly 12(special issue):171–7.

Dahlgren G and Whitehead M (1991) *Policies and Strategies to Promote Social Equity in Health*. Stockholm: Institute for Future Studies.

DH (2006) *Our Health, Our Care, Our Say: A New Direction for Community Services*. London: Department of Health.

DH (2007) *Management of Medicines—A Resource to Support Implementation of the Wider Aspects of Medicines Management for the National Service Frameworks for Diabetes, Renal Services and Long-Term Conditions*. London: Department of Health.

DH (2008) *A High Quality Workforce: NHS Next Stage Review.* London: Department of Health.

DH (2010) *Advanced Level Nursing: A Position Statement.* London: Department of Health.

Dossey BM and Guzzetta CE (2005) Holistic nursing practice. In Dossey BM, Keegan L and Guzzetta CE (eds) *Holistic Nursing: A Handbook for Practice*, 4th edn. Boston: Jones & Bartlett, pp. 5–40.

Ewles L and Simnett I (1999) *Promoting Health: A Practical Guide to Health Education*, 4th edn. Edinburgh: Harcourt Publishers, cited In Naidoo J and Wills J (2000) *Health Promotion Foundations for Practice* Edinburgh: Harcourt Publishers Limited.

Foot C, Gilburt H, Dunn P et al. (2014) *People in Control of their Own Health and Care: The State of Involvement.* London: King's Fund.

Fox C (2003) The holistic assessment of a patient with leg ulceration. *British Journal of Community Nursing Wound Care* March:26–30.

Freeman J (2005) Towards a definition of holism. *British Journal of General Practice* February:154–5.

Gough H (2008) Plugging the gaps and getting assessment right: A new holistic assessment framework for the community practitioner nurse prescriber. Care 2:24–40. www.gcu.ac.uk/care.

Harper C and Ajao A (2010) Pendleton's consultation model: Assessing a patient. British Journal of Community Nursing 15:38–43.

Hastings A (2006) Assessing and improving the consultation skills of nurses. Nurse Prescribing 4:418–22.

Haworth S and Dluhy N (2001) Holistic symptom management: Modelling the interactive phase. Journal of Advanced Nursing 36:302–10.

Irving K, Treacy M, Scott A et al. (2006) Discursive practices in the documentation of patient assessment. Journal of Advanced Nursing 51:151–9.

Kennedy CM (2004) A typology of knowledge for district nursing practice. Journal of Advanced Nursing 45:401–9.

Kenny, J.W. (2009) Theory based advanced nursing practice. In *Advanced Practice Nursing: Essential Knowledge for the Profession*. London: Jones & Bartlett, pp. 379–396.

King's Fund (2009) Patient Centred Care. (Accessed 12 November 2010) www.king's fund.org.uk/topics/patientcentred_care/#keypoints.

Maher D and Hemming L (2005) Understanding patient and family: Holistic assessment in palliative care. British Journal of Community Nursing 10:318–22.

McCormack B and McCance T (2010) *Person-centred Nursing: Theory and Practice.* Chichester: Wiley-Blackwell.

Muncey T (2002). In Muncey T and Parker A (eds) *Chronic Disease Management: A Practical Guide.* Basingstoke: Palgrave.

National Prescribing Centre (NPC) (1991) Signposts for prescribing nurses—General principles of good prescribing. *Nurse Prescribing Bulletin* 1:1–4.

NHS England and Local Government Association (2013) *Statement on the Health and Social Care Integration Transformation Fund.* Redditch: NHS England Publications.

Nursing and Midwifery Council (NMC) (2015) *The Code: Professional Standards of Practice and Behavior for Nurses and Midwives.* London: NMC.

Pearson H (2013) Science and intuition: Do both have a place in clinical decision making. *British Journal of Nursing* 22(4):212–5.

Roper N, Logan WW and Tierney A (1990) *The Elements of Nursing: A Model of Nursing Based on a Model of Living*, 3rd edn. Edinburgh: Churchill Livingstone.

Royal College of Nursing (2006) *Caring in Partnership: Older People and Nursing Staff Working Towards the Future*. London: ECN.

Royal College of Nursing (2014) *EHealth Technology in Practice: Nursing Content of eHealth Records*. London: RCN.

Rushworth H (2009) *Assessment Made Incredibly Easy*. Philadelphia, PA: Lippincott Williams, Wilkins.

Scottish Executive (2005) *Building a Health Service Fit for the Future: A National Framework for Service Change in the NHS in Scotland*. Edinburgh: Scottish Executive.

Scottish Government (2007) *Better Health, Better Care: Planning Tomorrow's Workforce Today*. Edinburgh: Scottish Government.

Scottish Government (2015) *Health and Social Care Integration Narrative*. Edinburgh: Scottish Government

Scottish Parliament (2013) *The Public Bodies (Joint Working) (Scotland Bill)*. Edinburgh: The Scottish Parliament.

The Health Foundation (2014) *Ideas into Action: Person Centred Care in Practice*. London: The Health Foundation.

UK Parliament (2013) *Select Committee on Public Service and Demographic Change Ready for Ageing Report?* London: The Stationary Office.

Whetsell MV, Gonzalez YM and Moreno-Ferguson ME (2011) Models and theories: Focused on a systems approach. In *Philosophies and Theories for Advanced Nursing Practice*. London: Jones & Bartlett Learning International, pp. 413–79.

Wilson SF and Giddens JF (2012) *Health Assessment for Nursing Practice*, 5th edn. St Louis, MO: Elsevier.

Worth A (2001) Assessment of the needs of older people by district nurses and social workers: A changing culture. Journal of Interprofessional Care 15:257–66.

Wright LM and Leahey M (2013) *Nurses and Families: A Guide to Family Assessment and Intervention*, 6th edn. Philadelphia, PA: FA Davis Company.

Young K and Duggan L (2010) Consulting with patients: The structure of history taking. *Journal of Community Nursing* 24:30–2.

Young K, Duggan L and Franklin P (2009) Effective consulting and history-taking skills for prescribing practice. *Journal of Nursing* 18:1056–61.

The role of the community nurse in mental health

INTRODUCTION

Community nurses are involved with a range of care provision including support and care for patients who are unwell, including those with end-of-life care needs, as well as supporting independence and self-care (Department of Health Public Health Nursing, 2013). This remit includes increasing the quality of life of people living with long-term conditions. In order to improve the quality of life for people living with a long-term condition, and their families, it is important that the district nurse is able to work collaboratively with other healthcare professionals and across health and social care (Queen's Nursing Institute & Queen's Nursing Institute Scotland, 2015). In 2008, the Department of Health reported that the number of people with a long-term condition would increase by 23% by 2033 (Department of Health, 2008b). Taking into consideration the increase in the number of people, this chapter examines the relationship between long-term conditions and mental health and examines the role of the community nurse.

The World Health Organization (WHO) states that

> Mental health can be conceptualised as a state of well-being in which the individual realizes his or her own abilities, can cope with the normal stresses of life, can work productively and fruitfully, and is able to make a contribution to his or her community.

(World Health Organization, 2007: 1)

Keyes (2002) identified six feelings that foster psychological well-being, see Box 8.1. It is perhaps unsurprising that living with one or more long-term conditions, which may impact upon independence and quality of life, can be linked to mental health challenges.

> **Box 8.1 Feelings that foster psychological well-being**
>
> • Self-acceptance
> • Positive relations with others
> • Autonomy (or ability to think for yourself)
> • Environmental mastery (the sense that you can change your circumstances for the better)
> • Life purpose (having goals and feeling helpful)
> • Personal growth (being able to learn from the stresses and challenges of life)
>
> *(Keyes, 2002)*

The evidence regarding the relationship between long-term conditions and mental health identifies that affective disorders such as depression and anxiety are more prevalent (Naylor et al., 2012). Furthermore, while depression and anxiety are experienced by people living with a long-term condition it is important to acknowledge that for some long-term conditions such as diabetes and cardiovascular disease there is also an increased risk of cognitive impairment including Alzheimer's and vascular dementia (Velayudhan et al., 2010).

The relationship between physical and mental health

An understanding of the link between physical and mental health is important for community nurses. Mental health problems are two to three more times likely to be experienced by people living with a long-term condition compared with the general population. Co-morbid mental health problems have a number of serious implications for people with long-term conditions, including poorer clinical outcomes, lower quality of life and reduced ability to manage physical symptoms effectively resulting in unhelpful health behaviours and poorer self-care (Naylor et al., 2012). There is a correlation between co-morbid mental health problems and the motivation and ability to manage self-care for people living with a long-term condition.

The mechanisms underlying the relationship between mental and physical health are complex, and evidence suggests that a combination of biological, psychosocial, environmental and behavioural factors may all be involved (Prince et al., 2007). The community nurse often providing care in the home setting is well placed to assess these aspects of patient-centred care in practice. Evidence suggests that quality of life, dietary control, relationships with healthcare professionals and carers alongside overall prognosis can be improved by consideration of the psychological needs of people with diabetes (NHS Diabetes and Diabetes UK, 2010). Mental health problems are experienced in a range of long-term conditions, see Table 8.1.

Anxiety and depression, in conjunction with reduced social skills and an impact upon concentration, are also components of a range of psychological distress experienced by people with a diagnosis of cancer (Macmillan Cancer Support, 2011). It is likely that anxiety and depression may also affect the families of people living with long-term conditions and cancer. While people with a long-term condition experience mental health problems, it is important to recognise that people with mental health problems have an increased risk of physical health problems. Consequently

Table 8.1 Research evidence on the prevalence of co-morbid mental health problems

Cardiovascular disease (CVD)	• Depression is two to three times more common in a range of CVD including stroke, angina, congestive cardiac failure and following a heart attack • Prevalence estimates vary between 20% and 50% • Anxiety problems also common in CVD
Diabetes	• Two to three times more likely to have depression than the general population • Also an independent association with anxiety
Chronic obstructive pulmonary disease	• Mental health problems three times more likely than the general population • Anxiety disorders particularly common, for example, panic disorder is 10 times more prevalent
Chronic musculo-skeletal disorders	• Up to 33% of women and more than 20% of men with arthritis may have a co-morbid depression • More than one in five people over the age of 55 with chronic arthritis of the knee have been reported to have a co-morbid depression

Source: Naylor C, Parsonage M, McDaid D et al., (2012) *Long-term Conditions and Mental Health The Cost of Co-morbidities.* London: King's Fund Centre for Mental Health (p. 4).

premature death from natural causes such as cardiovascular disease is two to four times more likely for people with mental health problems (Eaton et al., 2008).

ACTIVITY 8.1

Take some time to reflect on two people whom you have worked with who have a long-term condition. In relation to each of the people you identify answer the following three questions:

1. Could they have been depressed or anxious?

2. How did you consider the impact of their long-term condition on their psychological well-being?

3. Did they raise the issue of their mental health with you?

Mental health assessment and the role of the community nurse

Having explored the relationship between physical and mental health, it is important to examine mental health assessment tools and consider how they can be used by community nurses. The Voluntary Standards for District Nurse Education and Practice identify the promotion of

> mental health and well-being of people and carers in conjunction with mental health professionals and GPs, identifying needs and mental capacity, using recognised assessment and referral pathways and best interest decision making and providing appropriate emotional support.
>
> *(Queen's Nursing Institute & Queen's Nursing Institute Scotland, 2015: 3)*

Primary care can play a key role in supporting people with mental health problems and is the main source of formal support for mental health problems with only 10% of individuals with a mental health problem being referred to specialist mental health services (Naylor et al., 2012). Primary care provision with support from specialist mental healthcare professionals if appropriate can support people's needs more appropriately. However, in a King's Fund report, looking at long-term conditions and mental health, a separation between physical and mental health in the delivery of healthcare provision was evident in the organisation of services, professional education and funding (Naylor et al., 2012). Consequently, the detection of co-morbid mental health problems is not done well, evidence suggests that in the majority of cases of people with a long-term condition who also have depression, the depression is not identified (Cepoiu et al., 2008). It is important to consider mental and physical health together as they are inextricably linked.

Coventry et al. (2011) undertook qualitative research to identify and explore the barriers to the management of depression in people with long-term conditions. They interviewed 19 healthcare professionals, mainly from a primary care background, and seven pairs of service users and carers. Their work identified that depression was considered to be a normal response to the long-term condition and as such was normal. Furthermore, there was a suggestion that using structured assessments, for example, those driven by quality framework requirements, could result in some aspects of case management being overlooked. The healthcare professionals interviewed suggested that patients rarely used the term *depression* to describe their low mood. This was supported by some service users who reported that they did not always tell their general practitioner (GP) (Coventry et al., 2011). The lack of sharing with the GP regarding low mood may be related to evidence that stigma has small to moderate impact on people seeking help for mental health problems; this is more prevalent among military and health professionals as well as ethnic minorities, young people and men (Clement et al., 2015). A study looking at the involvement of district nurses' contact with and involvement in mental health identified that 45% of nursing staff had been asked about depression and antidepressant treatments by patients occasionally, with only 15% being asked more frequently (Haddad et al., 2005). This, alongside the impact of stigma with regards to mental health, would suggest that community nurses need to raise the issue of mental health with patients by asking direct questions using familiar language rather than the language of healthcare professionals. More recently, a qualitative study in Sweden identified that the district nurses interviewed ($n = 25$) felt that mental health promotion and the management of mental health challenges was important. However the study identified that in practice the district nurses did not include mental health promotion within care plans and that collaboration with other services was key (Grundberg et al., 2016).

The guidelines for depression in adults with a chronic physical health problem (NICE, 2009) use the *Diagnostic and Statistical Manual of Mental Disorders*, 4th edition (*DSM-IV*) diagnostic system, see Table 8.2, as the majority of the evidence reviewed had utilised this diagnostic system. Diagnosis of depression requires consideration of three areas: severity, duration and course. In practice some of the symptoms of a long-term condition and depression, such as fatigue, can be present in both illnesses. For community nurses working in partnership with people with long-term conditions, consideration of the individual as a whole person, including their social and psychological circumstances and history will strengthen the ability to appropriately diagnose depression. Recognition of depression and an understanding of the diagnostic system enables the community nurses to address the situation and if necessary refer on to the general practitioner or mental health services.

Table 8.2 Depression definitions

Subthreshold depressive symptoms	Fewer than five symptoms of depression
Mild depression	Few, if any, symptoms in excess of five required to make the diagnosis, and symptoms result in only minor functional impairment
Moderate depression	Symptoms or functional impairment are between 'mild' and 'severe'
Severe depression	Most symptoms, and the symptoms markedly interfere with functioning; can occur with or without psychotic symptoms

Source: Taken from the *Diagnostic and Statistical Manual of Mental Disorders, 4th edition, DSM-IV.* For more information see National Institute for Health and Care Excellence (2009) *Depression in Adults with a Chronic Physical Health Problem NICE CG91.* Manchester: NICE (p. 11).

Community nurses can utilise two focused questions, set out in the National Institute for Health and Care Excellence (NICE) guidelines (NICE, 2009) when they suspect that the individual with whom they are working may have depression:

1 During the last month, have you been bothered by feeling down, depressed or hopeless?

2 During the last month, have you been bothered by having little interest in doing things?

One of the challenges of identifying and managing depression in people living with a long-term conditions is the complexity of symptoms that could be related to the long-term condition or depression. For example, sleep disturbances, weight gain and loss, fatigue and reduced appetite while symptoms of depression could also be indicative of poor management of diabetes (Egede and Ellis, 2010). The signs and symptoms of depression can be found in Box 8.2.

Box 8.2 Signs and symptoms of depression (adapted from Gurney, 2013)

Key symptoms

- Sadness or constantly low in mood
- Considerably reduced pleasure in activities or hobbies normally enjoyed
- Other common symptoms
- Ability to think, concentrate, remember or make decisions is impaired, with even simple tasks seeming to be difficult
- Fluctuations in appetite with under- or overeating
- Altered sleep patterns
- Behaviour that is distressed or slowed down
- Lethargy, weariness and reduced energy, aches or pains, headaches, cramps or digestive problems that do not ease with treatment
- Feelings of worthlessness, hopelessness, helplessness or disproportionate or inappropriate guilt
- Thoughts of death or suicide (with or without a specific plan) or a suicide attempt

The community nurse may not have specialist mental health skills and knowledge but is likely to know the individual circumstances of the person and their family and is well placed to undertake an initial assessment and identify the level of need. An understanding of the NICE guidelines and the *DSM-IV* definitions for depression will enable the community nurse to identify co-morbid depression and gain access for the person living with a long-term condition to specialist mental health services as appropriate (NICE, 2009).

ACTIVITY 8.2

Having examined the *DSM-IV* definitions of depression and the helpful list of signs and symptoms and recommended action take some time to review the assessment and care of the two people you identified in Activity 8.1. How could the NICE (2009) guidelines support assessment and decision making in each case?

While depression is often experienced by people living with a long-term condition it is also likely that community nurses will be involved in working with individuals who have dementia. The National Dementia Strategy for England and Northern Ireland (Department of Health, 2008a) identifies that assessment and diagnosis are the 'gateway to care'. The importance of assessment is also identified on the Scottish Dementia Strategy which identifies the development of person-centred assessment and care as one of the 10 key actions (Scottish Government, 2013). Early identification of dementia can be challenging as the symptoms overlap with those of depression and delirium (McCrae, 2013). The use of a recognised assessment tool can enable the community nurse to identify where there may be changes in cognition in order to refer on to the general practitioner for further investigation. A toolkit produced to help clinicians assess cognition provides a choice of cognitive tests (Alzheimer's Society, 2015). The toolkit recommends three cognitive assessment tests for use in primary care, each of which can also be used in care homes with an additional cognitive assessment test for care homes. The assessment tests are recommend when a person's daily life has been affected as a result of forgetfulness. One of the recommended tests, for both primary care and care homes is the Abbreviated Mental Test Score (AMTS) which is composed of 10 questions and can be completed in approximately 5 minutes.

ACTIVITY 8.3

Access the Helping You to Assess Cognition toolkit (www.alzheimers.org.uk/site/scripts/download_info.php?downloadID=1045 accessed 29.10.2015) and review the cognitive assessment tools for primary care and care homes.

Consider how the use of recognised cognitive assessment tools could enable the community nurse team to facilitate appropriate and timely referral to specialist services.

When working with individuals who have dementia and their families it is important to ensure that the care is person centred. Nolan et al., (2004) identified the need to consider both the person with dementia and their carer with services supporting key relationships and valuing the contribution of all. Nolan et al., (2004) developed the Six Senses Framework as a guide for maintaining effective relationships. The Six Senses Framework, see Figure 8.1, provides a focus on the importance of the individuals and their families, retaining the focus on relationships and respect. Each of the six aspects of the framework are considered for older people, family carers and staff. For example, with regard to a sense of belonging older people need to be able to maintain and form relationships and be part of the community, for family carers it is important that they can maintain relationships and are able to feel that they are not alone in the caring role. For staff, Nolan et al., (2004) identify the importance of being part of a team where their contribution and value are recognised.

When there is concern about an individual's ability to make decisions about their own treatment and healthcare, perhaps as a result of Alzheimer's or dementia, community nurses must consider if the individual has the capacity for decision making. The Mental Capacity Act 2005 sets out a number of principles to ensure that the interests of individuals remain the focus of decision making (Callaghan et al., 2009). These principles include the assumption that an individual has capacity until proved otherwise, all practicable steps must be taken to support the individual with decision making before lack of capacity is considered and any decision taken on behalf of someone who lacks capacity must be in that person's best interests. The Mental Capacity Act (MCA, 2005) sets out a framework for assessing decision-making capacity, see Figure 8.2.

Having asked about mental health, community nurses need to engage in the management of mental health difficulties, for example, depression and anxiety. It is important that the management of depression and other mental health difficulties is undertaken by the appropriately skilled healthcare professionals. The National

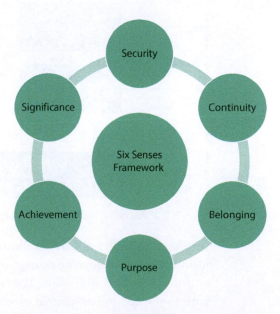

Figure 8.1 The Six Senses Framework. (Nolan et al., 2004.)

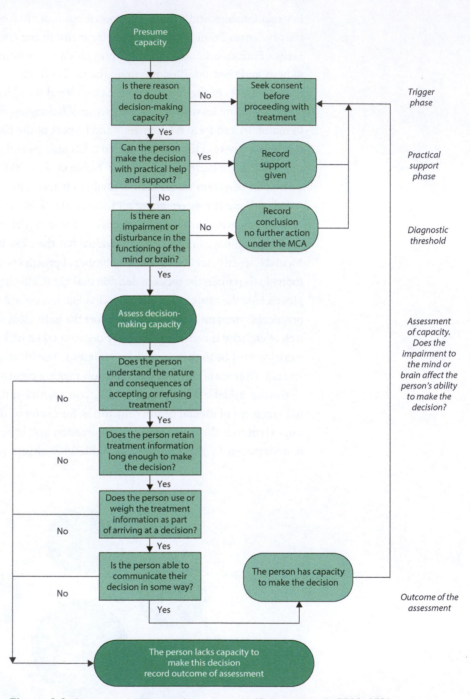

Figure 8.2 Assessing decision-making capacity. (Callaghan et al., 2009: 159.)

Institute for Health and Care Excellence (2009) provide a helpful framework for the identification of appropriate management, see Table 8.3.

If the individual with whom the community nurse is working in partnership with to provide patient-centred care requires general advice and monitoring or more active treatment in primary care there are a number of possible treatment options available.

Table 8.3 Appropriate management of depression

1	Factors that favour general advice and active monitoring	• Four or fewer symptoms of depression • Symptoms intermittent, or less than 2 weeks in duration • Recent onset with identified stressor • No past or family history of depression • Social support available • Lack of suicidal thoughts
2	Factors that favour more active treatment in primary care	• Five or more symptoms with associated disability • Persistent or long-standing symptoms • Personal or family history of depression • Low social support • Occasional suicidal thoughts
3	Factors that favour referral to mental health professionals	• Inadequate or incomplete response to two or more interventions • Recurrent episode within 1 year of last one • History suggestive of bipolar disorder • Patient with depression or relatives request referral • More persistent suicidal thoughts • Self-neglect
4	Factors that favour urgent referral to specialist mental health services	• Active suicidal ideas or plans • Psychotic symptoms • Severe agitation accompanying severe symptoms • Severe self-neglect

Source: National Institute for Health and Care Excellence (2009) *Depression in Adults with a Chronic Physical Health Problem NICE CG91.* Manchester: NICE (pp. 51–52).

Mental health interventions

Pharmacological treatment for depression in people with one or more long-term conditions is not necessarily the treatment of choice. For example, people with chronic obstructive pulmonary disease can benefit from education which increases their ability to exercise choice and self-manage their care, furthermore cognitive behavioural therapy and counselling are treatment options that can be used in conjunction with education (Heslop, 2014). The use of cognitive behavioural therapy (CBT) can be effective both in the management of some long-term conditions, for example, diabetes, and the treatment of depression (Egede and Ellis, 2010). A recent systematic review identified that people with co-morbid mental health problems benefit greatly from inclusion in self-management programmes for chronic disease (Harrison et al., 2011). The range of options and an indication of where they are appropriate are provided in the stepped-care model, see Table 8.4.

Referral to specialist mental health services is important for patients who have an inadequate response to treatment or severe and complex depression as identified in Steps 3 and 4. There are a number of options for people with known or suspected depression and mild to moderate depression at Steps 1 and 2. The principles of these varied psychological approaches can be used by community nurses working. Motivational interviewing which is also referred to in Chapters 2 and 13 is one approach to working with patients who wish to do something indifferent to improve their health (Ryrie, 2013a).

Table 8.4 The stepped-care model

Focus of the intervention	Nature of the intervention
Step 4: Severe and complex depression[a]; risk to life, severe self-neglect	Medication, high-intensity psychological interventions, electroconvulsive therapy, crisis service, combined treatments, multiprofessional and inpatient care
Step 3: Persistent subthreshold depressive symptoms or mild to moderate depression with inadequate response to initial interventions; moderate to severe depression	Medication, high-intensity psychological interventions, combined treatments, collaborative care[b] and referral for further assessment and interventions
Step 2: Persistent subthreshold depressive symptoms; mild to moderate depression	Low-intensity psychosocial interventions, psychological interventions, medication and referral for further assessment and interventions
Step 1: All known and suspected presentations of depression	Assessment, support, psychoeducation, active monitoring and referral for further assessment and interventions

Source: National Institute for Health and Care Excellence (2009) *Depression in Adults with a Chronic Physical Health Problem NICE CG91*. Manchester: NICE (p. 16).
[a] Complex depression includes depression that shows an inadequate response to multiple treatments, is complicated by psychotic symptoms and/or is associated with significant psychiatric co-morbidity or psychosocial factors.
[b] Only for depression where the person also has a chronic physical health problem and associated functional impairment.

Central to motivational interviewing is the philosophy that underpins the approach of healthcare practitioners as they engage in discussion with patients that is collaborative, evocative and honours patient autonomy (Rollnick et al., 2008). Change regarding health can only be actioned by the patient; taking this into consideration, it is important that the partnership working between the community nurse and patient is collaborative and decisions are made jointly. When utilising motivational interviewing skills the community nurse should draw out, evoke, the patient's reasons for change, thus identifying the motivators for making a change. Mindful of the fact that only the patient can make a change, it is important that the community nurse respects patient autonomy (Ryrie, 2013a). This philosophy of motivational interviewing is reflected in the principles which have been arranged into the acronym RULE: resist the righting reflex, understand the motivations of the patient, listen to patients and empower patients (Rollnick et al., 2008).

The core skills required for motivational interviewing – asking, listening and informing – are within the repertoire of expert communication skills utilised by community nurses. Open questions can be used to ask about the challenge and gain a shared understanding of the situation to identify the motivation for change. This could be explored further by asking what is good and what is not so good about the situation. If there is to be a shared understanding it is important that the community is actively engaged in reflective listening (Miller and Rollnick, 2002). By effectively listening it may be possible to identify how the patient is talking about change. Rollnick et al., (2008) identify six types of change talk, see Table 8.5. Alongside

Table 8.5 Types of change talk

Type	Statements about
Desire	Inclination for change; for example, I want, wish, like to
Ability	About capability; for example, I could, can, might be able to
Reasons	Explicit reasons for change; for example, I would probably feel better if
Need	Obliged to change, for example, I must, should
Commitment	Probability of change, for example, I am going to, I will
Taking steps	Action taken; for example, I tried.., I have…

Source: Ryrie (2013a: 362).

asking open questions and listening reflectively, the third core skill of motivational interviewing is informing; this may require permission before sharing information about the situation the patient finds himself or herself in, this needs to be balanced with asking and listening, if too much information is conveyed the patient may become resistant to the discussion (Ryrie, 2013a).

Motivational interviewing can also be used effectively to help people with a long-term condition self-care. In a recently reported study across 16 primary care centres it was found that motivational interviewing provides a patient-centred approach that improved older people's medication adherence (Moral et al., 2015).

Solution-focused therapy is a form of brief therapy that considers the present time for the individual and focuses on specific goals that can be reached (Ryrie, 2013b). This works by enabling people to identify how they want to be different and the strengths the individual has that can be utilised to achieve the goal. While community nurses are unlikely to be trained solution-focused therapists, the approach taken in solution-focused therapy of considering people as being unable to manage their problems rather than being unwell can be used to empower people living with a long-term condition (Webster, 2009). The types of questions that can lead to considering solutions rather than focusing on the problem are set out in Table 8.6.

The use of questions to support people to change enables patients to identify when they have been able to overcome the problem and to utilise the resources, both social and personal, that are linked to the exceptions when they overcame the

Table 8.6 Solution versus problem discourse

Solution discourse	Problem discourse
What would you like to change?	How can I help you?
Can we discover exceptions to the problem?	Can you tell me more about the problem?
What will the future look like without the problem?	How has this problem arisen in light of your past?

Source: Ryrie I (2013b) In Norman I and Ryrie I (eds) *The Art and Science of Mental Health Nursing Principles and Practice*, 3rd edn. Maidenhead: Open University Press, p. 349.

problem. This enables the person to imagine a future without the problem and identify the small steps required to change the situation (Ryrie, 2013b). This is described as a forward-looking process that empowers people without becoming trapped within the problem (De Shazer, 1985). While this section of the chapter has explored two possible approaches that can be used to work in partnership with patients and carers, it is important to acknowledge that the community nurse may at times need to refer to and work collaboratively with specialist mental health services. This would include occasions when the patient has not responded to treatment for mild to moderate depression or has severe and complex depression, see Table 8.4.

Collaborative working

The Transforming Community Services programme has resulted in a number of mental health providers taking responsibilities in some areas for community services for people with physical health problems. This in turn provides an opportunity for further developing integrated working between community nurses involved in working with individuals with long-term conditions and mental health staff. In order to deliver effective care for people with long-term conditions, effective multi-disciplinary team working is key. Working in partnership with patients to provide patient-centred care requires the expertise and competence of a range of healthcare professionals, for example, chronic obstructive pulmonary disease requires the identification and management of depression and anxiety, alongside advice regarding relaxation techniques (NICE, 2010). Collaborative case management focusing on controlling risk factors by a nurse has also been found to improve control of the long-term condition and depression outcomes in patients with diabetes and CVD (Katon et al., 2008).

ACTIVITY 8.4

Take some time to review depression in adults with a chronic physical health problem NICE CG91. You may find it helpful to discuss the role of the community nurse at a team meeting.

• How does the team view their role in terms of depression in long-term condition care?

• Is there collaboration with the wider healthcare team, especially the GP?

• What processes support effective working between the primary healthcare team, mental health professionals and other statutory and nonstatutory agencies?

Integrating physical and mental healthcare is more effective than adding mental healthcare and can result in a reduction of service use with the concomitant improved physical health. Collaborative care is one way in which people with a long-term condition and depression can benefit from equal consideration of physical and mental health challenges. Collaborative care requires a multi-professional approach to patient care with the use of structured patient management plans. This is further supported by scheduled follow-up and effective interprofessional communication (Gunn et al., 2006). Inevitably an understanding of the signs and symptoms, assessment tools and guidelines for mental health challenges experienced by people living with a long-term condition will enhance interprofessional communication and access to specialist mental health service. A qualitative evaluation of collaborative care for people with long-term conditions and depression found that case managers, practice nurses and GPs identified improved co-ordination of physical and mental healthcare. This resulted in increased confidence in managing the care for individuals with complex physical and mental health needs. Patients reported that the collaborative approach enabled them to access mental healthcare that they had previously been unable to access as physical health needs had been prioritised (Knowles et al., 2015).

Reflection point

Scenario

Emily Hobbs is 68 years old and was referred to the district nursing team by her GP following a home visit. Emily had developed a sacral pressure ulcer. The team have been for visiting for 4 weeks to dress the Grade 3 pressure ulcer and have referred Emily for an assessment by the occupational therapist. The initial assessment identified that Emily has been finding it more and more difficult to manage as a result of an exacerbation in her chronic obstructive pulmonary disease (COPD). Over the 4 weeks, it has been noted that Emily is increasingly reluctant to make eye contact and is withdrawn when any of the nurses visit. When asked she is not sleeping well and it would appear that she may have lost some weight.

Reflection

Take some time to consider what aspects the community nurse should consider and what steps could be taken for Emily.

There are several factors that you may have identified when considering Emily and her care. It may be that prior to the exacerbation of her COPD she was able to get out and manage fairly independently. The deterioration of her COPD and the consequent reduced mobility may have resulted in a reduction in autonomy, and feeling of helplessness. These are two of the factors that Keyes (2002) identified as fostering psychological well-being. Reluctance to make eye contact, being withdrawn, not sleeping well and weight loss are four of the signs and symptoms of depression (Gurney, 2013). The community nurse should ask Emily the focused questions identified by NICE (2009), for example, during the last month, have you been bothered by feeling down, depressed or hopeless?

It is important that depression is considered and action taken when Emily is exhibiting subthreshold depressive symptoms to prevent further deterioration. The NICE (2009) stepped-care model identifies that the community nurse should undertake an assessment, active monitoring and consider referral for further assessment and interventions. For Emily solution-focused therapy could be a useful tool to support Emily to adapt her lifestyle in response to her COPD.

CONCLUSION

It is evident that there is a strong relationship between physical and mental health. In order to deliver effective quality care to people in their own homes and their care, community nurses need an awareness of mental health challenges in order to sign-post services and on occasion facilitate referral and access to mental health services. This chapter has provided an overview of the role of the community nurse in mental health assessment and examined some mental health skills that can be used in practice by community nurses. By developing an awareness of these issues community nurses are better able to engage in effective interprofessional working, collaborative care and referral to specialist services to meet the complex needs of people with complex physical and mental health needs.

REFERENCES

Alzheimer's Society (2015) *Helping You to Assess Cognition; A Practical Toolkit for Clinicans.* London: Alzheimer's Society.

Callaghan P, Playle J and Cooper L (2009) *Mental Health Nursing Skills.* Oxford: Oxford University Press.

Cepoiu M, McCusker J, Cole M et al. (2008) Recognition of depression by non-psychiatrict physicians – A systematic literature review and meta-analysis. *Journal of General Internal Medicine* 23:25–36.

Clement S, Schauman O, Graham T et al. (2015) What is the impact if mental health-related stigma on help-seeking? A systematic review of quantitative and qualitative studies. *Psychological Medicine* 45:11–27

Coventry P, Hays R, Dickens C et al. (2011) Talking about depression: Barriers to managing depression in people with long term conditions in primary care. *BMC Family Practice* 12:10.

De Shazer S (1985) *Keys to Solutions in Brief Therapy.* New York, NY: WW Norton.

Department of Health (2008a) *Living Well with Dementia: A National Strategy.* London: Department of Health.

Department of Health (2008b) *Ten Things You Need to Know About Long-term Conditions.* London: Department of Health.

Department of Health Public Health Nursing (2013) *Care in Local Communities–District Nurse Vision and Model.* Leeds: Department of Health.

Eaton WM, Martins SS, Nestadt G, Bienvenu O, et al. (2008) The burden of mental disorders. *Epidemiologic Reviews* 30:1–14.

Egede L and Ellis C (2010): Diabetes and depression: Global perspectives *Diabetes Research and Clinical Practice* 87:302–12.

Gunn J, Diggens J, Hegarty K and Blashki G (2006) A systematic review if comploex system interventions designed to increase recovery from depression in primary care. *BMC Helth Services Research* 6: 88.

Gurney S (2013) The person who experiences depression. In Norman I and Ryrie I (eds) *The Art and Science of Mental Health Nursing Principles and Practice*, 3rd edn. Maidenhead: Open University Press, pp. 541–54.

Grundberg A, Hansson A, Hilleras P and Religa D (2016) District nurses' perspectives on detecting mental health problems and promoting mental health among community-dwelling seniors with multi-morbidity. *Journal of Clinical Nursing*. doi:10.1111/jocn.13302.

Haddad M, Plummer S, Taverner A et al. (2005) District nurses' involvement and attitudes to mental health problems: A three-area cross-sectional study. *Journal of Clinical Nursing* 14:976-85.

Harrison M, Reeves D, Harkness E et al. (2011) A secondary analysis of teh moderating effects of depression and mulitmorbidity on the effectiveness of a chronic disease self-management programme. *Patient Education and Counselling* 87(1):67–73.

Heslop K (2014) Non-pharmacological treatement of anxiety and depression in COPD. *Nurse Prescribing* 12:43–7.

Katon W, Russon J, Von Korff M et al. (2008) Long-term effects on medical cosots of impriving depression outcomes in patients with depresion and diabetes. *Diabetes Care* 31:1155–9.

Keyes C (2002) The mental health continuum: From languishing to flourishing in life. *Journal of Health and Social Research* 43:207-22.

Knowles S, Chew-Graham C, Adeyemi I et al. (2015) Managing depression in people with mulitmorbidity: A qualitative evaluation of an intergrated collaborative care model. *BMC Family Practice* 16:32.

Macmillan Cancer Support (2011) *Psycholgical and Emotional Support Provided by Macmillan Professionals: An Evidence Review.* London: Macmillan Cancer Support.

McCrae N (2013) Older people with demenita. In Norman I and Ryrie I (eds.) *The Art and Science of Mental Health Nursing Principles and Practice.* Maidenhead: Open University Press, pp. 503–20.

Miller W and Rollnick S (2002) *Motivational Interviewing: Preparing Pweople to Change Addictive Behaviuor,* 2nd edn. New York, NY: Guilford Press.

Moral R, de Toorres L, Oretga L et al. (2015) Effectiveness of motivational interviewing to improve therpeutuc adeherence in patients over 65 years old with chronic diseases: A cluster randomized clinical trial in primary care. *Patient Education and Counselling* 98: 977–83.

National Insitutue for Health and Care Excellence (2010) *Chronic Obstructive Pulmonary Disease: Management of Chronic Obstructive Pulmonary Disease in Adults in Primary and Secondary Care. NICE CG101.* London: NICE.

National Institute for Health and Care Excellence (2009) *Depression in Adults with a Chronic Physical Health Problem NICE CG91.* Manchester: NICE.

Naylor C, Parsonage M, McDaid D et al. (2012) *Long-Term Conditions and Mental Health The Cost of Co-morbidities.* London: King's Fund Centre for Mental Health.

NHS Diabetes and Diabetes UK (2010) *Emotional and Psychological Care and Treatement in Diabetes.* London, UK: Diabetes.

Nolan M, Davies S, Brown J et al. (2004) Beyond 'person-centred'care: A new vision for gerontological nursing. *Journal of Clinical Nursing* 13:45–53.

Prince M, Patel V, Saxena S et al. (2007) No health without mental health. *Lancet* 370:859–77.

Queen's Nursing Institute & Scotland QsNI (2015) *The QNI/QNIS Voluntary Standards for District Nurse Education and Practice.* London: QNI/QNIS.

Rollnick S, Miller W and Butler C (2008) *Motivational Interviewing in Health Care*. New York: Guilford Press.

Ryrie I (2013a) Motivational Interviewing. In Norman I and Ryrie I (eds) *The Art and Science of Mental Health Nursing Principles and Practice*, 3rd edn. Maidenhead: Open University Press, pp. 356–66.

Ryrie I (2013b) Solution-focused approaches. In Norman I and Ryrie I (eds) *The Art and Science of Mental Health Nursing Principles and Practice*, 3rd edn. Maidenhead: Open University Press, pp. 347–55.

Scottish Government (2013) *Scotland's National Demntia Strategy 2013–2016*. Edinburgh: Scottish Government.

Velayudhan L, Poppe M, Archer N et al. (2010). Risk of developing dementia in people with diabetes and mild cognitive impairment. *British Journal of Psychiatry* 196(1):36–40.

Webster D (2009) Using Solution-focused approaches. In Barker P (ed.) *Psychaitric and Mental Health Nursing: The Craft of Caring*, 2nd edn. London: Edward Arnold.

World Health Organization (2007) Mental Health: Strengthening mental health promotion FactSheet Number 220, September 2007 (WHO ed.).

Carers: The keystone of communities and families

Sally Sprung and Fiona Baguley

LEARNING OUTCOMES

• Gain an understanding of carer identity – who is a carer?
• Critically explore the impact of caring on young carers and adult carers.
• Reflect on the financial and practical support needs of carers.
• Recognise areas of community nursing support for carers.

INTRODUCTION

Carers are now acknowledged as an essential component of community care (McNamara and Rosenwax, 2010), but there still exists some confusion around who we are referring to when we talk about carers. In this chapter, the definition of 'carer' in the United Kingdom will be examined along with the role and contribution carers make to society.

The exhaustive nature of the caring role will be highlighted along with the financial and practical impact that the caring role has upon young and adult carers. The role community nurses have in the identification, assessment and support of carers will also be made clear.

It has been predicted that by 2021, the number of people aged over 75 years in the United Kingdom will have increased by 75% and the percentage of young people will have fallen by 20%. People will be living longer and also living with long-term conditions for a significant part of their lives (DH, 2008). The need for carers is projected to increase and the situation now is not unusual where two older people live together, one caring for the other, but neither with good health.

It is in response to these changes that the UK government wish to increase the relationship between primary healthcare, social services, charities and the acute sector. There will be a continuing emphasis on the development of new models of care in the community with a greater provider role for primary care, health promotion and sustaining people at home (Department of Health, 2014a).

Each country in the United Kingdom has produced its own carer strategies and policies (see Further Reading). However, the aims and requirements of all UK countries are broadly the same, as are the needs of carers. Whether a carer fulfils the criteria to receive benefits or not, the focus for community nursing teams is to improve the effective identification of carers, increase the uptake and quality of carer assessment and provide information and advice. Carers' health, well-being and support can be enhanced by assisting them to contact voluntary agencies, promoting short breaks (previously called respite) and providing education with skills such as moving and handling. Health and social care professionals working closer together with other appropriate local services can provide and participate in partnership training. General practitioners (GPs) are being encouraged to advocate regular health checks for carers between the ages of 40 and 65 years. This provides the opportunity for the community nurse to assess how the carer is coping with the caring role. The ability of the carer to cope and continue to provide care impacts on the district nurses' role in terms of time and team capacity.

Carers' recognition and the rights of carers have increased greatly across Europe in the last 10 years, and the UK Care Act (Department of Health, 2014a) gives local authorities a responsibility to assess a carer's need for support, where the carer appears to have such need. In Scotland the Carer's Strategy (Scottish Government, 2010) calls for early intervention and a preventative approach to prevent crises. The government in England recognises the valuable contribution of carers who support the independence of other people, and they seek to empower this hidden group by supporting key national organisations such as Carers UK and Carers Trust (DH, 2010a). However, contemporary government papers emphasise the use of integrated care with strategic needs assessment and a strong personalisation agenda based on emerging evidence of effective early intervention in identifying, involving and supporting carers (DH, 2010b, 2012, 2013a,b, 2014b).

The carer's assessment is carried out by Social Services, or a Single Shared Assessment by Social Services and the National Health Service together (Department of Health, 2014a; Scottish Government, 2014). These tools are used to assess the carer's experience, his or her ability or willingness to cope and the carer's quality of life.

ACTIVITY 9.1

Reflection point
There are many reasons why adult and young carers have remained hidden and often unsupported when taking on levels of care that they have not been trained to provide even though national UK health policy advocates and emphasises carer support in care throughout a patient's illness and death (Laing and Sprung, 2014).
• What do you think the reasons are?

WHO IS A CARER?

In the United Kingdom a carer is someone who provides a substantial amount of unpaid care, on a regular basis, to an adult or child who may not be able to manage daily activities because of frailty, illness or disability (Carer UK, 2014a). A carer can be an adult or a child. Others who provide care, for example, care workers who work for local authority or a private agency that provides personal care, are often also referred to as carers. However, these people are employed to provide care and receive payment for doing so. To differentiate between paid and unpaid carers the terms 'formal carer' and 'informal carer' are often used to denote the difference between paid care and unpaid care. This chapter focusses on the 'informal carer'.

Anyone might become an informal carer during their lifetime, sometimes caring for several people at once, or perhaps fulfilling the informal carer role on more than one occasion, for example, a mother who cares for her own mother, then later is the carer for her father-in-law. Carers can be family members, who perhaps switch between several roles at once, who may have learning disabilities or be physically frail themselves. Carers can be under 16 years of age; they can be migrants or asylum seekers. Carers may also be part of a fixed or travelling community. Young carers are specifically defined as *children and young people under the age of 18 years who provide regular and ongoing care and emotional support to a family member who is physically or mentally ill, disabled or misuses substances* (Association of Directors of Adult Social Services [ADASS] and the Association of Directors for Children's Services [ADCS] 2009). It is important to make the distinction between young carers in their juvenile years between 16 and 17 years, and those young adult carers aged 18–24 years as the former are legally classed as children and the latter are legally classed as adults. Sprung and Laing (2015) suggest that there are major implications for policy development and commissioning of services for those carers who are legally considered children (under 16 years) and those who are legally considered adults (over 18 years).

ACTIVITY 9.2

Reflection point
It is important to make the distinction between young carers in their juvenile years between 16 and 17 years, and those young adult carers aged 18–24 years as the former are legally classed as children and the latter are legally classed as adults.
• Why is it important?

According to Carers UK (2014b), approximately 10% of the population is a carer in the United Kingdom and Northern Ireland. In the United Kingdom, there are currently 6.5 million carers; this figure is predicted to rise by 3.4 million by 2045 (Carers UK, 2014b). It is projected that 174,995 people under 18 years of age in the United Kingdom and Northern Ireland are carers, just over 13,000 of whom provide more than 50 hours of care a week. It is anticipated that by 2031 the working age population in the United Kingdom will have reduced from five to three people for every person over the age of 65. These demographic predictions have implications for the availability of carers and the future of health and social care in the community setting, which will impact on the role and responsibilities of healthcare practitioners (Carers UK, 2014b).

There are several reasons that adult and young carers are often difficult to identify and define. They might not recognise or may be unwilling to recognise themselves as carers for many complex reasons. This can result in them receiving little or no support from other agencies or professionals. Recognition, definition and appropriate use of the term 'carer' are important in enabling the identification of both adult and young carers throughout the country, publicising the support needed for those carers and directing the appropriate advice and financial provision to them.

The need for carers to take on a caring responsibility will continue to increase as the population ages and more people live longer with long-term conditions. The UK-wide Health Service focus on preventative, anticipatory care will only be possible if carers become equal partners in care delivery. The potential cost to health and social services if this informal care situation breaks down is highly significant for the future economic sustainability of society (Jarvis, 2011). District nurses and community nursing teams often work in partnership with carers and are invaluable in identifying, supporting and assessing carer needs.

ACTIVITY 9.3

Reflection point

Consider the role of a carer you have known, either in the clinical area or personally.

• What support did that carer receive?

• What other life commitments did that carer have to manage?

• What are your thoughts on the definition of the terms 'formal carer' and 'informal carer'?

THE IMPACT OF CARING

Carers of older people and those with long-term conditions in the community are often the spouses of the people they care for and are older people themselves. Jack and O'Brien (2010) highlight the exhaustive nature of the caring role, and it is suggested that it is this very group who cope least well with the responsibility of caring, physically and emotionally, for a dependent person. A lack of support, education, ability or willingness can often result in carer depression and illness, fatigue and mortality. It is reported in the United Kingdom that carers can feel isolated, particularly partner carers, who might live alone with their dependent spouse and often in poverty, or carers who live in a rural remote situation. Sometimes carers exhibit reluctance to admit that they are having difficulty coping because they are unaware of the help and support that can be offered to assist in the home situation (Lawrence et al., 2008). The effective identification of carers and appropriate assessment and interventions can ease the role of caring for those who are struggling, it can avoid hospital admission and reduce isolation and burnout, thus promoting quality of life for the carer as well as sustaining the carer relationship and quality of life for the dependent person.

Forty percent of carers have health problems (Royal College of General Practitioners, 2011). Yet although the health and ability of the carer to cope are essential to enable the dependent person to stay at home and receive the assistance he or she needs, it is not uncommon for carers to dismiss their own health and well-being in order to fulfil the caring role. In 2015, the value of healthcare spending will be £134 billion compared to the cost of the unpaid care we provide for friends and family in the United Kingdom which is £132 billion, compared to just £68 billion in 2001 (Carers UK, 2015). The majority of carers have no income coming into the home except for benefits. Four hundred thousand carers balance full-time work, while also providing over 20 hours of care per week. Working carers have been found to compromise their career prospects because of their caring responsibilities, and according to Milne et al. (2013) two-thirds of carers give up work to care on a full-time basis and this incurs financial loss.

Financial and emotional impact of caring

Nearly 8 out of 10 families caring for someone say it has had an impact on their finances (Carer UK, 2014b). Loss of earnings and the day-to-day financial costs of caring can increase by simple daily life expenditure, for example, higher laundry bills, greater heating costs and transportation expenses and this increase in expenses can lead to carer poverty. This may lead to carers having to make drastic compromises, for example, in their daily diet and use and consumption of fuel. Accumulation of debt in order to survive at a basic level can have an impact on a carer's health.

The benefit system is complicated and has been subject to a lot of change in recent years. The main financial assistance available to carers is Carer's Allowance and carers may be eligible if they provide care for someone for 35 hours a week or more. There are also benefits to help with the long-term costs of living with illness or disability as shown in Table 9.1.

As the number of people caring continues to rise, it is vital that carers are signposted to the correct information and advice on financial and practical support. Many are unaware of their rights, leaving millions of pounds in carers' benefits to go unclaimed. Carers UK have a telephone advice line and an online benefits checker to enable carers to claim the benefits they are entitled to (see Further Resources). Face-to-face appointments are available from local statutory and voluntary services in most UK areas. Special rules apply to some groups of people such as students, those under 18 years, people living permanently in residential care, UK nationals living overseas and people who are not British or Irish nationals (Carers UK, 2014a). Some further financial assistance and benefits are shown in Table 9.2.

National Insurance credit contributions are paid for every week that Carers Allowance is paid. Carers Credits are also available for carers who are not eligible for Carers Allowance but who may be entitled to claim National Insurance contribution credits (Carers UK, 2014a). Other financial help available is shown in Table 9.3.

Table 9.1 Carers allowance

Carer's allowance	For those who care for someone for 35 hours a week or more
Personal Independence Payment (PIP)	For people aged 16–64 years old
Disability Living Allowance (DLA)	For children aged under 16 years old
Attendance Allowance	For people aged 65 years and over

Source: Carers UK (2014a) Carers Rights Guide 2014/15 Looking After Someone. London: Carers.

Table 9.2 Other financial assistance and benefits

Other financial assistance and benefits
• Council tax reduction – Available from your local authority council benefits department
• Disabled facilities grant – For people who may need to adapt the home to make it suitable for a disabled person
• Disability reduction scheme – This scheme may apply when the home environment has had work carried out on it to help you or someone else living at the property live there with a disability
• Council tax discounts – People who live alone qualify for a 25% Council Tax discount

Source: Carers UK (2014a) *Carers Rights Guide 2014/15 Looking After* Someone. London: Carers.

Table 9.3 Other financial help

Other financial help	
Winter Fuel Payments	Those of qualifying age may be entitled to £100–300 Winter Fuel Payment to help pay winter bills.
Warm Home Discount	The Warm Home Discount scheme means you could get a discount on your electricity bill if you meet certain criteria.
Cold Weather Payments	Those in receipt of certain benefits may be able to get a Cold Weather Payment for each week that the local average temperature is at freezing or below.

Source: Carers UK (2014a) *Carers Rights Guide 2014/15 Looking After* Someone. London: Carers.

For those in receipt of certain benefits, help with other costs is available such as:

NHS health costs – this includes free prescriptions, free dental treatment, free NHS eye tests and vouchers to help with the cost of glasses/contact lenses. Fares to hospital for treatment can be claimed in some instances when travelling as a companion with someone who needs to travel for medical reasons.

Other grants and loans which were previously available from the Social Fund have been abolished and replaced with local provision from local councils.

Under new arrangements, community care assessments are available for people who require care from someone else to determine what help is needed and how social services can help. Community care assessments look at the role of the carer and the help the carer provides.

Carers' assessments are available from social services for people who provide 'regular and substantial' care for someone else such as a partner, friend or relative. These assessments are available from April 2015 for anyone who feels that the care they provide will impact on their life, work and family.

The government is moving towards enabling people to choose and control the support services they receive through direct payments and personal budgets. Direct payments and personal budgets are made instead of community social care services and are designed to give the person needing care more choice and control, allowing them to purchase their own service providers (Carers UK, 2014a).

ACTIVITY 9.4

Reflection point
- What criteria do a carer need to meet to be eligible for Carers Allowance?
  - What other financial assistance and benefits may be available to carers to help them meet long-term costs?
  - What other financial assistance and benefits may a carer be eligible for?
- Carer assessments are available for those who provide 'regular and substantial' care for someone else. What constitutes 'regular and substantial' care?

The impact of caring on adult and young carers

For older people, generational beliefs about their role as a spouse, confusion between caring for and caring about their partner, shame and the fear of change can stop carers who are exposed to repeated difficulties from seeking the help and support they need. Research conducted by Rees et al. (2001) states that when they analysed the data on carer assessment, the quality of life of the carer tended to be 'worse than that of the patient'.

For the community nurse assessing the situation and establishing a balance between the carer getting the support he or she needs to care for the dependent person and establishing that the carer is doing so because he or she wants to is essential. Buhr et al. (2006) identified that the quality of life and health status of the carer in the year prior to the dependent person being admitted to a residential placement predicts the likelihood of admission of the cared-for person into institutional care. Any extra pressure on the carer or perceived extra pressure by the carer may eventually lead to the breakdown of a care situation. This is a particularly important issue when the carer is hidden and no one has any insight into the carer's needs or the treatment the disabled/unwell person is receiving. It is essential for community nurses therefore to understand different groups of carers and different carer experiences if they are to offer the support that carers need to fulfil the role they have in today's society. It is important to identify the 'hidden carers': carers who are in the majority, who receive no help, no support, are not aware what help they are entitled to and do not know how to access assistance and/or services. In some areas of the United Kingdom, this is being done through the creation of a 'carers point' in the local general hospital, where carers can go to identify themselves, get advice and information. General Practice is also identifying carers in the GP surgery, while the acute sector admission and assessment process now documents if someone is a carer, or if someone depends on a carer.

It is important for community practitioners to have effective working relationships and regular communication with the wider multidisciplinary team. Interprofessional appreciation of roles and responsibilities and what each can offer and what they can offer together will effectively use resources to highlight and help more known and unidentified carers.

Carers from ethnic minority populations have traditionally been less likely to access health or social services (Laing and Sprung, 2013). It could be argued that it is those populations who cope best with the caring role, identifying it as a natural and expected role, especially in marital or parental relationships. This positive perspective helps to balance out feelings of carer strain, isolation and fear. For many carers, whatever their relationship or background, the role of carer can be viewed as one that gives satisfaction and fulfilment. It can be perceived as being virtuous in nature. There is some evidence to suggest that those who cope less well with the caring role and find it more difficult to adapt to are white, well-educated women (Lawrence et al., 2008). However, it is the white, well-educated women who are also the most able to voice their needs and difficulties and gain access to health and social services in order to acquire support. For those adult children who now care for parents, there might be a desire to give back the care and support shown to them as they were growing up.

The change in relationship between carer and the cared-for person is one of the most complex areas for the community nurse to offer support with. Often there has been some role reversal or a dramatic change in role (e.g. a child caring for a parent, husband caring for his wife). Each situation has to be assessed individually. Some carers will be reluctant to perform personal tasks, while others feel quite comfortable with the role. For some carers, the change in roles and relationships as one person becomes more dependent on another is acceptable, whereas for others it represents the end of the relationship that was (Laing and Sprung, 2013).

For all carers the unpredictable nature of the role means that they focus on coping with the daily activities of caring and have little emotional or mental support to plan for the future (e.g. plan a holiday). Most carers who live with the person they are caring for find the constant need to be present and vigilant the most taxing characteristic of the role.

It can be difficult for a carer to take a step back and put plans in place to take a short break, arrange day care or find a carers' support group. The community nursing team can be invaluable in providing advice, objectivity, empathy and direction to give some balance to the carer's life and identity.

Some carers look after a dependent person because they see residential and nursing home care as a last resort and one that has negative connotations (Neville et al., 2015). However, the use of respite care and other services can positively enhance the carer's experience and enable the care situation at home to continue for longer, perhaps avoiding a crisis.

Perceptions of whether caring is predominantly a burden or has some reward are closely tied with cultural background, as has already been mentioned, and also religious beliefs and life expectations. Carer empowerment through education, support and recognition is a significant part of the community nursing team role.

Adult carers provide care because they want to help the people they care about and because their child, partner, relative or friend could not manage without that help. They often have to juggle the support and care they give with other responsibilities, in a difficult balancing act. However, for young carers it is often a way of life that develops insidiously and these young children/young adults often don't realise that they are carers (The Children's Society, 2013). Despite the emphasis on the use of integrated care with strategic needs assessment and a strong personalisation agenda based on emerging evidence of effective early intervention in identifying, involving and supporting carers, for many young carers, looking after their own health, combining caring with schooling, or getting access to training, or simply having time to take a break or go away for the weekend can be a major challenge (Department of Health, 2010a,b, 2012, 2013a,b). It is these aspects of a young carer's needs that could be better supported and navigated with the assistance of the community nursing team, teachers and other health and social care professionals that they come into contact with (Sprung and Laing, 2015).

The young carer populations are more predisposed to having problems at school with attendance, engaging in work and in attaining qualifications. They are often isolated from their peer group or bullied. Young carers feel that their difficulties are not understood, and they feel unsupported by professionals from healthcare, social care and education. They can experience feelings of guilt and resentment because of the conflict between the needs of the person they are caring for and their own lifestyle, emotional and recreational needs. This all accumulates, and problems often occur when they move into adulthood, finding employment, living independently and establishing relationships (The Children's Society, 2013).

The difficulties that young carers can experience can be expressed through disruptive or antisocial behaviour, drug taking, depression, ill health, and so forth. Although it cannot be said that young people should not be in a caring role at all, because each situation is unique, the community nursing team does have an important role to play in the identification, assessment and support of young carers, together with local authority, education and voluntary services. The difficulty is that one of the issues of caregiving that can be ignored or hidden is that carers experience difficult behaviours on a frequent and regular basis, leading to carer anxiety, grief and a breakdown in the caring relationship.

The definition of difficult behaviours is not clear – it can range from something as simple as the frustration created by the dependent person refusing to eat after requesting something specific for lunch, or it can be as extreme as violence, spitting, deliberate defeacation, and so forth. Difficult behaviour that is repeated in the home environment is a stress that may well contribute to the challenge of caring. If one person becomes more dependent on the other and the balance of the close relationship, such as a partner or spousal relationship, changes, the carer's patience and care satisfaction can be lowered when he or she is subject to difficult behaviours (Laing and Sprung, 2013).

Carers sometimes do not identify themselves as being subject to abusive behaviours because of the perceived lack of intention to harm by the perpetrator, for example, in dementia/mental illness (Mowlam et al., 2007). In a study by Zink et al. (2006) looking at the mistreatment of older partner female carers, it was identified that mistreatment of a carer often takes place in relationships when relational change occurs, for example, the spouse becomes a carer and the relationship status and balance are altered. In relationships where historically there has been evidence of physical or sexual mistreatment from the dependent person, the abusive behaviour continues, but often changes in nature. Also as spousal carers age, they may actually become more psychologically vulnerable than before.

ACTIVITY 9.5

Reflection point
Identify and reflect on the rewards of caring as well as the difficulties –
considering the emotional, physical and financial features of the carer role.

SUPPORTING CARERS

In community nursing there is generally a good understanding of the importance
of carrying out health needs assessments as discussed in Chapter 1, where the
assessment of need can be carried out for individuals, families, carers and communities in any situation that the community nurse encounters. Much of the emphasis
on nursing assessment has traditionally been on the patient/individual rather than
the family and the carer, although some assessment tools do include the needs of
family and carer.

Carers are often asked to make proxy decisions on behalf of patients, and their
own interests and perceptions of the situation and the choices available to them can
significantly influence these judgements. It is important therefore for the community nurse to be aware of this in order to protect the dependent person and be an
advocate for the dependent person. A specific carer assessment will often help community nurses and healthcare professionals to understand carers' experiences and
the support that carers need to fulfil the role (Laing and Sprung, 2013).

Something to note is that the community nurse or healthcare professional carrying out the assessment should not assume that the carer wants to continue in the
caring role. Sometimes carers can think that if they do not care for the dependent
person it will be assumed that they also do not care about the dependent person,
resulting in them taking on a responsibility they are not able or willing to carry out,
to the detriment of all concerned. Any assessment or support tool will require professional sensitivity and well-developed communication skills, enabling a relationship of trust and honesty to develop. The development of a trusting relationship and
support building take time, investment and effort.

Areas of community nursing support for carers

A series of systematic reviews of the literature by Laing and Sprung (2013) and
Sprung and Laing (2015) commissioned by the Queen's Nursing Institute aimed to
appraise the published evidence base relating to adult and young carers' needs when
providing care to patients in the community. They concluded with the following
key findings.

Research has consistently reported carers' requirements for practical nursing
support and nursing-based information provision (Peeters et al., 2010; Gort, 2007).
The lack of carers' knowledge was also identified as a key concern in carers' evaluations of their nursing care abilities and worries about these have been found in the
context of general patient care issues. There are also concerns because of a lack of
knowledge of the medications that carers are expected to administer (Caress et al.,
2009; O'Brien et al., 2012).

A number of studies purported that family carers were not necessarily recipients of district nursing support in their own right but were dependent upon the cared-for person receiving nursing care (Walsh et al., 2007; O'Brien et al., 2012; Gerrish, 2008). Their access to support is conditional upon others, for example, GPs and hospital staff making appropriate patient referrals to district nursing and community nursing teams. This issue is a key area to be addressed in the future if carers are to receive the support they need to maintain their own health and well-being. The literature reviewed did contain a strong theme of carers feeling that they were being excluded from information and decision making which led to a sense of little worth and value in partnership and social isolation, with potential financial hardship and loss of employment. The professional advocacy role to support carers was seen as a significant aspect of support and control for patients and carers, ensuring they do have a sense of worth and value in partnering care with professionals.

Other studies also indicated that community and district nursing teams need to take a more active stance in providing family carer support by adopting a broader family approach, rather than solely a patient-focused approach in order that family carers might be supported more effectively (Bullard, 2007; Plank et al., 2012; Pattenden et al., 2007; Gerrish, 2008). This advice/support is especially required in a constantly changing world of modern technologies that are more frequently used to support care at home.

Overall, these findings relating to the needs of adult carers (see Chapter 17) were reported by Laing and Sprung (2014) following the appraisal of 23 journal articles. The results of the studies included in this literature review suggest insufficient preparation and education of community and hospital staff to support carers and this could potentially have a substantial impact on carer health and well-being. Informal caregivers often experience a negative health and financial impact as a result of their caring responsibilities (Carmichael and Hulme, 2008; Lévesque et al., 2010). In particular, carers who find it difficult to access support services report feelings of burnout and exhaustion (Bullard, 2007; Freer, 2010). Without adequate provision of information, families can feel out of control, disempowered to make decisions and unable to cope with the physical care of a relative on a day-to-day basis (Zwaanswijk et al., 2010; O'Brien et al., 2012). Many studies also highlight that, in the absence of adequate support or guidance, many carers learn to cope with unpaid caregiving through a process of 'trial and error' with day-to-day tasks, with carers assuming a significant emotional component with the prospect of performing unfamiliar nursing tasks inducing stress in many carers (O'Brien et al., 2012; Freer, 2010; Carmichael and Hulme, 2008; Caress et al., 2009).

Some key studies identified that professionals acted on the assumption that family carers would, by choice or default, provide care (Bullard, 2007; Plank et al., 2012; Pattenden et al., 2007). This notion of the family or carer being used as a means of promoting 'self-care' appeared to be conflated with the notion that the patient no longer needed community services. The families' ability to care for the patient, thereby reducing the patient's dependence from nursing services has been conflated to give a rationale for withdrawal of community services. The literature has indicated that the decision for providing family carer support appears to be based largely on service capacity rather than on carer needs and preferences (Gerrish, 2008; Taggart et al., 2012; Tan et al., 2012).

Education and training related to emotional support and medication management were identified as key concerns for carers. Studies that examined health professionals' perspectives also acknowledged deficits in caregiver preparation. District nurses and community nurses typically viewed carers as ill-prepared both for the fundamental nursing care aspects and the far-reaching nature of the role (Jack and O'Brien, 2010; Gerrish, 2008; Greenwood and Mackenzie, 2010). District nurses and community nurses also emphasised the psychological consequences of inadequate caregiver knowledge, which induced carer anxiety and its impact on caregiver confidence (Whitehead et al., 2012; Walsh et al., 2007).

A number of publications considered the district and community-nursing role in supporting patients who had been discharged at a much earlier point of the care pathway. This pressure on carers and district and community nursing teams was accelerated by an increase of faster throughput of hospital patients mostly with an emphasis on end-of-life care for patients in their own homes (Jack and O'Brien, 2010; Whitehead et al., 2012). The work by Laing and Sprung (2013) and Sprung and Laing (2015) also highlights the issue that there has been very little research around carer support needs. However, they identified specific recommendations in relation to the characteristics of district nursing support for carers to include enabling, supporting, mediating, care substitution, crisis prevention and crisis intervention.

A number of key themes emerged as helpful for community and district nursing teams to better support carers' needs in areas as shown in Table 9.4. These issues highlight areas for education and training for community and district nursing teams.

It is evident from the literature that a high proportion of carers have significant health problems themselves, often exacerbated by their caring role. However, the needs of this group are incredibly under-researched when compared with the paid workforce or patient groups themselves. Key difficulties experienced by carers are feelings of being excluded and loss of control, social isolation, financial hardship and loss of employment as well as their own emotional and health problems. Within the context of carers' support requirements a major gap in the literature around the area of how professionals can best support carers with these needs has been

Table 9.4 Key themes to better support the needs of carers

- Assessment of needs to include emotional anxieties
- Trust and partnership relationships with healthcare staff to ensure continuity of care
- Communication and understanding around disease process and prognosis
- Knowledge and understanding around medication and medication administration
- Support with personal care and routine nursing tasks
- Referral to carer groups, volunteer services and social opportunities
- Benefits advice and signposting
- Reduction in bureaucracy, easier navigation of services
- Recognising carer stress and burnout

Source: Laing M and Sprung S (2013) *The Queen's Nursing Institute Carers Project Literature Review: Working with Health Care Professionals to Increase Carer Awareness, Identification and Referral.* London: QNI.

highlighted. There is evidence that carers need support, guidance and signposting assistance, and there is no consideration in the literature of what education, training and skills staff may need to provide this support to carers. Further research is indicated. However, over recent years the government has charged the organisations Skills for Health and Skills for Care with identifying some resources for staff and carers' activities and support (Skills for Health, 2011).

One of the key problems faced is that carers do not often recognise themselves as carers. A caring role can develop gradually over a long period and the first step in the process of carer identification and referral is now being identified by formal agencies such as GPs and hospitals (Fraser, 2012). A recommendation from Fraser's work is that there needs to be other proactive opportunities for carer identification, assessment of needs and access to services through simple routine assessment processes by community and district nursing teams resulting in information sharing with support agencies and appropriate signposting.

The review of the literature indicates that professional, voluntary services and family carers need to work together effectively, with a clear role for nurses in undertaking assessments, giving information and providing other support (Zwaanswijk et al., 2010; O'Brien et al., 2012). Many health professionals feel unprepared for understanding the experience of carers and conversations around long-term conditions or end-of-life care can be challenging for staff. There is also evidence that the transitions into and out of care settings are managed poorly, and this increases the demands on carers (Whitehead et al., 2012; Walsh et al., 2007). As government policy supports and enables more people to be nursed at home, district and community nurses could be instrumental in managing these transitions to reduce stress and disruption to patients and carers. District nurses in particular are uniquely placed to play a critical role in minimising the strain on carers and families as they have the ability to ensure integration between home caring and professional support (QNI, 2013).

The topic of carer identification, information and support within district and community nursing services appears to be under-researched. It is timely for a major review of the models to support carers in assisting with the nursing and personal care needs of patients. This would in turn lead to a better understanding of the tools and resources district and community nursing teams working in primary care need to successfully engage with carers to support them in this unique and challenging role (DH, 2013a). In summary there is a lack of publications that robustly examine the differential roles of district nurses and other community nursing services to ensure carers' needs in community nursing teams are being supported adequately. A review of the literature also identifies a distinct gap in service and a lack of leadership and knowledge about the needs of carers and how carers can be appropriately supported to avoid carer breakdown (Laing and Sprung, 2013).

District and community nurses express concerns about their confidence to give the right support to carers, and this clearly indicates that they have education needs of their own (Jack and O'Brien, 2010; Whitehead et al., 2012). They do, however, have a unique position to make an enormous difference to the carers' experience by providing the link between carer organisations, education, benefits and support.

This could mean a real difference to a carer on the brink of burnout and not being able to cope towards having a happy healthy life allowing the carer to continue to do what he or she wants to do, care for his or her loved ones.

Agencies

A voluntary agency, usually a charity or grant-funded body, provides help to people with a particular need. The Princess Royal Trust for Carers would be an example of a voluntary agency that provides help for carers. The aim of voluntary and charitable agencies in relation to carers is to make a practical and positive difference through the provision of useful information, carer relief, a listening ear, support groups, respite care and everyday support to all carers who need it. These agencies have the carer and the dependent person at the centre of their philosophy and are often run by carers themselves or their representatives. This gives a significant and informed insight into the needs of carers.

Voluntary and charitable organisations are ideally placed to empower carers. However, as the carer role increases the skills that carers need, such as moving and handling training, health education, definition of carer role and responsibilities, will be provided. One of the overall benefits of voluntary agencies is that they are less bureaucratic and able to respond to need quickly.

A statutory agency (or in Scotland Public Body) is one provided under law and is usually the responsibility of a Local Authority or Central Government department. These agencies (voluntary, charitable, statutory and public) work slightly differently from country to country and between localities. However, it remains important, especially in the ever-changing face of healthcare provision, that agencies work together for the common good of the patient. They need to share information, communicate effectively and be aware of the others' roles and responsibilities.

ACTIVITY 9.6

Reflection point

Sue and Mike have been married for 18 years and have two children, Chloe aged 10 and Caitlin aged 14. Mike was a successful businessman until recently, when he was forced to sell the business because he was unable to manage it. Mike was diagnosed with multiple sclerosis 13 years ago. His mobility is reduced and he mobilises using an electric wheelchair, requiring assistance from his wife Sue to maintain personal hygiene and to dress, and he requires significant emotional support. Mike has recently become anxious and emotional, which Sue says has had an impact on the children.

The district nurse has been called in to discuss intermittent catheterisation with Mike. She has not met the family before because Jean has tried to protect the home environment from medical and healthcare equipment and personnel.

Sue does not recognise herself as a carer because she thinks that in doing so it will confirm her husband's frailty, while also confirming to her that he is deteriorating. She fears it may also change their relationship.

ACTIVITY 9.6

- What assessments need to be carried out in this home?
- What support would you suggest introducing to this family?
- What other agencies in your area would be appropriate to help Sue, Mike and the children?
- What skills, values and behaviours would the district nurse need to apply in this situation?

CONCLUSION

The future of caring in the community, with an ageing population and more people living with long-term conditions, mental health issues or substance misuse, is being taken seriously by government and service providers throughout Europe.

The important issues of carer identification, assessment, education and collaborative partnership have been acknowledged in this chapter, along with an exploration of the definition of 'carer'. There has been opportunity to gain an understanding of carer identity and appreciate who may become a carer. There has also been a chance to consider some aspects of the caring role and consider the financial and emotional impacts that caring has on young and adult carers.

The role and contribution carers make to society and the personal and financial issues they experience have been explored. The exhaustive nature of the caring role has been highlighted along with recognition of the importance of the community nurse's role in the identification, assessment and support of carers.

The role of assessment and support by an educated, skilled multiprofessional health and social care team is valued as fundamental in meeting the needs of carers and promoting the carer's ability to cope. Governments are funding and championing charities and voluntary organisations which are essential providers of services and support for carers. Although the picture can seem daunting, there are constant changes taking place in the world of technology with telehealth, social networking and electronic care applications and packages making care at home more feasible and the responsibility of caring lighter, enabling carers and patients, although physically isolated, to access support and maintain communication with the world around them.

FURTHER READING

Carers' Strategy for Wales UK – Action Plan. 2007. http://www.asdinfowales.co.uk/resource/9_0_carers_strategy-e.pdf (Accessed 14/6/17).

Carers UK (2014) Carers Rights Guide 2014/15 *Looking After Someone*. Carers UK.

Department of Health (1998) '*They Look After their Own, Don't They?' Inspection of Community Care Services for Black and Ethnic Minority Older People*. London: The Department of Health Publications.

Mutch K (2010) In sickness and in health: Experience of caring for a spouse with MS. *British Journal of Nursing* 19:214–9.

Obadina S (2012) Parental mental illness: Effects on young carers. *British Journal of School Nursing* 3:135–9.

Rees J, O'Boyle C and MacDonagh R (2001) Quality of life: Impact of chronic illness on the partner. *Journal of the Royal Society of Medicine* 94:563–6.

The Scottish Government (2010) Carers Strategy. http://www.gov.scot/Publications/2010/07/23153304/0 (Accessed 14/06/17).

FURTHER RESOURCES

http://alzheimers.org.uk/site/index.php

www.ageuk.org.uk

www.barnardos.org.uk/what_we_do/our_projects/young_carers.htm

www.carersuk.org

www.carersinformation.org.uk

www.diabetes.org.uk

www.dementiacarer.net/#

www.gov.uk/government/uploads/system/uploads/attachment_data/file/329867/Carers_Pathway.pdf

www.gov.uk/government/uploads/system/uploads/attachment_data/file/299270/Young_Carers_pathway_Interactive_FINAL.pdf

www.macmillan.org.uk/Cancerinformation/Ifsomeoneelsehascancer/CaringForSomeone.aspx

www.macmillan.org.uk/Cancerinformation/Ifsomeoneelsehascancer/Youngcarers/Youngcarers.aspx

www.mssociety.org.uk

www.magonlinelibrary.com/doi/full/10.12968/bjcn.2014.19.7.346

https://professionals.carers.org/working-mental-health-carers/triangle-care-mental-health

www.qni.org.uk/supporting_carers/carers_project_resources

www.qni.org.uk/docs/Young_Carers_Lit_Review.pdf

www.qni.org.uk/docs/Carers_Literature_Review.doc

www.schoolhealthstreet.co.uk/

www.youngcarers.net

REFERENCES

Association of Directors of Adult Social Services (ADASS) and the Association of Directors for Children's Services (ADCS) (2009) *Working Together to Support Young Carers—A Model Local Memorandum of Understanding between Statutory Directors for Children's Services and Adult Social Services.* ADASS and ADCS.

Buhr GT, Kuchibhatla M and Clipp EC (2006) Caregivers' reasons for nursing home placement: Clues for improving discussions with families prior to the transition. *Gerontologist* 46:52–61.

Bullard R (2007) A little oasis. *Community Care* 1696:28–9.

Carers UK (2014a) *Carers Rights Guide 2014/15 Looking After Someone.* London: Carers.

Carers UK (2014b) *State of Caring 2014.* London: Carers.

Carers UK (2015) Making life better for carers. (Accessed 14 November 2015) www.carersuk.org/?gclid=CMyZpMaVkMkCFYoEwwodaP8GhA.

Caress A, Luker K, Chalmers K and Salmon M (2009) A review of the information and support needs of family carers of patients with chronic obstructive pulmonary disease. *Journal of Clinical Nursing* 18(4):479–91.

Carmichael F and Hulme C (2008) Are the needs of carers being met? *Journal of Community Nursing* 22(8–9):4.

Department of Health (2008) *Carers at the Heart of 21st Century Families and Communities: A Caring System on Your Side, A Life of Your Own.* London: Department of Health Publications.

Department of Health (2010a) Recognised, valued and supported: Next steps for the Carers Strategy. (Accessed 14 November 2015) http://tinyurl.com/l5bvnov.

Department of Health (2010b) *Personalising Services and Support for Carers.* London: Department of Health.

Department of Health (2012) *Compassion in Practice: Nursing, Midwifery and Care Staff Our Vision and Strategy.* London: Department of Health.

Department of Health (2013a) *Care in Local Communities: A New Vision and Model for District Nursing.* London: Department of Health.

Department of Health (2013b) *Helping Carers to Stay Healthy.* London: Department of Health.

Department of Health (2014a) *The Care Act.* London: Department of Health.

Department of Health (2014b) *Five Year Forward View.* London: Department of Health.

Fraser M (2012) Involving carers makes a difference to outcomes for all. *British Journal of Cardiology Nursing* 7(10):500–1.

Freer S (2010) Motor neurone disease: Insight into experience of family carers. *End of Life Journal* 4(1):54–62.

Gerrish K (2008) Caring for the carers: The characteristics of district nursing support for family carers. *Primary Health Care Research and Development* 9(1):14–24.

Gort A, Mingot M, Gomez X et al. (2007) Use of the Zarit scale for assessing caregiver burden and collapse in caregiving at home in dementias. *International Journal of Geriatric Psychiatry* 22(10):957–62.

Greenwood N and Mackenzie A (2010) An exploratory study of anxiety in carers of stroke survivors. *Journal of Clinical Nursing* 19(13–14):2032–8.

Jack B and O'Brien M (2010) Dying at home: Community nurses views on the impact of informal carers on cancer patients. *European Journal of Cancer Care* 19(5):636–42.

Jarvis A (2011) Working with carers in the next decade: The challenges. *British Journal of Community Nursing* 15:125–8.

Laing M and Sprung S (2013) *The Queen's Nursing Institute Carers Project Literature Review: Working with Health Care Professionals to Increase Carer Awareness, Identification and Referral.* London: QNI.

Laing M and Sprung S (2014) Enabling the health and well-being of carers through district nursing support. *British Journal of Community Nursing* 19(7):346–51.

Lawrence V, Murray J, Samsi K and Banerjee S (2008) Attitudes and support needs of Black Caribbean, South Asian and White British carers of people with dementia in the UK. *The British Journal of Psychiatry* 193:240–6.

Lévesque L, Ducharme F, Caron C et al. (2010) A partnership approach to service needs assessment with family caregivers of an aging relative living at home: A qualitative analysis of the experiences of caregivers and practitioners. *International Journal of Nursing Studies* 47(7):876–87.

McNamara B and Rosenwax L (2010) Which carers of family members at the end of life need more support from health services and why? *Social Science and Medicine* 70:1035–41.

Milne A, Palmer A, Brigden C. and Konta E (2013) The intersection of work and care: Evidence from a local case study. *European Journal of Social Work* 16(5):651–70.

Mowlam A, Tennant R, Dixon J and McCreadie C (2007) UK Study of Abuse and Neglect of Older People: Qualitative Findings. National Centre of Social Research and Kings College, London, pp. 8–80.

Neville C, Beattie E, Fielding E and MacAndrew M (2015) Literature review: Use of respite by carers of people with dementia. *Health and Social Care in the Community* 23(1):51–63.

O'Brien MR, Whitehead B, Murphy PN et al. (2012) Social services homecare for people with motor neurone disease/amyotrophic lateral sclerosis: Why are such services used or refused? *Palliative Medicine* 26(2):123–31.

Pattenden JF, Roberts H and Lewin RJ (2007) Living with heart failure; patient and carer perspectives. *European Journal of Cardiovascular Nursing* 6(4):273–9.

Peeters JM, Van Beek AP, Meerveld JH et al. (2010) Informal caregivers of persons with dementia, their use of and needs for specific professional support: A survey of the National Dementia Programme. *BMC Nursing* 9:9.

Plank A, Mazzoni V and Cavada L (2012) Becoming a caregiver: New family carers' experience during the transition from hospital to home. *Journal of Clinical Nursing* 21(13–14):2072–82.

Queen's Nursing Institute (2013) Report on District Nurse Education in England, Wales and Northern Ireland. QNI, London.

Rees J, O'Boyle C and MacDonagh R (2001) Quality of life: Impact of chronic Illness on the partner. *Journal of the Royal Society of Medicine* 94:563–6.

Royal College of General Practitioners (2011) *Supporting Carers: An Action Guide for General Practitioners and Their Teams.* London: Royal College of General Practitioners.

Scottish Government (2010) *Caring Together: The Carers Strategy for Scotland 2010–2015.* Edinburgh: Scottish Government.

Scottish Government (2014) *Public Bodies (Joint Working) (Scotland) Act.* Edinburgh: Scottish Government.

Skills for Health (2011) Carers matter (3 parts) skills for care and skills for health. Skills for Health. http://www.skillsforhealth.org.uk/resources/service-area/22-carers?highlight= WyJjYXJlcnMiLCInY2FyZXJzIiwibWF0dGVyIiwiY2FyZXJzIG1hdHRlciJd (Accessed 14/6/17).

Sprung S and Laing M (2015) *The Queen's Nursing Institute Young Carers Project Literature Review: Working with Health Care Professionals to Increase Young Carer Awareness, Identification and Referral.* London: QNI.

Taggart L, Truesdale-Kennedy M, Ryan A and McConkey R (2012) Examining the support needs of ageing family carers in developing future plans for a relative with an intellectual disability. *Journal of Intellectual Disabilities* 16(3):217–34.

Tan SB, Williams AF and Morris ME (2012) Experiences of caregivers of people with Parkinson's disease in Singapore: A qualitative analysis. *Journal of Clinical Nursing* 21(15–16):2235–46.

The Children's Society (2013) *Hidden From View: The Experiences of Young Carers in England.* The Children's Society. https://www.childrenssociety.org.uk/sites/default/ files/tcs/report_hidden-from-view_young-carers_final.pdf (Accessed (14/6/17).

Walsh K, Jones L, Tookman A et al. (2007) Reducing emotional distress in people caring for patients receiving specialist palliative care. *British Journal of Psychiatry* 190:142–7.

Whitehead B, O'Brien MR, Jack BA and Mitchell D (2012) Experiences of dying, death and bereavement in motor neurone disease: A qualitative study. *Palliative Medicine* 26(4):368–78.

Zink T, Jacobson J and Regan S (2006) Older women's descriptions and understandings of their abusers. *Violence Against Women* 12:851.

Zwaanswijk M, Van Beek AP, Peeters J et al. (2010) Problems and needs of informal caregivers of persons with dementia: A comparison between the initial stage and subsequent stages of the illness process. *Tijdschr Gerontology Geriatric* 41(4):162–71.

10

Spirituality: A neglected aspect of care

Ann Clarridge

LEARNING OUTCOMES

- Critically discuss the concept of 'spirituality' and spiritual care within nursing.
- Describe the principles underpinning spiritual assessment and appraise the associated tools and interventions available.
- Explore the concept of 'self-awareness'.
- Critically discuss how, as a community nurse, developing self-awareness can enhance the spiritual assessment of patients/clients.

INTRODUCTION

This chapter is concerned with the concept of spirituality in the care provided by nursing professionals. Reference is made to some of the relevant research and literary reviews which offer a useful context for this complex subject area. Some definitions of spirituality are outlined and the place of spirituality within community nursing is considered. The consequent implications in terms of spiritual assessment and possible interventions are discussed. The need for self-awareness and its development in nurses is explored. Finally, the competence of nurses to deal with the spiritual aspects of care is considered together with the importance of observational skills and communication, essential tools in the repertoire of all nursing professionals.

LITERATURE REVIEW AND RESEARCH

There is a growing interest surrounding the place of spiritual care in nursing, and this is supported by a plethora of literature.

MacKinlay and Hudson (2008) undertook an extensive review of the literature. From their findings, seven main themes on spirituality and ageing emerged that highlighted issues relevant to spiritual care and to practice in nursing older people. The themes were spirituality concept development and models, spirituality and chronic illness, promoting spiritual health and wellbeing, spirituality and dying, cross-cultural and multi-faith issues, spiritual assessment and ethics (MacKinlay and Hudson, 2008: 143).

Ross (2006) also undertook a thorough and comprehensive review of research on spiritual care in nursing. The results of this review provided insight into how nurses, clients and their carers perceive spirituality and spiritual care with relevance to clinical practice. It would seem that nurses identify spiritual needs not only from specific religious requests made by clients but also from their non-verbal cues such as anxiety, depression and being withdrawn (Ross, 2006). Some nurses do not always respond to those needs because of feelings of inadequacy and lack of preparation. The nurses who reported feeling confident to meet spiritual needs were those who were aware of their own spirituality, beliefs and values. Most nurses, however, were happy to listen to clients or simply be present with a client. Clients who expressed particular needs were often referred to another experienced professional, for example, a chaplain or appropriate religious leader dependent upon the client's preference (Ross, 2006).

More recently the Royal College of Nursing (RCN) undertook a survey of all its members in response to the identification by nurses themselves of their 'uncertainty and hesitancy in engaging with the spiritual dimension of their profession' and of their need for guidance. The survey consisted of a five-part questionnaire, incorporating the Spirituality and Spiritual Care Rating Scale (SSCRS), to explore perceptions of spirituality and the delivery of spiritual care (Executive summary. RCN Spirituality Survey, 2010).

Ross et al. (2014) carried out a study of the perceptions of spirituality and spiritual care together with the perceived competence required for its delivery. The study was based on information gathered from undergraduate nurses and midwives from six universities in four European countries in 2010. The findings were positive within the limitations of the study, the student sample being predominantly Christian and female. The attributes rated most highly by the students when considering the importance of both spiritual and personal care were their 'sense of connectedness to others and their sense of life/self-responsibility' (Ross et al., 2014: 701). Within the context of regulatory body guidelines such attributes should be a necessary feature in the profile of any professional seeking to deliver truly holistic care.

Two further studies undertaken within the field of education have revealed a growing awareness of the need to understand the problems that emerge regarding how, what, where and when spiritual care is to be taught and by whom and how these problems might be addressed.

Prentis et al. used a mixed-method, small-scale explorative online survey initially to identify what healthcare teaching staff understood by 'spirituality' and how they were able to integrate it into their teaching practice. A further aim was to explore how nursing practice might be improved in terms of the assessment of patient care needs (Prentis et al., 2014: 44). The results of the study affirmed a considerable level of interest within healthcare education and the willingness of providers to include aspects of spirituality in their educational programmes. However the whole issue of the development and evaluation of resources for use in teaching still remains.

Timmins et al. (2015) sampled 543 books from the Nursing and Midwifery Core Collection list (UK) and analysed the data using a Spirituality Textbook Analysis Tool specifically designed for the study. The findings revealed that while there are specific texts for nursing and spiritual care, there is little evidence of spiritual care in key nursing textbooks. It is suggested by Timmins et al. that spirituality and spiritual care should not be 'sequestered' to specialised texts but integrated into all textbooks where relevant so that care and nursing practice would indeed be 'holistic'.

The overall conclusions to be drawn from this extensive review point to the need for further, systematic and co-ordinated research, particularly in the area of preparation of nurses in the assessment and provision of spiritual care. The overriding problems that emerge are how, what, where and when spiritual care should be taught and who should teach it.

ACTIVITY 10.1

Reflection point

Consider the following questions:

• What is your experience of being taught about spiritual care?
• Would you have found it helpful if spirituality had been included in your education and training?
• What knowledge and skills would be helpful to enable you to explore a patient's spiritual needs with confidence?

DEFINING SPIRITUALITY

The concept of spiritual care is equivocal. There is a need to define spirituality and consider how it relates to nursing care.

The terms *spiritual* and *religious* are often used to mean the same thing, and although there is an overlap between the two, not everyone would agree that an individual needs to be religious in order to be spiritual, or vice versa (Clarke, 2009). Koenig et al. (2001) mark very distinct differences and define religion as 'an organised system of beliefs, practices, rituals and symbols' and spirituality as the personal quest for understanding answers to ultimate questions about life, about meaning, and about relationship to the sacred or transcendent which may or may not lead to or arise from the development of religious rituals and the formation of community (Koenig et al., 2001, cited in MacKinlay and Hudson, 2008: 140).

Thus, it could be argued 'that the practice of religion is a way that humans relate to the sacred, to otherness' and that all humans have a spiritual dimension but not all humans practice religion (MacKinlay and Hudson, 2008: 140).

'Spiritual but not religious' is a phrase used by many people to express the belief that real spirituality is the concern of the individual (Sulmasy, 2009). Those who hold this view will affirm that their individual experience is one thing and institutionalised religion is another (Jamison, 2006: 142). On one side, classical religion, including all the main world religions each with its own specific doctrine, rituals and beliefs, 'offers us an educative process that helps us to see the whole of life in a different way' (Jamison, 2006: 146). On the other side, modern spirituality might well be defined as 'psychological well-being combined with the moral golden rule – do unto others as you would have them do unto you' (Jamison, 2006: 143). Chochinov (2006a) suggests that spirituality is to 'invoke a sense of searching or yearning for significance or meaning in life' (Chochinov, 2006b: 88).

Spirituality outside religion often signifies a believer whose *faith* is personal, more open to new ideas and numerous influences than the *dogmatic* faith of mature religions. Such believers tend to regard spirituality not as a religion but as the active and vital connection to a force, power or energy, or a sense of the deep *self*. It can also signify the personal nature of the relationship or connection with the god(s) or *belief system*(s) of a believer as opposed to the general relationship with a *deity* and the rites of group worship shared by members of a given faith. Those who claim that they are spiritual but not religious often believe in the existence of many 'spiritual paths' and would refute that there is an *objectively* definable best path to follow. They often emphasise the importance of finding one's individual path to the divine and may or may not believe in the supernatural. Where there is such a belief and a relationship with supernatural beings represents the foundation of happiness then that will form the basis of spiritual practice. Where there is no such belief, a different form of practice provides the way to manage thoughts and emotions which otherwise would prevent happiness (Sulmasy, 2009).

Definitions of spirituality are constantly evolving so it would seem appropriate, therefore, in the context of this chapter to accept Chochinov's (2006a) simple definition without necessarily invoking religion. Thus spirituality may be understood to be that search for inner peace and the foundation of happiness which requires some form of spiritual practice but which is essential for the promotion of personal well being. Chochinov identifies a client who speaks of loss of hope, feelings of being a burden to others, loss of dignity or loss of the will to live as being one who is experiencing spiritual distress. Many techniques and practices have been explored and developed in religious contexts, such as meditation or contemplative reading, and are immensely valuable in themselves as skills for managing aspects of the inner life.

ACTIVITY 10.2

Reflection point

Consider the following questions:

- What does spirituality mean to me? How would I define it for myself?
- What does it mean when an individual is said to be 'spiritual'?

SPIRITUALITY AND COMMUNITY NURSING

Spirituality and all its associated vocabulary are terms much in vogue: they sound significant, with a touch of mystery. As with all jargon, however, it provides us with a language that enables us to think and talk about issues and concepts which are otherwise difficult to articulate. Individual spirituality as an important element in nursing practice is now being generally and officially recognised. The importance of addressing a person's spiritual needs with an emphasis on competence in spiritual care is placed firmly within the professional regulatory body in *The Code: Professional Standards of Practice and Behaviour for Nurses and Midwives* (NMC, 2015).

More recently, the Royal College of Nursing (RCN) has identified four key priorities one of which is the need 'through liaison and collaboration with the

Nursing and Midwifery Council (NMC) and the government health departments to build on existing work and advance the area of spirituality within nursing and health care' (RCN, 2010: 28). Health boards and government policies also support the importance of meeting the spiritual needs of patients. The International Council of Nurses (ICN) specifies 'an environment in which the human rights, values, customs and spiritual beliefs of the individual, family and community are respected' (ICN Code of Ethics, 2000: 5). The Department of Health (2002) in its guidelines for Chaplaincy and Spiritual Care in the NHS in Scotland includes an aim 'to develop and implement spiritual care policies' which are appropriate to our 'increasingly multi-cultural society' (MacLaren, 2004: 457). 'Spiritual nursing can be an opportunity for nurses to enquire into that which is fundamental about the human condition and to give truly whole person care in a multi-faith society' (MacLaren, 2004: 461).

Community nurses need a definition of the context for the care they provide. The term *community* frequently describes a wide range of patterns of relationships but generally includes two important characteristics. The first describes those who share values and a sense of purpose and who encourage and support each other in the challenges of daily life. 'The giving and receiving of love is an important element for this community of people' and such a community might be the local church, neighbours or family (Runcorn, 2006: 55). The second describes shared work, special circumstances or interests.

It would seem at first glance that community nursing could be defined through shared work and special circumstances. However, a closer look at what actually underpins nursing – *The Code: Professional Standards of Practice and Behaviour for Nurses and Midwives* (NMC, 2015), for example – suggests that community nursing may well be identified by the first characteristic – the shared values and sense of purpose. So, in effect, both descriptions could be said to apply to the work of the community nurse.

Nurses who work within the context of a community as opposed to an institution fulfil a specific role. They care for individuals and families with a variety of conditions in their own homes or in homely settings. They are involved with people from different ethnic backgrounds, with those who have and with those who do not have an expressed religious faith. In every case, the nurse needs to be aware of the spiritual dimension of each individual no matter how it finds expression. In 1964 Jean Vanier (1989) established a community where people with various physical and learning difficulties could live as equals with able-bodied people. He asserted that 'the fundamental right of each person includes amongst the right to life and care, the right to a spiritual life' (L'Arche Charter, in Runcorn, 2006: 55).

Community nurses find themselves in the role of 'key players', able to recognise and meet the spiritual needs of clients and their families (McSherry and Ross, 2010). The QNI/QNIS voluntary standards for District Nursing Education and Practice (2015) encompass all aspects of holistic care as provided by the district nurse. Community nurses would argue that holistic care of the individual and not just physical need has always been their concern. Indeed their claim is justly supported by the plethora of nursing models of care. A holistic approach to care reflects the underlying principles and philosophy that all nurses draw upon to shape the way in which they act and carry out their nursing practice. Although conceptual models of nursing differ quite considerably because nurses have different ideas about what nursing means for them, fundamental to most models is the person or the individual. Each model has something to say about this key element, especially in the assessment for proposed care. It is here, within this area of the model, that the spiritual needs of the patient can be addressed (Smith, 2004).

Research undertaken by Perry (2005) identified four areas that were of importance to nurses: 'affirming the value of the person, defending dignity, enabling hope and helping patients find meaning' (Perry, 2005, in McSherry and Ross, 2010: 155). Neuman (1995) and Roper et al. (2000) revised their nursing theories to include spirituality, thus seeking to provide true holistic care (Smith, 2004).

In times of illness or loss of independence patients will frequently raise fundamental questions concerning the meaning or purpose of life wherever they may be on the spectrum of religious belief. It is the experience of community nurses that at such times patients turn to those who are caring for them for answers, help and support. Spiritual care may be said to be 'that care which recognises and responds to the needs of the human spirit when faced with trauma, ill health or sadness and can include the need for meaning, for selfworth, to express oneself, for faith support, perhaps for rites or prayer or sacrament, or simply for a sensitive listener' (Department of Health, 2009; 6).

Research literature suggests that nurses need to be aware of their own beliefs and values in order to best meet the spiritual care needs of patients. The RCN survey (2010) has raised some pertinent issues relating to the personal and professional boundaries that need to be drawn by nurses when providing spiritual care. Many nurses expressed the need for help when distinguishing between their own values and their professional judgments as providers of care. Nurses need to be clear about how they express their beliefs in their own lives, whether through doctrine, ritual or membership of a religious community. Such clarity is essential if they are to remain objective when assessing, planning and delivering holistic patient care. Those nurses who professed to a personal belief were aware of the need for objectivity and that while providing support to the patient they should not allow their own values and beliefs to impinge upon or influence the patient in any way. Nurses would then be in a position to demonstrate an interest in and a willingness to discuss issues of a spiritual nature with patients without the necessity of a wide-ranging knowledge of the doctrines, rituals and practices of the many religions. A review of research established that the level and amount of spiritual care given by a nurse were related to the amount of time available for listening and the possession of spiritual awareness, sensitivity and communication skills of the nurse (Ross, 2006).

ACTIVITY 10.3

Reflection and action point

To explore your spiritual beliefs and feelings about other people's beliefs (adapted from Burnard, 1992: 16,17)

Write a short passage that sums up what you believe in.

Some helpful questions:

- Do you believe in God, and if so what does your concept of God involve?
- If you do not believe in God, what do you think about people who do?
- What do you consider to be the purpose of your life?
- How did you develop your beliefs and where have they come from?
- How might you respond if colleagues said (1) they did not believe in God, (2) tried to convince you of their belief?
- How might you respond if a patient were to tell you that life is meaningless or hopeless?
- You might like to discuss what you have written or discuss the questions with a friend.
- Share your thoughts and ideas and note the degree to which you agree or disagree with each other.
- Consider what it might be like to take the opposite approach to the one that you hold and what that might mean to you.

SPIRITUAL ASSESSMENT AND INTERVENTION

The importance of assessment in the approach to client care is paramount, with the inclusion of the spiritual needs of the client as an integral element of an holistic approach. There are a number of guidelines and strategies within the discipline of social work and family therapy for assessing spiritual needs of families (Hodge, 2001). In the past there have been fewer within nursing literature but the situation is changing. Most health and nursing care assessments include a question regarding religious affiliation (Orem, 1980; Peplau, 1988). In recognition of the importance of a patient's spirituality, the number of published guidelines and models in the nursing and spirituality literature is now increasing (Narayanasamy, 2006a; McSherry, 2006; Koenig, 2007). Tanyi (2006) suggests that when assessing the needs of clients and their families, there are three major goals to spiritual assessment:

- To support and enhance families' spiritual well-being and development
- To discern spiritual distress and its effect on overall family health
- To ascertain ways to incorporate family spirituality when providing care

(Tanyi, 2006: 289)

However, the nurse must feel comfortable and have already established a relationship of trust with the client before being able to undertake a thorough spiritual assessment and plan appropriate care (see Chapter 5). Tanyi (2006: 289–90) provides a series of questions and spiritual interventions that can be adapted and used as a guide by nurses to undertake a spiritual assessment and to plan patient care (Box 10.1).

> **Box 10.1 Guideline questions for spiritual assessment**
>
> **Strengths**
> • What has helped you in the past to deal with crisis?
> • What gives you strength?
> • What do you do to rebuild your strength?
>
> **Meaning and purpose**
> • In your daily life, what gives you meaning?
> • What gives you peace, joy and satisfaction?
>
> **Relationships**
> • Who is the most important person in your life?
> • To whom do you turn when you need help?
>
> **Beliefs**
> • Do you have a relationship with God/deity, universe, or other?
> • If yes, how would you describe it and what does it mean to your health?
> • Do you practice rituals such as prayer, worship or meditation?
>
> **Personal spirituality and preference for spiritual care**
> • How do you express/describe your spirituality?
>   • Do you consider anyone as your spiritual leader and if necessary can this person be contacted?
>
> These questions are provided as a general guide and can be adapted for use according to the individual and the nurse's preference.
>
> *(Tanyi, 2006; McSherry and Ross, 2010)*

The RCN has responded to the findings of the study by producing a 'pocket-sised' book which provides guidance for nurses when assessing patients' spiritual needs: *Preparing to Give Spiritual Care*

Just as you would assess your patients' physical needs, an initial assessment of their spiritual concerns is important. You may find questions such as these helpful:

• Do you have a way of making sense of the things that happen to you?
• What sources of support/help do you look to when life is difficult?
• Would you like to see someone who can help you?
• Would you like to see someone who can help you talk or think through the impact of this illness/life event? (You don't have to be religious to talk to them.) (RCN, 2010)

(See Further Reading for a full text of the guidelines to spiritual assessment and interventions for families.)

McSherry (2006: 905) offers a model that includes a number of components ('the principal components model') and suggests that familiarity with it is likely to give nurses the confidence to tackle some of the difficulties inherent in undertaking spiritual care. For example, it is recognised that when assessing a client's spiritual needs the nurse must develop a relationship of trust which takes time – the very commodity not always available to busy nurses. If sufficient resources are to be made available to enable nurses to support clients appropriately, it is necessary for the medical practice or other directing 'organisation' to recognise the value of the relationship and to credit as worthwhile the time spent in listening (McSherry, 2006).

The patient's spiritual history is a critical element in the background information that needs to be taken into account when planning nursing care. It ensures an understanding and recognition of the patient's own beliefs and value systems. In particular, religious beliefs and practices are clarified, so that any intervention by the professional is appropriate. By identifying individual spiritual needs the patient is given a clear message of the respect that will be shown in the delivery of the proposed care. Furthermore, significant information may be gathered that sheds light upon the motivation underpinning the patient's behaviour. Such information can provide a useful resource when identifying the patient's support network, with the added potential of identifying the patient's ability to comply with care. Additionally, the information provides a baseline from which the situation can be monitored (Koenig, 2007).

Koenig (2007) suggests a number of criteria to be considered when choosing an appropriate model. Perhaps the most important is that questions should be open and brief, focused upon the beliefs and value systems of the patients and not of the nurses. Hodge (2001) identified this as an important aspect of assessment recognising the value of 'personal and environmental strengths being central to the helping process' (Hodge, 2001: 204). Based upon this premise, Koenig (2007: 44) offers a single question: 'Do you have any spiritual needs or concerns related to your health?' This simple question acknowledges to the patient that this is an area of importance for the professional. At this point, however, one might take issue with Koenig. An individual who is in need of care from a nursing professional almost certainly will have spiritual concerns related to health without necessarily being able to articulate them in such terms in response to a blunt question. By listening to what is said and by hearing what is left unsaid, it is for the professional to tease out the spiritual concerns of the patient.

The use of a mnemonic can provide the nurse with a helpful tool when making an assessment based on a series of questions that explores 'spiritual and religious themes' within an 'empathic dialogue' (Hodge, 2001: 205). The following examples of FICAA (adapted by Koenig (2007: 44) and HOPE (Puchalski, 2002 in McSherry and Ross, 2010: 87) when suited to the linguistic register of the patient could prove to be useful as a mental blueprint:

F—Faith	What is your faith tradition?
I—Important	How important is your faith to you?
C—Church	What is your church or community of faith?
A—Apply	How do your religious and spiritual beliefs apply to your health?
A—Address	How might we address your spiritual needs?

H—Hope	What are your sources of hope, strength, meaning, peace?
O—Organised religion	What role does organised religion have for you?
P—Personal	What is your personal spirituality and does it involve any specific practices?
E—Effects	Does your spirituality affect your decisions regarding medical care?

A more appropriate alternative to taking a spiritual history might be the use of a diagrammatic representation (Hodge, 2001). Genograms and maps as used within the field of family therapy are designed to show psychological and emotional relationships within the family. A genogram can provide a picture of family structure and offers a useful way to organise information (Carter and McGoldrick, 1980). Genograms are also discussed in Chapter 7. Inviting a patient to draw a spiritual genogram or a spiritual map may have a greater appeal than responding to a series of questions. In this way patients can be encouraged to draw a timeline or tree plotting significant spiritual experiences, history, books and events that have added to their spiritual history and development.

Building upon their earlier work in this field, McSherry and Ross (2010) have devised a model for 'actioning spiritual care using a systematic approach' (McSherry and Ross, 2010: 164). See Further Reading for the 'model for actioning spiritual care'.

ACTIVITY 10.4

Action point

Try using the mnemonic FICAA or HOPE with a friend or colleague.

Draw a spiritual genogram, map or tree for yourself detailing your spiritual history and development. Include the significant people, books and experiences that have influenced that development. You may find the following website a useful resource for this activity: www.sociology.org.uk/as4fm3a.doc.

SELF-AWARENESS

Who we are, what we are like and what other people think of us are all questions that relate to our 'self'. We are made up of many parts, 'our bodies, our thoughts, our feelings, our perceptions of ourselves, our beliefs and our actions' (Burnard, 1992: 6). The more we come to know our 'self' – that is, the greater our self-awareness – the more integrated we become as people and the more able we are to offer effective spiritual care.

Gardner suggests that 'practitioners need to be aware of their own spirituality and the assumptions they may make from their own experience' and that 'we are less likely to be able to hear about other people's if we are not aware of our own' (Gardner, 2011: 89). Thus it might be concluded that nurses above all professionals should have a highly developed sense of self-awareness if they are to function successfully.

Reflection is a commonly used term in the education of nursing and provides a useful way to learn about oneself. Much has been written on the subject that is particularly valuable in the development of self-awareness when applied to the richness of experience in nursing practice. Nurses are able to observe the effect they have on patients and the impact of treatment and care. A vital tool in the nurse's repertoire must be the ability to keep feelings and thoughts from private life separate from the issues of the workplace. Although personal experiences can enrich and enhance a nurse's empathy for a patient's situation they should not impinge on decisions taken relating to assessment or care. Rather they should inform and guide responses to situations in practice, especially when approaching a sensitive area such as undertaking a spiritual assessment.

Becoming self-aware, according to Rungapadiachy (1999), is essential to effectiveness and comprises three interrelated perspectives: thinking, feeling and acting. If nurses are to be effective practitioners they need to include patients' spiritual needs when addressing all other aspects of patient care. Therefore, it is essential that they are clear about their own spiritual beliefs and are able to avoid the pitfall of assuming that everyone else thinks about things spiritual in the same way that they do. Nurses who have little understanding of their own spirituality and feel uncomfortable discussing such issues are more likely to avoid conversations concerning a client's spiritual needs, whereas those who are secure in their beliefs are less likely to be uneasy when faced with a patient expressing anxieties about the meaning of life and the loss of a sense of purpose (Burnard, 1992). In a professional situation, a nurse has a duty of care to the patient but it does not include trying to influence or change the beliefs and values of the patient (Burnard, 1992). Spirituality is a very personal matter: individuals reach their own understanding of what it means for them in the context of their own lives.

This was one of the areas of particular interest to be addressed by the RCN and was investigated in an exploration between 'the associations that may exist between religious belief and the RCN members' understandings of spirituality and the provision of spiritual care' (RCN, 2010: 6). Among the conclusions was the statement that 'many of the qualitative responses indicate nurses are acutely aware of the need not to impose their own personal beliefs and values on patients' (RCN, 2010: 27).

However, nurses are in a privileged position and those who have considered their own beliefs and values are more able to help others to think and talk through theirs (Burnard, 1992). While recognising limitations (Gardner, 2011) such self-knowledge gives the nurse the opportunity to be prepared and plan ahead for those situations where clients need to express their fundamental concerns in the face of a crisis of illness. It enables the nurse when providing care for clients and their families to develop the necessary coping skills rather than evasive strategies.

Effective communication with clients is crucial and most nurses would state that they feel very skilled in this area. Furthermore, when challenged most nurses would be able to give examples of how and when they had been successful in communicating with a patient. They might also be able to state with honesty that they had blocked a conversation with a client when they felt the level of disclosure by the client was entering an area in which they were not comfortable. When confronted by a client who might wish to express anger or fear concerning their current situation or to question the ultimate meaning of life, the nurse with a well-founded knowledge of self would be better equipped to respond to the client's needs (Koenig et al., 2001).

Ross et al. (2014) when considering 'spiritual care competency' within nursing found several studies that raised fundamental questions regarding the extent to which spiritual care is indeed influenced by the personal characteristics of the carer. Furthermore, Ross acknowledged the importance of self-awareness and the ability to clarify personal values and beliefs.

Self-awareness is not a state that can be attained completely (Burnard, 1988) but is rather an ongoing journey of enlightenment. Narayanasamy (2006b) undertook an empirical study relating to the impact of spirituality and culture on nurse education. The resulting model incorporates 'communication – verbal and non-verbal; cultural negotiation – being sensitive to and aware of aspects of other people's culture and an understanding of clients' views; establishing respect and rapport and enabling clients to feel culturally 'safe' (Narayanasamy, 2006a: 841). An adaptation of the original model by Ellis and Narayanasamy (2009) offers a valuable approach to the consideration of a nurse's own self-awareness and spirituality in a way that is helpful and open to adaptation (Box 10.2). Thus may a nurse be encouraged to greater confidence when undertaking and identifying a patient's spiritual needs.

Box 10.2 Guideline questions for self-awareness and spiritual nursing

Strengths
- What are my personal beliefs, values, prejudices, assumptions and feelings?
- Am I aware how these might influence the way in which I care for a patient?

Beliefs
- What is the extent of my knowledge and understanding of the rituals and practices of different religious or non-religious beliefs and is it important that I know?

Relationship
- Am I enabling a patient to express their spiritual beliefs?
- Am I providing a supportive and trusting relationship within 'outside' constraints?
- Do I involve other professionals when appropriate to meet the spiritual needs of the patient?

Meaning and purpose
- Do I enable a patient to find meaning and purpose in their illness?
- What is my response to a patient who speaks of fear of the unknown, loneliness or hopelessness?
- These questions are provided as a general guide and can be adapted for use according to individual preference.

(Adapted from Ellis and Narayanasamy, 2009)

For further source/guidance/reading, see 'Exploring Spirituality and Practice' (Gardner, 2011: 92).

If we wish to become more self-aware and therefore more effective practitioners, Rungapadiachy (1999) suggests that there are three layers of self-awareness that we should consider. The first layer is superficial and related to acknowledgement and awareness of our age and our gender. The next layer is more in-depth and is related to those elements of which we need to be aware if we are to be effective, such as our appearance and attitudes and how they affect our behaviour. The third layer is the deepest and represents those issues that are known only to ourselves, our deepest secrets and thoughts.

A way to explore these layers is by means of the Johari window (Luft, 1969, in Smith, 2007: 50). The 'window' comprises four areas of the 'self': open, blind, hidden and unknown. The 'open' area covers what is known to me and to others: feelings, attitudes and behaviours, likes and dislikes. In the 'blind' area is what is not known to me but might be revealed by others: mannerisms or habits of which I am not aware. The 'hidden' area is concerned with those things which I know about myself but would not wish to disclose to others. In the 'unknown' area, there are those aspects of the self which are within my deepest self and not brought to the surface except when unexpectedly triggered by a word or circumstance: for example, a sudden irrational anger felt following a comment made by another (Smith, 2007: 50) (Table 10.1).

ACTIVITY 10.5

Action point

Draw a Johari window and fill in each of the quadrants.

You might wish to discuss your observations with a friend or colleague, particularly noting how your view of yourself differs from that of your friend/ colleague, recognising that your own view may be the one that you think you should have rather than the one that is truly you.

Make notes on what you have learned about yourself and how this is relevant for practice.

NURSING COMPETENCE AND SPIRITUAL CARE

In an extensive study undertaken by Van Leeuwen et al. (2006: 878) a patient noted that it was not possible 'to expect a nurse to be an all-rounder' and questioned 'whether a nurse should be an expert in psychology and religion as well as health care'.

The data for the study were collected from focus group interviews with patients, nurses and hospital chaplains. Certain limitations were acknowledged by the team in that many of the participants were interested in the topic and so were very willing to join the study. In addition, the participants were not culturally or religiously diverse so could not be said to reflect a representative cross section of the population. However, within these limitations some interesting factors emerged that have particular relevance to spirituality and spiritual care.

Table 10.1 Johari window

	Known to self	Not known to self
Known to others	Open area *Example:* This is what I know about myself and what others know of me, for example – I am a nurse and hard working	Blind area *Example:* My friends may have a view of me of which I am unaware. I can uncover these views if others tell me about them. This will increase my 'open' area. For example – my friends may think I do not actively listen to them and I am unaware of this fact.
Not known to others	Hidden area *Example:* This is what I know about myself but hide from others. As I disclose more about myself, within a safe environment, my 'open' area will become larger and I may learn more about myself in the process. For example – I am finding my work very tiring.	Unknown area *Example:* This is the area that is unknown to me and to others. As we tell others more about ourselves and receive feedback this area will decrease in size. We will become more self-aware.

Source: Adapted from Luft (1969) in Smith (2007).

Patients in general required a nurse who could provide good professional skills in physical care. There was also an expectation that the nurse would 'be there' for patients, would have time for them, be sensitive to their needs and would enable them to express emotions. It is interesting to note that in relation to conversations between nurses and patients these frequently started spontaneously and were often initiated by the patients. Of equal importance to these conversations was whether or not the patients and the nurses 'shared the same ideology' and the same 'religious language'. When asked about actions taken in the area of spiritual care, nurses emphasised how important it was that they did not breach the boundary of an individual's personal limits, their own or the patient's. Praying with a patient was found to be acceptable but only at the patient's request and if the nurse felt able to do so. It must be emphasised that nurses should not initiate a process that they cannot then follow through (Van Leeuwen et al., 2006).

Prentis et al. (2014) in considering healthcare lecturers' perceptions of spirituality in education found that 'development of the intellect, emotion and spirit is an essential component of good teaching' and that 'spirituality involves more than subject knowledge; it implies personal development for students and lecturers' (Prentis et al., 2014: 49). This conclusion underlines the values and perceptions already identified in the RCN survey (2010).

It has been established that the goal of spiritual care in nursing is to help patients find meaning and purpose during times of illness. Unfortunately, spiritual care cannot be administered like a dose of medicine but depends on the quality and success of the relationship between the client and the professional. It is for the nurse a privileged situation to be able to support another in a time of distress (MacKinlay and Hudson, 2008: 21).

It has already been concluded that if they are to deliver spiritual care in a professional manner nurses must be competent (Stern and James, 2006). The literature and research on the provision of competencies through education and practice are limited (Baldacchino, 2006: 885). The nurse who wishes to deliver professional spiritual care is required to exhibit the four nursing competencies identified by Baldacchino (2006):

- Role of the nurse as a professional and as an individual person
- Delivery of spiritual care by the nursing process
- Communication with patients, the interdisciplinary team and clinical/educational organisations
- Safeguarding of ethical issues in care

(Baldacchino, 2006: 889)

To assist in the difficult task of delivering spiritual care there is a need to explore Baldacchino's identified competencies in a little more detail, taking first the role of the nurse as a professional and as an individual. Baldacchino's study was undertaken with nurses whose patients had had a myocardial infarction. Some nurses reported that they were prepared and felt competent in their knowledge, both physiological and medical, but did not feel confident or competent to deal with the spiritual aspect of their patients' care. As a result they were more inclined to leave that aspect to the chaplain, especially when a patient had expressed anxieties about life and the life-threatening nature of the illness. Those nurses who considered themselves to be well developed in terms of both their clinical and their life experiences stated that they felt competent in undertaking spiritual care. However, they also indicated that the support of the chaplain was important to them as well as their professional support. On the basis of these findings, there is clearly a need to include in their training an opportunity for nurses to develop their skills to meet the spiritual needs of their patients. MacKinlay (2010: 20) confirms this need when referring to the required sensitivity of nurses when providing spiritual care 'with all its variations according to culture and religion'.

The second competency refers to the delivery of spiritual care by the nursing process.

The use of a structured approach to care has long been advocated within the nursing profession. Certainly, the processes of physiological and medical assessment, planning, implementation and evaluation are relatively straightforward. However, it is more problematic to apply a structured approach when a patient who may be experiencing spiritual distress speaks of fear of the unknown, loneliness or hopelessness. In the study undertaken by Baldacchino (2006), it was found that it was difficult to evaluate the effectiveness of any spiritual care given because patients did not necessarily give feedback to nurses regarding their state of wellbeing. What is possible to evaluate is whether or not nurses were able to spend time developing a trusting relationship with patients listening to their expressed anxieties in a private environment. Here the issues depend upon the communication skills of the nurses and their ability to facilitate strategies or rituals for coping with spiritual dilemmas.

The remaining competencies refer to the involvement of other professionals and the relevant ethical issues of care. The involvement of other professionals, religious or not, at the right time and in the right manner is another sensitive issue (Baldacchino, 2006). A number of nurses in the study reported that they felt it was the role of chaplains to undertake the spiritual dimension of patient care since they did not feel themselves to be sufficiently well prepared. A further difficulty that was reported was how to document a patient's spiritual concerns without breaking the trust and confidentiality that build between a patient and a nurse: a fundamental issue within *The Code of Conduct, Standards and Ethics for Nurses and Midwives* (NMC, 2015). This then becomes an issue of ethics and presents the problem of how much should a nurse 'hand over' to other professionals where the spiritual status of the patient is concerned.

CONCLUSION

The place of spirituality in the holistic care of patients, whether in hospital or in the community, has been an acknowledged fact for a number of years. Information garnered from recent research has emphasised the pressing need felt by nurses for relevant training in spiritual care. Further research will inevitably continue to clarify the issues surrounding the content and provision of such training in future educational programmes.

FURTHER READING

Gardner F (2011) *Critical Spirituality. A Holistic Approach to Contemporary Practice*. England: Ashgate Publishing Company.

McSherry W and Ross L (eds) (2010) *Spiritual Assessment in Healthcare Practice*. Cumbria: M&K Publishers.

O'Brien ME (2014) *Spirituality in Nursing: Standing on Holy Ground*, 5th edn. Burlington, MA: Jones & Bartlett Learning.

Rempel GR, Neufeld A and Kushner KE (2007) Interactive use of genograms and ecomaps in family caregiving research. *Journal of Family Nursing* 13:403–19.

REFERENCES

Baldacchino DR (2006) Nursing competencies for spiritual care. *Journal of Clinical Nursing* 15:885–96.

Burnard P (1988) Self-evaluation methods in nurse education. *Nurse Education Today* 8:4229–33.

Burnard P (1992) *Know Yourself: Self Awareness Activities for Nurses*. London: Scutari Press.

Carter EA and McGoldrick M (eds) (1980) *The Family Life Cycle. A Framework for Family Therapy*. New York, NY: Gardner Press.

Chochinov HM (2006a) Dying, dignity, and new horizons in palliative end-of-life care. *CA: A Cancer Journal for Clinicians* 56:84–103.

Chochinov HM (2006b) In Ellis HK and Narayanasamy A. (2009) An investigation into the role of spirituality in nursing. *British Journal of Nursing* 18:886–90.

Clarke J (2009) A critical view of how nursing has defined spirituality. *Journal of Clinical Nursing* 18:1666–73.

Department of Health (2002) *Guidelines of Chaplaincy and Spiritual Care in the NHS in Scotland*. Edinburgh: Scottish Executive.

Department of Health (2009) *NHS Education for Scotland*. Edinburgh: Scottish Executive.

Ellis HK and Narayanasamy A (2009) An investigation into the role of spirituality in nursing. *British Journal of Nursing* 18:886–90.

Gardner F (2011) *Critical Spirituality. A Holistic Approach to Contemporary Practice*. England: Ashgate Publishing Company.

Hodge DR (2001) Spiritual assessment: A review of major qualitative methods and a new framework for assessing spirituality. *Social Work* 46(3):203–14.

International Council of Nurses (2000) *Code of Ethics for Nurses*. Geneva: ICN.

Jamison CA (2006) *Finding Sanctuary. Monastic Steps for Everyday Life*. Collegeville, MN: Liturgical Press.

Koenig HG (2007) *Spirituality in Patient Care*. Philadelphia, PA: Templeton Foundation Press.

Luft J (1969) *Of Human Interaction*. Palo Alto, CA: National Press.

MacKinlay E (2010) *Ageing and Spirituality Across Faiths and Cultures*. London: Jessica Kingsley Publishers.

MacKinlay E and Hudson R (2008) A review of the literature in 2006. *International Journal of Older People Nursing* 3:139–44.

MacLaren J (2004) A kaleidoscope of understandings: Spiritual nursing in a multi-faith society. *Journal of Advanced Nursing* 45:457–64.

McSherry W (2006) The principal components model: A model for advancing spirituality and spiritual care within nursing and health care practice. *Journal of Clinical Nursing* 15:905–17.

McSherry W and Ross L (eds) (2010) *Spiritual Assessment in Healthcare Practice*. Cumbria: M&K Publishers.

Narayanasamy A (2006a) The impact of empirical studies of spirituality and culture on nurse education. *Journal of Clinical Nursing* 15:840–51.

Narayanasamy A (2006b) *Spiritual Care and Transcultural Care Research*. London: Quay Books.

Neuman B (1995) *The Neuman Systems Model*, 3rd edn. Norwalk, CT: Appleton and Lange.

Nursing and Midwifery Council (NMC) (2015) *The Code: Professional Standards of Practice and Behaviour for Nurses and Midwives*. London: NMC.

Orem DE (1980) *Nursing: Concepts of Practice*. New York, NY: McGraw-Hill.

Peplau HE (1988) *Interpersonal Relations in Nursing*. Basingstoke: Macmillan Education.

Prentis S, Rogers M, Wattis J et al. (2014) Healthcare lecturers' perceptions of spirituality in education. *Nursing Standard* 29(3):44–52.

Puchalski C (2002) In McSherry W and Ross L (eds) *Spiritual Assessment in Healthcare Practice*. Cumbria: M&K Publishers.

Queen's Nursing Institute/Queen's Nursing Institute Scotland (2015) *Voluntary Standards for District Nursing Education and Practice*. London: QNI/QNIS.

Roper N, Logan WW and Tierney AJ (2000) *Roper-Logan-Tierney Model of Nursing: The Activities of Living Model*. Edinburgh: Churchill Livingstone.

Ross L (2006) Spiritual care in nursing: An overview of the research to date. *Journal of Clinical Nursing* 15:852–62.

Ross L, van Leeuwen R, Baldacchino D et al. (2014) Student nurses perceptions of spirituality and competence in delivering spiritual care: A European pilot study. *Nurse Education Today* 34:697–702.

Royal College of Nursing (2010) Executive Summary, Spirituality Survey.

Runcorn D (2006) *Spirituality Workbook: A Guide for Explorers, Pilgrims and Seekers.* Great Britain: SPCK.

Rungapadiachy DM (1999) *Interpersonal Communication and Psychology for Health Care Professionals.* Edinburgh: Elsevier.

Smith JK (2007) Promoting self-awareness in nurses to improve nursing practice. *Nursing Standard* 21:47–52.

Smith M (2004) Nursing in the Community. In *An Essential Guide to Practice*, Chilton S, Melling K, Drew D, and Clarridge A (eds). London: Hodder Arnold Oxford University Press.

Stern J and James S (2006) Every person matters: Enabling spirituality education for nurses. *Journal of Clinical Nursing* 15:897–904.

Sulmasy DP (2009) Spirituality, religion, and clinical care. *CHEST Journal of the American College of Chest Physicians* 135:1634–42.

Tanyi RA (2006) Spirituality and family nursing: Spiritual assessment and interventions for families. *Journal of Advanced Nursing* 53:287–94.

Timmins F, Murphy M, Neill F et al. (2015) An exploration of the extent of inclusion of spirituality and spiritual care concepts in core nursing textbooks. *Nurse Education Today* 35:277–82.

Van Leeuwen R, Tiesinga LJ, Post D and Jochemsen H (2006) Spiritual care: Implications for nurses. *Journal of Clinical Nursing* 15:875–84.

Vanier J (1989) *Community and Growth*. New York, NY: Paulist Press. In Runcorn (2006) *Spirituality Workbook. A Guide for Explorers, Pilgrims and Seekers*. Great Britain: SPCK.

Collaborative working: Benefits and barriers

Sally Sprung and Sue Harness

LEARNING OUTCOMES

• Critically explore the political drivers that influence collaborative working.
• Critically examine the concepts of collaborative working.
• Critically reflect on interprofessional relationships, and consider the challenges that can affect collaborative working.

INTRODUCTION

This chapter examines the relevance of collaborative working from the nursing perspective. Included is a brief outline of the UK political drivers that are influencing health and social care professionals to work in collaboration with an emphasis on understanding core concepts. In order to capture the complexity of this phenomenon, the factors needed for successful collaboration are discussed. To support the learning from this chapter there is a scenario of a patient named Jenny who has been diagnosed with breast cancer with widespread metastases and has recently completed her final chemotherapy treatment. This scenario demonstrates how important it is to work collaboratively with a wide range of health and social care professionals including other agencies to provide the best care for Jenny and her family. The health needs of patients like Jenny are increasing in complexity and the need to work collaboratively to deliver care is crucial to reduce fragmentation and improve positive patient outcomes.

POLITICAL DRIVERS

Although successive governments have recognised the importance of collaborative working and joined-up thinking to improve care, it should be acknowledged that collaboration and team working across the professions is not a new phenomenon. However, the current prominence around the integration of health and social care services signifies the need for collaborative working and consequently the substantial reorientation of professional working practices.

From a historical perspective, since the 1990s, the UK government health and social policies have focused on developing an integrated approach to improving health and tackling health inequalities. A leading aim of 'A Vision for the Future'

(Department of Health, 1995) was targeted towards health professionals and the need to work collaboratively in achieving common goals. The Primary Care Act (Department of Health, 1997) underlined seven areas for action; one of these identified that health and social care professionals including other agencies needed to form effective working partnerships and encouraged collaborative working. Another influential UK government policy was The NHS Plan (Department of Health, 2000), which stimulated the agenda for health and social care professionals to collaborate to reduce fragmented care and improve patient outcomes. One of the overriding criticisms that came out of this fundamental policy was that it described the National Health Service (NHS) as *'old fashioned in its approach to care delivery and organisation'.* In particular, it identified poor team working as a huge contributor to past failings within the NHS. Regrettably, and in spite of these government policies, there were three significant inquiries with the Bristol Royal Infirmary (Kennedy, 2001), Victoria Climbie (Department of Health, 2003) and Baby P (Ofsted, 2008), which all found catastrophic failures in the organisational management of two different clinical areas related to health and social care. Some core recommendations emerged from all three inquiries, including the need for health and social care professionals to have an improved network of communication and an ethos based on teamwork.

The next decade moved towards a UK government wanting to promote principles of choice and control for users within a seamless service (Equity and Excellence: Liberating the NHS, Department of Health, 2010). This policy recognised that patients' care needs are increasingly complex and that no one profession could meet all of these. The government's aim was to provide a genuinely patient-centred service that required health and social care professionals to work collaboratively and as a team. This policy advocated achieving quality and outcomes needed to be *'the best in the world'* (Department of Health, 2010a: 8). This policy recognised that when professionals are committed to working collaboratively in a supportive organisation that empowers its staff then this can overcome obstacles to collaborative working and could lead to less fragmented care and better patient outcomes.

More recently, the agenda for collaborative working is gathering importance. The UK government has aspired to the improvement of the quality of healthcare through encouraging inter-professional collaboration within acts of parliament (Health and Social Care Act, 2012) and policy documents from the four UK nations (Five Year Forward View, Department of Health, 2014; NHS Wales, 2013; Scottish Government, 2014; Department of Health, Social Services and Public Safety, 2012) as integrated care is increasingly being implemented within healthcare services. The focus will be for health and social care professionals to work in partnership in order that services can be co-ordinated around the needs of the patient and family. The UK government is instituting a shift of ambitious changes together with financial investment to improve collaboration among health and social care professionals.

Within the Five Year Forward View (Department of Health, 2014: 6) the policy declared that barriers, which can prevent collaboration, need to be broken down articulating an ambition that

Artificial boundaries need to be broken down between hospitals and primary care, between health and social care and between generalists and specialists—all of which get in the way of care that is genuinely co-ordinated around what people need and want.

The King's Fund responded to the poor co-ordination of services and fragmentation within health and social care with the 'Place-based systems of care' paper (King's Fund, 2015) and argued that providers of services should work together to improve health and social care for the populations they serve. The need to consider the overbearing level of financial deficit that the NHS finds itself means that it will be necessary for organisations to collaborate in order to manage the common resources available to them. From a strategic perspective, Ham (2014) argued that the transformation of primary care services will depend on better collaboration between health and social care professionals to develop integrated care teams which focus on the patient at the centre of care. Earlier, the World Health Organisation (2010) stated their vision that a

> cultural shift is needed in working practices so that health and social care professionals, voluntary agencies and networks may collaborate to reduce fragmentation of care and meet the needs of patients and families.
>
> *(WHO, 2010: 64)*

It is this cultural shift around working practices between different professional groups and voluntary agencies that may act as a constraint and challenges the success of collaborative working. A lack of understanding of others' roles and responsibilities may lead to barriers in collaborative working even when professionals are delivering health and social care to the same patient. The need to communicate and develop a greater understanding is crucial in order that these barriers may be broken down. By enabling all services to work together this may increase the efficiency around the management and delivery of care and lead to positive outcomes for the patient and family.

Increasingly, there is a need to focus on planning and implementing patient-centred care that is seamless, less fragmented and cost effective. The Five Year Forward View (Department of Health, 2014; NHS Wales, 2013; Scottish Government, 2014; Department of Health, Social Services and Public Safety, 2012) requires healthcare professionals to change outdated mind-sets and overcome resistance in working together to achieve common goals for the good of the patient. This will empower others to work collaboratively and actively contribute to ensuring the highest quality of care that can be delivered. Collectively, these visionary policies identify that continuity of care requires health and social care professionals to work collaboratively which is crucial at a time of increased patient demand, complexity of health and care needs, together with the challenge of financial constraints around health and social care budgets.

An understanding of what is meant by collaborative working

Due to the nature of increasing complexity of health problems, it is imperative that all health and social care providers acknowledge and develop new and innovative ways to working collaboratively so that care delivered to patients and service users may be improved. Throughout our working lives there are collective environments with sustained interactions with other health and social care professionals and voluntary agencies. The idea that we share collective action by working towards a common purpose in a supportive trusting environment with other professionals is representative of effective collaborative working.

Henneman et al. (1995: 103) concluded within their concept analysis on collaboration that this was a complex phenomenon and significant to nursing. Makowsky et al. (2009: 169) defined collaborative working as a

> joint communicating and decision-making process with the goal of satisfying the patient's wellness and illness needs while respecting the unique abilities of each professional.

Oandasan et al. (2006) asserted that each health and social care professional needed to combine their efforts and work collaboratively. They acknowledged that resources are scarce and together with an increased workload were crucial to avoid delivering care that was potentially unsafe and staff could be at risk of burnout.

A common thread running through these concepts is that of collective efficacy – that is, a shared objective being the necessity for group members to believe that the combined group efforts are not only necessary to obtain the desired goal but also that each member is capable of and willing to do their share of the work. However, the term collaborative working can often be misinterpreted. Collaborative working is often considered synonymous with other modes of interaction such as co-operation, compromise, teamwork, alliancing, and joint planning, inter-multidisciplinary, inter-professional, multi-agency and intersectoral. This ambiguity has resulted in the term *collaborative working* sometimes being used inappropriately. For example, it is often considered on equal terms as co-operation or compromise, which could be interpreted as having a negative meaning and may actually be counterproductive. If health and social care professionals do not fully understand the concept, this may contribute to a lack of collaboration when working with patients and families.

The concept of collaboration is complex which requires time and energy from all participants. Health and social care professionals need to invest in developing a relationship with members being confident in their own abilities and competent and confident in their level of expertise. Members need to consider each of these themes (Figure 11.1) when beginning to work collaboratively. Crucially, each member needs to respect and value each contribution from the perspective of each discipline to enable collaboration to be successful.

MODELS AND THEORIES OF COLLABORATIVE WORKING

From the definitions in the previous section it is fair to assume that collaborative working is a complex activity with success based upon many factors. Needless to say, there is not one single model or framework that can explain this phenomenon. Gajda (2004: 69) in Figure 11.2 classifies working collaboratively across a continuum of integration by suggesting that the first spectrum of *co-operation* could be seen as weak or

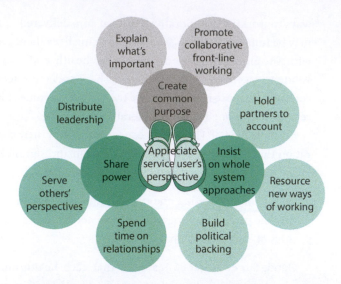

FIGURE 11.1 Collaborative working from the service user's perspective.

Defining strategic alliances across a continuum of integration			
Co-operation	Co-ordination	Collaboration	Co-adunation
Shared information and mutual support	Common tasks and compatible goals	Integrated strategies and collective purpose	Unified structure and combined cultures

Low   Formal integration   High

FIGURE 11.2 System of classification. (From Gajda, R., *American Journal of Evaluation*, 25(1), 65–77, 2004.)

limited progressing through to moderate *co-ordination* and *collaboration* then ultimately strong collaborative working relationships in the form of *co-adunation* where Gajda (2004: 69) implies '*the complete relinquishment of autonomy of at least one partnering entity in an effort to strengthen a surviving organisation*'.

Other models refer to the process of collaborative working by examining the type of partnership within the group as in Figure 11.3 (Gray, 1989: 241).

The model by Pratt et al. (1999: 100) examines different behaviours of partnership working with the horizontal axis representing different goals from an individual to the collective and the vertical axis measuring the extent to which the purpose and the behaviour are needed for success in the form of degrees of predictability (Figure 11.4).

Competition is most appropriate where there is clear consensus on the nature of success. This requires independence from others and motivation by self-interest.

Exploratory	Leads to heightened awareness of interdependence; establishing trust and good faith; clarifying parameters of problem domain
Advisory	Lead to agreement to analyse and agree on options for dealing with a problem
Confederative	Adopt and implement consensual agreements reached by the stakeholders; co-operative exchanges of resources; co-ordination of behaviours
Contractual	Institutionalised; contractual agreements enforceable in law

FIGURE 11.3 Four categories of collaborative arrangements. (From Gray, B., *Collaborating, Jossey-Bass*, San Francisco, CA, 1989.)

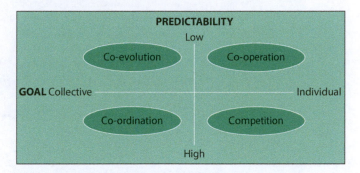

FIGURE 11.4 Model of partnership behaviour. (From Pratt et al., *Working Whole Systems*, King's Fund, London, 1995.)

Co-operation is best, even though organisations are motivated by self-interest, especially where the landscape is rugged and uncertain. Members try to influence each other and perhaps achieve win-win outcomes.

Co-ordination is where solutions are knowable but goals are shared and not individual. Because the strategy is overt and a collective goal must be agreed, various co-ordinating structures are set up. The driving force may be to reduce duplication, pool resources or fit different parts of a service together.

Co-evolution is where the goal is collective but the landscape very rugged which requires new and innovative solutions. Members need to co-design something for a shared purpose. It is not about consensus but lifting the game to a new level where future action is not knowable and the timeframe is convoluted.

Wilson and Charlton (1997: 16) represent five stages within their linear model that in reality may depict groups travelling back and forth through each stage of the process (Figure 11.5).

These models and theories are a sample and are not an exhaustive list as there are many diverse theories to explain collaborative working.

FACTORS FOR SUCCESSFUL COLLABORATION

In order for collaboration to occur there are a number of factors to consider. In the qualitative study by Croker et al. (2012: 19), they recognised that a number of influences and attributes are essential for collaborative working and these provide a

STAGE	ACTIVITIES
1	Partners come together through mutual recognition of a common need, or in a joint effort to obtain public funds.
	If they have not worked together before, the partners begin the process of overcoming differences in backgrounds and approach, building trust and respect.
	There may be a need for training, building each partner's capacity to operate effectively in this new organisation.
2	Through a process of dialogue and discussion, the partners establish the common ground and work towards agreeing on a vision and mission statement for the initiative.
	The original core group might agree on the need to involve more individuals and organisations in the initiative.
	The partners develop mechanisms for assessing needs and quantifying the size of the task they propose to undertake.
	The initiative combines the information generated by the needs assessment excercise with the vision and mission statement to produce and agenda for action.
3	The formal framework and organisational structure of the partnership is designed and put in place.
	The partners set specific goals, targets and objectives linked to the agenda for action.
	Where appropriate, the executive arm of the partnership selects or appoints a management team to oversee the work of the initiative.
4	The partnership delivers to its action plan, whether this be service provision or some other function.
	The executive arm seeks to maintain the involvement of all partners, formulates policy decisions and ensures the continuing accountability of the partnership.
	There is an ongoing process of assessing, evaluating and refining the operations of the partnership.
5	Where appropriate, the partners should plan their exit strategy. This involves developing a new set of goals for the survival and continuation of the work of the initiative in some form.
	They should seek to create 'life after death' by transferring the assets of the partnership back into the community with which they work.

FIGURE 11.5 Stages in the partnership process. (From Wilson and Charlton, *Making Partnerships Work*, JRF, New York, 1997.)

foundation upon which professionals may reflect upon and decide to '*consciously and deliberatively develop their collaborative practice*'. Successful collaboration depends on participants sharing power with values placed on knowledge and expertise rather than on status in a role within the organisation or hierarchy. The value of working in a trusting and honest environment is recognised as facilitating good collaborative working relationships. It is important that the group recognise the collective accomplishments rather than individual effort. Effective communication is essential between participants so that issues can be discussed and debated in order that the plan and delivery of services are agreed so that patients receive the highest quality care.

Collaborative working requires each participant to communicate effectively with each member (Connolly et al., 2010; Rothberg et al., 2011) with trust being an essential component (Magalhães and Fidalgo, 2010). Successful collaboration allows participants to discuss issues, check understanding and share good practice. According to Andvig et al. (2014), this allows each professional to be able to acknowledge each other's roles and responsibilities in order that common goals and decisions are made, which may improve health outcomes for patients and families. Fortune and Fitzgerald (2009) advocate the need for the entire healthcare team to identify and articulate the benefits of working in partnership so that the needs of the patient can be met.

In Figure 11.6, Mattessich and Monsey (1992: 12) identified a model based upon types of factors that influenced the success of collaborative working.

Successful collaborative working is dependent on participants feeling supported within an environment that encourages individuals to share their expertise. A crucial element is that initially each individual needs to be receptive to the idea of working in collaboration. The success of this may depend on each individual's past experience of working closely with other professionals and agencies. From an individual perspective, their own emotional intelligence, confidence in their expertise and maturity in their role together with how other members within the wider team recognise and value their professional input can influence the overall success of collaborative working.

Factors related to the ENVIRONMENT

History of collaboration or co-operation in the community

Collaborative group seen as a leader in the community

Political/social climate favourable

Factors related to MEMBERSHIP CHARACTERISTICS

Mutual respect, understanding and trust

Appropriate cross section of members

Members see collaboration as in their self-interest

Ability to compromise

Factors related to PROCESS/STRUCTURE

Members share a stake in both process and outcome

Multiple layers of decision making

Flexibility

Development of clear roles and policy guidelines

Adaptability

Factors related to COMMUNICATION

Open and frequent communication

Established informal and formal communication links

Factors related to PURPOSE

Concrete, attainable goals and objectives

Shared vision

Unique purpose

Factors related to RESOURCES

Sufficient funds

Skilled convenor

FIGURE 11.6 Factors influencing the success of a collaboration. (Mattessich and Monsey, *Collaboration: What Makes it Work*, Amherst H. Wilder Foundation, St. Paul, MN, 1992.)

CASE STUDY

Jenny Jacobs, a nurse, is 45 years old with newly diagnosed breast cancer with widespread metastases. Her husband Chris is her main carer; he works as a self-employed builder. Jenny and Chris have two children. Luke, aged 14 years, has recently been playing truant from school and complaining of headaches. Each morning, Chris has struggled to get Luke motivated and finds that he is reluctant to go to school.

Lucy, aged 8 years, has always enjoyed school and belongs to a small group of friends. However, her teacher has noticed that Lucy has recently become withdrawn and weepy in class and in the playground.

The family are owner-occupiers of a three-bedroomed semi-detached house. Situated in an urban area, the family have a small group of close neighbours with whom they are friendly. Jenny's parents live over 200 miles away, although Chris's parents live in the next town.

Jenny has completed her final chemotherapy treatment and has been told by her consultant that active treatment is no longer an option available to her.

For the past week, Jenny has complained of severe headaches with some visual disturbances, which have been quite distressing. Jenny has not had much appetite recently and her clothes are becoming quite loose. She is also feeling tired due to not sleeping and is worried for her family.

As the main carer for Jenny, Chris is finding it difficult to cope, both emotionally and financially. He has also found it difficult to support both children, and has recently discovered Luke has been self-harming. Luke appears angry and refuses to talk to his Dad. Chris has not spoken to Jenny about this for fear of upsetting and worrying her further.

The benefits of working collaboratively are well recognised (D'Amour et al., 2005; Lynne et al. 2009; Reeves et al., 2009). This reinforces competence and the value of their contribution to the planning and delivery of care to the patient and family. Successful collaboration can facilitate a win-win situation for the health and social care team and the patient with a sense of accomplishment and job satisfaction that by working collaboratively enriches respect for each other's roles.

THE INTERFACE OF COLLABORATIVE CARE

Jenny, Chris, Luke and Lucy will all have individual health needs. The diverse well-being of multiple-generation family members is rarely delivered by one provider.

Therefore, in managing the healthcare of this family, it is essential to include all the relevant health, social and voluntary services that they may need, which can be identified through ongoing holistic assessment.

The World Health Organization believes that collaboration occurs when 'multiple health workers from different professional backgrounds work together with patients, families, carers and communities to deliver the highest quality of care' (WHO, 2010: 13). The level of intervention provided by health and allied services will depend on the tangible requirements of the personal healthcare needed by the Jacobs family.

Reflection point

Reflect on the case study. What care services do you think Jenny, Chris, Luke and Lucy may require?

The Department of Health (2012) identified the importance of nursing values in interprofessional collaboration. Weis and Schank (2000) indicate a list of such values as the 'hallmark' of professionalism – caregiving, accountability, integrity, trust, freedom, safety and knowledge. In relation to the Jacobs family, these features of professionalism can be used to guide and inform the collaborative process.

Caregiving is about working together for patients. The Nursing and Midwifery Council states that a nurse must 'work in partnership with people to make sure you deliver care effectively' (NMC, 2015).

You may have identified several healthcare providers or *caregivers* required by the family – district nurse, general practitioner (GP), community mental health nurse, health visitor, school nurse, Macmillan nurse, practice nurse, hospital teams and social workers. This list is not exhaustive, however; to maintain a continuity of appropriate care, it is essential for the practitioner to have an awareness of the roles and responsibilities of others required to meet the expectations of an integrated care approach. Carefully matching the patient care requirements to the service provider who can best meet these needs is fundamental to collaborative care management (King's Fund, 2013).

As the clinical care manager, the district nurse is likely to include the GP for advice and support and anticipatory prescriptions for Jenny. The GP will be informed of the progress of all family members but the GP might not necessarily be directly involved in care. Discussions with the health visitor and school nurse will initiate any care needs required by the children, Luke and Lucy. The health visitor might know the family and could provide additional help and support. The school nurse will be able to liaise with teachers and see that the children's wellbeing in the school environment is met. The Macmillan nurse is central to providing advice and support to the multi-professional team involved in an end-of-life episode of care. However, like the GP, the Macmillan team may not necessarily be required to see Jenny and her family. The level of interaction and engagement will vary depending on the requirements of Jenny, Chris and their children. The community mental health nurse can support Chris and Luke (and the wider health team) to enable them to be of assistance in recognising and understanding the difficulties experienced by them.

Accountability is a professional requirement for all personnel involved in the care of Jenny and her family. For example, the district nurse must be able to account for why he or she has involved others in the care of this family. Practitioners are personally accountable for practice and must be able to defend clinical decision making (NMC, 2015; Health and Care Professions Council [HCPC], 2016). It is likely that multiple services will be involved (as listed above); however, the consent of each family member must be sought to enable a good working relationship and constructive interaction to occur.

McDonald and McCallin (2010) recognise that complex scenarios involving the wider healthcare context, of Jenny and her family for example, are the driving force for interprofessional collaboration. Team interactions are required here for effective and efficient patient-centred care to take place as the knowledge and skills of many services will be required.

Appreciation of roles and respect for colleagues are paramount if healthy collaboration is to work (Lemetti et al., 2017). For example, Chris has confided that he is experiencing financial difficulties. He is unable to work because he is the main carer for Jenny. The social worker may be able to assist him to claim for benefits he could be entitled to. During your discussions with Chris, he agrees for you to make a referral. At this point, it would be unwise for you to make any promise or pinpoint a date and time that the social worker would visit as you are unaware of the social worker's priorities and workload. This information can be provided once there has been some dialogue with the social worker involved.

Integrity places the Jacobs family needs first. The family must be able to trust the practitioner with their health and wellbeing. This means treating them as individuals and respecting their dignity when working with others to promote health (NMC, 2015). Jenny will rely on you to access the knowledge and skills of a variety of experts for herself and her family. However, McDonald and McCallin (2010) warn of the risk of the identification of superfluous problems, purely since a collaborative team is accessible. Ongoing holistic assessment will guide the practitioner to make appropriate referrals based on need.

While Jenny's condition is stable, it is useful to examine her wishes for a 'good death'. This requires well-developed communication skills. Impending death is a difficult topic to talk about. This topic can be initiated at an appropriate time when Jenny is ready, and preferably when the conversation can take place in private without interruption. Jenny's hopes, fears, requests and expectations must be respected and documented to inform an advanced care directive. As Jenny's condition deteriorates, it is the role of the practitioner to advocate for Jenny to ensure that her recorded wishes are met (NMC, 2015). *Actions for End of Life Care: 2014–16* (NHS England, 2014) requires all services to work in partnership to respond positively to patients' needs in line with NICE guidelines (NICE, 2015).

Trust involves having a firm belief in the reliability of a person, and in this case Jenny will develop trust in the interprofessional team as long as they demonstrate appropriate and sensitive interpersonal skills and a good communication manner. recognises that partnership working usually occurs within teams. In this scenario, the team is a wider group of people than the community nursing team. Placing the patient and family at the centre of a care plan relies on the patient being involved in the collaborative process at every level.

Veracity and openness form the basis of a good working relationship with patients, within teams and the wider interprofessional team (Beauchamp and Childress, 2012). It is essential that Jenny and her family are kept fully informed and have their questions answered openly and honestly.

Freedom is the quality of not being controlled. Although it is important to provide a firm evidence base to support the care plan designed for Jenny, it is important that she has the freedom to make personal choices (King's Fund, 2013). Collaborating with Jenny means working with her to meet her personal needs, not taking over, and not avoiding sensitive difficult areas of discussion. Decisions should be supported and not made on behalf of patients unless the patient lacks the capacity to make decisions. In this situation, the fourth principle of the Mental Capacity Act (2005) – 'best interests' – will apply, unless an advanced directive has been drawn up. If an advanced directive exists that applies to the situation which has arisen, the advanced directive decision will prevail (Dimond, 2015).

Safety is the key feature for patient care and a shared objective for all involved (Lemetti, 2015). Risks can be obvious or hidden. They can relate to people or environments and can be the result or consequence of acts and omissions. Rigorous risk assessment is essential to maintain the wellbeing of Jenny and her family. It is also required to safeguard the visiting services who may be involved in the care of Jenny and her family. All healthcare providers are bound by policy and guidance to minimise risk and promote safety (NMC, 2015; HCPC, 2016). For example, if any risks are identified that may pose harm, this information must accompany the referral made to other services.

There are known risks associated with chemotherapy. The practitioner can provide advice and support for Jenny in relation to this. Additionally, vulnerable visiting staff must be aware of any issues that may pose a hazard or risk, for example, to a pregnant member of staff. As Jenny's disease process progresses, it is vital that the risk assessment is evaluated and updated along with the care plan. Any changes will need to be disseminated to all those involved in visiting the Jacobs family.

Knowledge is the theoretical or practical understanding of a subject. In relation to Jenny and her family, it applies to the utilisation of widely accepted evidence-based practice performed by a variety of professional and allied healthcarers. All direct clinical interventions, advice, support and education must be evidence based and from a valid and reliable source (Ellis, 2016). When working with patients like Jenny, sometimes they access information online that may not be from a recognised reliable source. In this context, the practitioner must encourage the use of widely accepted reliable information sources such as NHS direct; however, they are still obliged to maintain a non-judgemental attitude if the patient chooses to use a non-evidence-based remedy that claims to be a miracle cure. They are not, however, obliged to administer any lotion, potion or any other treatment that is not prescribed by a doctor or nurse prescriber. When patients make such requests, this should be clearly documented in the care plan along with any advice given. This will safeguard the patient and guide other staff visiting the family (NMC, 2015; HCPC, 2016).

SKILLS NEEDED TO COLLABORATE EFFECTIVELY

Healthcare context drives interprofessional collaboration with referrals made to others' services, usually as the result of a holistic health needs assessment. Collaboration therefore is purposive. It is a process that produces the result that no single service provider could achieve autonomously (Lemetti, 2015).

Communication is an essential component of collaboration (Lord Laming, 2003). Poor communication between services and personnel was cited as a fundamental flaw by Lord Laming, who reported on the Victoria Climbié inquiry. Communication was also highlighted as a vital factor for collaborative working by Lord Francis (2013) who investigated failings in healthcare in Mid Staffordshire. During this inquiry, *Compassion in Practice: Nursing, Midwifery and Care Staff – Our Vision and Strategy* (Department of Health, 2012) was published to set out an approach for high-quality compassionate care built on a set of six enduring values and behaviours known as the 6Cs. Each of these values and behaviours shares equivalent significance when working with patients.

The six fundamental values – The six Cs (6Cs)

- Care
- Compassion
- Competence
- Communication
- Courage
- Commitment

(Department of Health, 2012)

In 2015, the regulator for Nursing and Midwifery published *The Code: Professional Standards of Practice and Behaviour for Nurses and Midwives* (NMC, 2015). The new set of standards puts the interests of patients first under four key headings.

The Code – The four Ps (4Ps)

- Prioritise people
- Practice effectively
- Preserve safety
- Promote professionalism and trust

(Nursing and Midwifery Council, 2015)

ACTIVITY 11.2

Considering your role as a community nurse – how do the 6Cs from the *Compassion in Practice* document relate to the 4Ps from the NMC *Code of Professional Standards of Practice and Behaviour for Nurses and Midwives*?

Sharing information with other services requires that we send and receive information; yet, communication is a multifarious concept. The two-way sharing of information can be face to face, but as teams and services are generally widely geographically spread, health professionals liaise in a face-to-face context less frequently. They increasingly rely on information technology where the interpersonal nature of verbal cues and body language are lost. Four dimensions of communication were described by Cox and Hill (2010) as:

- *Mechanistic* – Transmitted where interpersonal skills are not required. However, this method is reliant on clear verbal or written information being provided for accurate interpretation by the recipient.
- *Psychological* – Emotionally charged dialogue that is written or spoken where emotive language can make clarity less factual and less objective.
- *Social constructivism* – Where the same problem can be interpreted in different ways, depending on the area that the health professional is working. Different priorities emerge as the health professionals involved interpret the need of the patient within the commissioning framework of their specific service delivery.
- *Systemic* – How communication is provided by an organisation, and within an organisation. Often there are differences in the way in which information is cascaded and shared both within an organisation and to other organisations and services.

ACTIVITY 11.3

In considering the care services required by Jenny, Chris, Luke and Lucy in the last exercise, now think about how those services will communicate with each other.

Using the four dimensions of communication discussed in the last paragraphs, examine how these dimensions are used by health professionals providing care for the Jacobs family.

Preceding sections of this chapter have discussed why healthcare professionals are required to work collaboratively, what it means to collaborate and with whom we are required to work. This section is about the skills required to collaborate effectively. Using the case study of Jenny, Chris, Luke and Lucy, scenarios will be drawn out to demonstrate the range of skills that are fundamental to effective collaboration.

COLLABORATIVE ATTITUDES

Collaboration is a word used widely in nursing and healthcare. Attitudes of those involved in team working can influence the collaborative process. Key attitudinal skills can make or break the sustenance and progression of a successful shared care episode. Clarridge and Ryder (2004) describe these professional attributes as relational skills.

Relational skills include readiness, willingness and trust, and these are thought to be the basic skills required for collaborative work (Pavord and Donnelly, 2015). However, an expansion on these core skills can include other communication features such as the following:

- *Listening* – Ensures understanding and is a requirement for both parties. Listening and checking that you have understood fully the information conveyed to you can help to reduce conflict and aggressive behaviours.
- *Use of suitable language* – Is a requirement from all responsible healthcare providers to ensure that communication is made in such a way that patients, other professionals and carers understand the information provided. Understanding each other is essential.
- *Respect* – Is also a requirement of all therapeutic relationships. Expressing opinions, the use of humour and making disclosures are all facets of communication that involve showing respect.
- *Fairness* – Is a feature of any good relationship. One example of when therapeutic communication requires the use of fairness is when the nurse or healthcare professional must refuse an unreasonable request.
- *Sensitivity* – Is required when supporting and managing patients and families who are anxious or distressed.
- *Empathy* – At the end of life is warmth of sympathy that enables patients, families and carers the opportunity to discuss their feelings, beliefs and attitudes in an open and honest way.
- *Courtesy* – Is required when there is confrontation and the nurse or healthcare provider is required to communicate in a professional manner.
- *Honesty/openness* – Aids the nurse/patient relationship and requires the healthcare provider to display genuineness in their approach towards developing a therapeutic relationship.

ACTIVITY 11.4

In terms of nurse–patient relational skills, what factors do you think contribute to the issues raised in the following scenario?

Jenny discovers that a lesion on her breast that she thought was a pimple has developed into a wound that is leaking odorous fluid. She tells the district nurse. The district nurse assesses the wound and tells Jenny that the wound is unlikely to heal and it will need to be re-dressed every day. During a subsequent outpatient appointment, another nurse tells Jenny that her breast is fungating and it is likely that the 'smell' could become a problem. Jenny becomes distressed and later in the day she rings the district nurse and indicates that she has had enough and wants to 'end it all'.

The district nurse visits Jenny and during their conversation reassures her that the wound can be managed to maintain her comfort and dignity. Jenny seems much happier with this information and advice.

You may have considered that the outpatient department nurse has provided too much information. However, this information may have been given in response to Jenny asking questions (Leadership Alliance for the Care of Dying People, 2014). Conversely, while maintaining good relational skills with patients, the nurse could have contacted the district nurse (as Jenny's care manager) to alert her to the sensitive nature of the conversation the nurse had had with Jenny.

All of these characteristics are required for the development and maintenance of professional relationships with patients, carers, healthcare professionals and organisations allied to health (Riley, 2015).

Although it is wholly appropriate to be open and honest, there is always the need to be sensitive and empathetic. Also, the use of therapeutic language can cause alarm to patients and perhaps if the word 'fungating' had been replaced with more suitable language, the distress caused to Jenny may have been minimised (Riley, 2015). However, both nurses work in different settings. Each will have a different job description, yet both will be working within the same professional code and striving to meet the same goals in meeting patients' needs. Therefore, there must be respect for the roles and responsibilities of others and relational skills apply to professional relationships, too (NMC, 2015; HCPC, 2016).

CONCLUSION

This chapter has offered an insight into the nature of collaborative working and how the scenario highlights that the delivery of care to patients can often be complex. It recognises that individual healthcare professionals involved in the scenario will use different skills but share a common goal of providing a comprehensive service tailored to meet the needs of the patient and family. The success of collaborative working will require that individuals must be able to acquire a vision and to develop common goals.

Policy initiatives and the needs of those who use services and resources will continue to steer the collaborative working agenda. In order for new policies to operate effectively they need the commitment of healthcare professionals to work collaboratively together with the ability to critically evaluate practice and work in partnership with patients and service users.

Critically evaluating your understanding of collaborative working within your practice and how this can be incorporated will help you to become an effective practitioner.

REFERENCES

Andvig E, Syse J and Severinsson E (2014) Interprofessional collaboration in the mental health services in Norway. *Nursing Research and Practice*. (Accessed 1 June 2016) doi:10.1155/2014/849375.

Beauchamp T and Childress J (2012) *Principles of Biomedical Ethics*, 7th edn. Oxford: Oxford University Press.

Clarridge A and Ryder E (2004) Working collaboratively. In Chilton S, Melling K, Drew D, and Clarridge A (eds) *Nursing in the Community: An Essential Guide to Practice*. London: Hodder Arnold.

Connolly M, Deaton C and Dodd M (2010) Discharge preparation: Do healthcare professionals differ in their opinions? *Journal of Interprofessional Care* 24(6):633–43. (Accessed 1 June 2016) http://content.ebscohost.com/ContentServer.asp?T=P&P=AN-&K=54098920&S=R&D=a9h&EbscoContent=dGJyMNLe80SeqK84yOvqOLCmr06ep7BSsqu4SLOWxWXS&ContentCustomer=dGJyMPGptkqyqLRMuePfgeyx44Dt6fIA.

Cox CL and Hill MC (2010) *Professional Issues in Primary Care Nursing.* Chichester: Wiley-Blackwell.

Croker A, Trede F and Higgs J (2012) Collaboration: What is it like?—Phenomenological interpretation of the experiencing of collaborating within rehabilitation teams. *Journal of Interprofessional Care* 26:13–20. (Accessed 1 June 2016) http://content. ebscohost.com/ContentServer.asp?T=P&P=AN&K=70231046&S=R&D=a9h&EbscoCo ntent=dGJyMMTo50SeqLA4yOvqOLCmr06ep69Ssqi4S7KWxWXS&ContentCustome r=dGJyMPGptkqyqLRMuePfgeyx44Dt6fIA.

D'Amour, Ferrada-Videla M, San Martin Rodriguez L, Beaulieu MD (2005) The conceptual basis for interprofessional collaboration: Core concepts and theoretical frameworks. *Journal of Interprofessional Care* 19 Suppl., 1:116–31.

Department of Health (1995) *A Vision for the Future.* London: HMSO.

Department of Health (1997) *National Health Service Primary Care Act.* London: HMSO. (Accessed 1 June 2016) https://www.gov.uk/government/uploads/system/uploads/ attachment_data/file/266003/newnhs.pdf.

Department of Health (2000) *The NHS Plan: A Plan for Investment, a Plan for Reform.* London: HMSO. (Accessed 1 June 2016) http://webarchive.nationalarchives.gov. uk/20130107105354/http://www.dh.gov.uk/prod_consum_dh/groups/dh_digitalas-sets/@dh/@en/@ps/documents/digitalasset/dh_118522.pdf.

Department of Health (2003) *The Victoria Climbie Inquiry: Report of an Inquiry by Lord Laming.* London: HMSO. (Accessed 1 June 2016) https://www.gov.uk/government/ uploads/system/uploads/attachment_data/file/273183/5730.pdf.

Department of Health (2010) *Equity and Excellence: Liberating the NHS.* HMSO: London. (Accessed 1 June 2016) https://www.gov.uk/government/uploads/system/uploads/ attachment_data/file/213823/dh_117794.pdf.

Department of Health (2012) *Compassion in Practice: Nursing, Midwifery and Care Staff Our Vision and Strategy.* Leeds: DH/NHS Commissioning Board.

Department of Health (2014) *Five Year Forward View.* London: NHS England. (Accessed 1 June 2016) https://www.england.nhs.uk/wp-content/uploads/ 2014/10/5yfv-web.pdf.

Department of Health, Social Services and Public Safety (2012) *Living with Long Term Conditions.* (Accessed 22 July 2016) https://www.health-ni.gov.uk/sites/default/files/ publications/dhssps/living-longterm-conditions.pdf.

Dimond B (2015) *Legal Aspects of Nursing,* 7th edn. Harlow: Pearson Education.

Ellis P (2016) *Evidence-based Practice in Nursing,* 3rd edn. London: Learning Matters.

Fortune T and Fitzgerald MH (2009) The challenge of interdisciplinary collaboration in acute psychiatry: Impacts on the occupational milieu. Australian Occupational Therapy 56(2):81–8. (Accessed 1 June 2016) http://content.ebscohost.com/Content-Server.asp?T=P&P=AN&K=37183898&S=R&D=a9h&EbscoContent=dGJyMNLe80Seq K84yOvqOLCmr06ep7FSrq64TbSWxWXS&ContentCustomer=dGJyMPGptkqyqLRM uePfgeyx44Dt6fIA.

Francis R (2013) *Report of the Mid Staffordshire NHS Foundation Trust Public Inquiry.* London: The Stationary Office.

Gajda R (2004) Utilising collaboration theory to evaluate strategic alliances. *American Journal of Evaluation* 25(1):65–77.

Gray B (1989) *Collaborating.* San Francisco, CA: Jossey-Bass.

Ham C (2014) *Reforming the NHS from Within: Beyond Hierarchy, Inspection and Markets.* London: King's Fund. (Accessed 1 June 2016) http://www.kingsfund.org.uk/time-to-think-differently/publications/reforming- nhs-within.pdf.

Health and Care Professions Council. (2016) Standards of conduct, performance and ethics. (Accessed 26 July 2016) http://www.hcpc-uk.org/assets/documents/10004EDFSt andardsofconduct,performanceandethics.pdf.

Health and Social Care Act (2012) *Health and Social Care Act.* http://www.legislation.gov.uk/ukpga/2012/7/pdfs/ukpga_20120007_en.pdf

Henneman EA, Lee JL and Cohen JI (1995) Collaboration a concept analysis. *Journal of Advanced Nursing* 21:103–9. (Accessed 1 June 2016) http://content.ebscohost.com/ContentServer.asp?T=P&P=AN&K=107405987&S=R&D=rzh&EbscoContent=dGJyM NLe80SeqK84yOvqOLCmr06ep7BSs6q4Sq%2BWxWXS&ContentCustomer=dGJyMP GptkqyqLRMuePfgeyx44Dt6fIA.

Kennedy I (2001) *Learning Form Bristol: The Report of the Public Inquiry into Children's Heart Surgery at the Bristol Royal Infirmary* 1984-1995. London: The Stationary Office. (Accessed 1 June 2016) http://webarchive.nationalarchives.gov.uk/20090811143745/http:/www.bristol-inquiry.org.uk/final_report/the_report.pdf.

King's Fund (2013) *Delivering Better Services for People with Long-Term Conditions. Building the House of Care.* London: King's Fund.

King's Fund (2015) *Place-based Systems of Care: A Way Forward for the NHS in England.* (Accessed 1 June 2016) http://www.kingsfund.org.uk/sites/files/kf/field/field_publication_file/Place-based-systems-of-care-Kings-Fund-Nov-2015_0.pdf.

Leadership Alliance for the Care of Dying People (2014) *One Change to Get It Right.* (Accessed 26 July 2016) https://www.gov.uk/government/uploads/system/uploads/attachment_data/file/323188/One_chance_to_get_it_right.pdf.

Lemetti T, Voutilainen P, Stolt M, Eloranta S, Suhonen S (2017) An enquiry into nurse-to-nurse collaboration within the older people care chain as part of the integrated care: A qualitative study. *International Journal of Integrated Care* 17(1): 1–11, DOI: https://doi.org/10.5334/ijic.2418.

Lord Laming (2003) *The Victoria Climbié Inquiry: Report of an Enquiry by Lord Laming.* (Accessed 26 July 2016) https://www.gov.uk/government/uploads/system/uploads/attachment_data/file/273183/5730.pdf.

Lynne B, Sinclair MA, Lorelei A, Lingard PhD, Ravindra N, and Mohabeer, PhD (2009) What's so great about rehabilitation teams? An ethnographic study of interprofessional collaboration in a rehabilitation unit. Archives of *Physical Medicine and Rehabilitation* 90: 1196–1201.

Makowsky MJ, Schindel TJ and Rosenthal M (2009) Collaboration between pharmacists, physicians and nurse practitioners: A qualitative investigation of working relationships in the inpatient setting. *Journal of Interprofessional Care* 23:169–84. (Accessed 1 June 2016) http://content.ebscohost.com/ContentServer.asp?T=P&P=AN&K=3-7154729&S=R&D=a9h&EbscoContent=dGJyMNLe80SeqK84yOvqOLCmr06ep7FSr6q 4SLGWxWXS&ContentCustomer=dGJyMPGptkqyqLRMuePfgeyx44Dt6fIA.

Mattessich PW and Monsey BR (1992) *Collaboration: What Makes it Work.* St. Paul, MN: Amherst H. Wilder Foundation.

McDonald C and McCallin A (2010) Interprofessional collaboration in palliative nursing: What is the patient-family role? *International Journal of Palliative Nursing* 16:285–8.

McInnes S, Peters K, Bonney A and Halcomb E (2015) An integrative review of facilitators and barriers influencing colaboreation and teamwork between general practitioners and nurses working in general practice. *Journal of Advanced Nursing* 7(199):1973–85.

Mental Capacity Act (2005) London: Department of Health, The Stationery Office.

NHS England (2014) *Actions for End of Life Care: 2014-2016.* Leeds: NHS England.

NHS Wales (2013) *Delivering Local Health Care: Accellarating the Pace of Change.* (Accessed 22 July 2016) http://gov.wales/docs/dhss/publications/131101planen.pdf.

NICE (2015) *Care of Dying Adults in the Last Days of Life.* (Accessed 26 July 2016) https://www.nice.org.uk/guidance/ng31/resources/care-of-dying-adults-in-the-last-days-of-life-1837387324357.

Nursing and Midwifery Council (2015) *The Code: Professional Standadrds of Practice and Behavior for Nurses and Midwives.* London: NMC.

Oandasan I, Baker GR, Barker K et al. (2006) *Teamwork in Healthcare: Promoting Effective Teamwork in Healthcare in Canada* (Accessed 24 June 2016) http://www.cfhi-fcass.ca/Home.aspx.

Ofsted (2008) *Report into the Death of Baby P in the London Borough of Haringey.* London: Ofsted. (Accessed 1 June 2016) http://dera.ioe.ac.uk/10510/1/Baby_Peter_report_FINAL_12_May_09_(2).pdf.

Pavord E and Donnelly E (2015) *Communication and Interprofessional Skills.* Banbury: Lantern Publishing.

Pratt J, Gordon P and Plampling D (1999) *Working Whole Systems.* London: King's Fund.

Reeves S, Zwarenstein M, Goldman J, Barr H, Freeth D, Hammick M, and Koppel I. (2009) Interprofessional education: Effects on professional practice and health care outcomes (review). *Cochrane Database Systematic Reviews* 1:1–21.

Riley J (2015) *Communication in Nursing,* 8th edn. Missouri: Elsevier.

Rothberg MB, Steele JR, Wheeler J et al. (2011) The relationship between time spent communicating and communication outcomes on a hospital medicine service. *Journal of General Internal Medicine* 27(2):185–9. doi: 10.1007/s11606-011-1857-8. (Accessed 1 June 2016) http://content.ebscohost.com/ContentServer.asp?T=P&P=AN&K=2-1922161&S=R&D=mnh&EbscoContent=dGJyMNLe80SeqK84yOvqOLCmr06ep7FSsKq4SLOWxWXS&ContentCustomer=dGJyMPGptkqyqLRMuePfgeyx44Dt6fIA.

Scottish Government (2013) *Everyone Matters: 2020 Workforce Vision.* http://www.gov.scot/Resource/0042/00424225.pdf.

Scottish Government (2014) *Health & Social Care Information Sharing—A Strategic Framework*: 2014–2020. (Accessed 22 July 2016) http://www.gov.scot/Resource/0046/00469375.pdf.

Weis D and Schank MJ (2000) An instrument to measure professional nursing values. Journal of Nursing Scholarship 32:201–4.

Wilson A and Charlton K (1997) *Making Partnerships Work.* New York, NY: JRF.

World Health Organization (2010) *Framework for Action on Interprofessional Education and Collaborative Practice.* (Accessed 26 July 2016) http://apps.who.int/iris/bitstream/10665/70185/1/WHO_HRH_HPN_10.3_eng.pdf?ua=1.

CHAPTER 12

Approaches to acute care in the community

Nicola Brownie

LEARNING OUTCOMES

- Explore the spectrum of conditions that might be considered acute in community care.
- Discuss and analyse theory and assessment tools required to support the community nurse caring for acute conditions.
- Identify and rationalise the skills required to support the community nurse caring for acute conditions.
- Recognise pharmacology knowledge and interventions to manage acute conditions.
- Discuss the concept and elements related to discharge planning and avoiding hospital admission.

INTRODUCTION

The aim of this chapter is to examine approaches to managing acute care in the community. Current healthcare policy drivers within the four UK countries highlight the desire to continue to expand the delivery of care within the community (Department of Health, 2014; Scottish Government, 2013, 2015; Department of Health, Social and Public Safety, 2011; Welsh Assembly Government, 2010). To achieve this vision, further and indeed continued development of community nursing is required to reach its fullest potential of service delivery, and this includes the use of technology, which is discussed further in Chapter 18 (Maybin et al., 2016; QNI/QNIS, 2015; Royal College of Nursing, 2013; Department of Health England, 2013).

Traditionally 'acute care' depicts how and where specialised healthcare is provided in the case of emergency situations or care as a result of referral for further investigation, surgical intervention, complex tests or other care, that historically has not been delivered or available in the community setting. Treatment was continued until the individual was well enough to be supported and cared for in the community again (Naylor et al., 2015). The shifting balance of care to the community setting as highlighted in policy requires this definition of acute care to be reconsidered and to consider acute care within community-based services, including the home setting. For the purpose of this chapter acute care in the community refers to a short episode of care for a new condition or an exacerbation of an existing long-term condition.

ACUTE CARE IN THE COMMUNITY SETTING

In many areas realignment of the current mind-set pertaining to the degree of acute care that was traditionally delivered in the hospital setting transferring to the community setting is required. Chapter 1 considered the community environment and the services required to deliver person-centred care. While government policy is explicit in its aim to deliver acute care in the community, much of the literature around moving care closer to home is in the grey literature rather than influenced from research studies (Scottish Government, 2016). However, governments are investing in a number of models of care to support moving healthcare into the community (Department of Health, 2014), and to prevent unplanned admissions to hospitals for acute episodes of illness or injury. It is envisaged that these initiatives will provide an evidence base for further redesign of future services.

Complexities of care needs delivered within the community setting are increasing and intensifying. In response to managing this group of patients effectively, the skills set of the community nurse must reflect this to meet service demands (Maybin et al., 2016; Edwards, 2014). Recognition must be given to the enormity of caring and managing complex patients within the community setting. It comes without the safeguard of a controlled environment as within a hospital setting (Royal College of Nursing, 2013); therefore, having staff with the appropriate skillset is pivotal.

Traditionally the responsibility of diagnosing and developing the management plan for acute episodes of care in the community has been with the general practitioner (GP), or alternatively the individual has sought care in the hospital setting, such as with an accident and emergency for a minor injury or minor illness. However, more recently it has been recognised that nurses and other health professionals have a potential role in managing episodes of acute care (Scottish Government, 2015, 2016; Department of Health, 2014).

In some areas 'hospital at home' services have been developed which refer to the delivery of an episode of care that traditionally would have been carried out within the hospital setting taking place at home. To enable this delivery of care to occur a consultant or equivalent specialist, for example, a GP with a special interest oversees and is responsible for the management of the patient, similarly, to the management of patients within the hospital setting. The multidisciplinary team will comprehensively assess and co-ordinate the delivery of hospital level care within the home setting (NHS Education for Scotland, 2016) and many would suggest that this could be co-ordinated within district nursing services with adequate resource (Royal College of Nursing, 2013). However, there are other community services and settings such as community hospitals, general practices, community pharmacies, schools, urgent care centres and out of hours care that could also be involved in the delivery of acute care (Naidoo and Wills, 2016; Royal College of Nursing, 2014).

ACUTE CARE IN THE HOME SETTING

To support the effective delivery of community services in line with the forementioned policy drivers the Royal College of Nursing (2013) devised three domains of care within district nursing practice: end-of-life care at home, complex care at home and acute care at home. The conceptual framework (Figure 12.1) adapted from Royal College of Nursing (2013) illustrates these elements.

Acute care at home can only be successfully implemented fully when the appropriate infrastructure has been embedded to support the delivery of acute care and the development of staff. Therefore, within the umbrella of acute care, it is important to consider healthcare systems and their ability to deliver within this remit (Royal College of Nursing, 2013). The boundaries of acute care delivery within the community will continually change as dictated by healthcare policy relevant to the needs of the service; therefore, it can be challenging for healthcare systems to keep up (Hewison, 2009). Nevertheless, an element of the professional role within practice is to question current practices and the impact on patient care, identifying gaps in care and developing concise and articulate evidence-based outlines as to how the gap can be addressed (Crumbie, 2008).

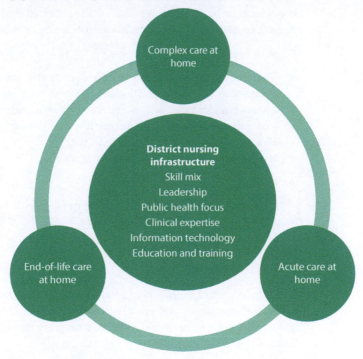

Figure 12.1 Three domains for effective care delivery. (From Royal College of Nursing, *District Nursing: Harnessing the Potential, The RCN's UK Position on District Nursing*, London, 2013.)

ACTIVITY 12.1

Reflection point

As a nurse working in the community, reflect upon your experiences of individuals who have presented as acutely unwell, but whose illness was not considered as life threatening. Then consider the necessary infrastructure within the framework above to manage their acute care at home:

• Do you have the required clinical leadership skills?

• Do you possess clinical expertise/advanced assessment skills to assess, diagnose and manage acute care?

- Is there an effective skill mix within your team to support the management of acute care?
- What opportunities are there to promote health and well-being when managing acute care at home or in other community settings?
- What information technology is available in your area to support your role?
- Do you have access to education and training to support your development?

SHORT EPISODE OF CARE FOR A NEW CONDITION

CASE STUDY

Reflect on the following scenario:

Mrs Smith is normally fit and well, she lives at home with her husband whom she cares for as he has Parkinson's disease. She attended the health centre and was diagnosed with a deep vein thrombosis (DVT) and commenced on to anticoagulants.

On your first visit to her,

- What knowledge and skills can you identify that would be required to assess and manage this patient's illness?
- What is your knowledge and understanding of anticoagulants?
- What are the risks of such treatment?
- What health education may be required?
- Review local and national treatment guidelines.

As her husband's main carer,

- What impact will this diagnosis have in relation to her ability to care for him?
- What psychological support may they need?
- Which members of the multi-disciplinary team can help to support this couple?
- Who leads the care delivery?

Initially, Mrs Smith is in a lot of pain which you have assessed using a validated pain assessment tool, and you discover that she is not taking the analgesia prescribed while in hospital as it makes her very drowsy and unable to help her husband.

- What tool could you use to ensure holistic pain assessment is completed?
- How does a patient's pain score help determine the level of analgesia required?
- Which types of analgesics are required when a patient has severe pain?

Discussion point
Discuss with your pharmacist:

- The range of opiate drugs available
- Which have less sedative effects
- How to safely manage renally impaired patients' analgesia

EXACERBATION OF A DISEASE

Nurses working in the community are often working with individuals who have one or more long-term conditions. These conditions often have the potential to develop an acute exacerbation in the community setting. Table 12.1 adapted from Information Service Division Scotland (2016) provides some examples.

Anticipatory care planning to avoid acute exacerbations

Purdy (2010) states that it is pivotal to distinguish which admissions are avoidable potentially, if adequate interventions are put into place to support the patient through the use of anticipatory care planning. With increasing pressures on the

Table 12.1 Conditions that have the potential to become an acute condition in the community setting

Women's health	Cancer	Chronic pain	Depression
Chronic obstructive pulmonary disease (COPD)	Cellulitis	Multiple sclerosis	Chronic kidney disease
Chest pain	Pyrexial child	Minor injuries	Thyrotoxicosis
Non-specific abdominal pain	Occluded lines	Hepatitis	Urinary incontinent
Respiratory tract infections	Catheters and feeding tubes	Hearing loss	Alcoholic liver disease
Minor head, neck and back injuries	Eye infections	Haemorrhoids	Arrhythmias
Pain	Skin and mouth	Glaucoma	Spina bifida
Asthma	Nausea and vomiting	General ear disease	Visual impairment
Cardiac disease	Deep vein thrombosis	Epilepsy	Inflammatory bowel disease
Arthritis	Epilepsy	Chronic fatigue syndrome	Hypertension
Mental health problems	Diabetes	Blood disease	Ulcer
Alzheimer's/dementia	Chromosomal disorders including Down's syndrome	Allergies	Warfarin therapy
Cerebrovascular	Hypothyroidism	Anaemia	Malnutrition
Joint disorders	Human immunodeficiency virus (HIV)	Bronchiectasis	Osteoporosis and bone metastases
Endocrine disorders	Obesity	Prostate hyperplasia	Diverticular disease
Drug and alcohol misuse	Osteomyelitis	Chronic tonsil disease	

Source: Information Service Division Scotland, http://www.isdscotland.org/index.asp, 2016.

National Health Service (NHS) because of increasingly complex patients with multiple co-morbidities, an aging population and funding limitations, advanced planning of care has become particularly topical. Approximately 20%–30% of emergency admissions may have been avoided had there been better management of their care prior to their admission (Health Foundation, 2013). This statistic highlights the need for effective anticipatory care planning.

The ethos of anticipatory care planning to look ahead and forward plan care was referred to in Chapter 13 looking at emerging issues in long-term conditions. Antcipatory care planning is most commonly completed for patients with long-term conditions or end-of-life care to identify at an early stage, any circumstances which may have a negative impact on their health or long-term conditions and to help avoid acute exacerbations (Baker et al., 2012).

The anticipatory care plan evolves through good communication, collaborative working and shared decision making with the patient to create a dynamic record. Contained within the plan are preferred responses, interventions and actions to be carried out in the presence of a clinical deterioration, crisis in care provision or circumstance. The plan needs to be reviewed on a regular basis to reflect changes in well-being, wishes or provision of care (Scottish Government, 2011).

ACTIVITY 12.2

Discussion point
Consider patients within the community whose medical condition has the potential to develop an acute exacerbation.
- Identify the pathophysiology of the illness and what happens during an exacerbation phase.
- Consider which assessment approach you would undertake to assess the patient.
- Reflect on your current knowledge and skills set and identify areas you wish to develop.
- Have you seen or are you using anticipatory care plans?
- Are they effectively updated to reflect changing circumstances?
- Do they support and empower patients?

CASE STUDY

Daniel Manson is 71 years old and has chronic obstructive pulmonary disease (COPD). He has experienced two episodes of an infective exacerbation of his COPD in the last 6 months; both episodes resulted in hospital admissions. He lives at home with his wife, both of whom are normally independent. They have three children, none of them or their families live local.

Consider the following:
- Who should be involved in developing the anticipatory care plan?
- How are the risk factors/circumstances that may cause deterioration/crisis identified?

CASE STUDY

- How familiar are you with the pathogenesis of COPD?
- How is the anticipatory care plan communicated and shared effectively between varying healthcare professionals?
- How often should they be reviewed and by whom?
- How can the effectiveness of the anticipatory care plan be assessed?

Daniel's condition deteriorates over time in line with the trajectory of disease and he enters the terminal phase of his illness.

Consider the following:

- Who should be involved in the review of the anticipatory care plan?
- Do additional healthcare professionals/agencies factor into the plan?
- How is the updated plan communicated?
- How often should it be reviewed now?

DETERIORATING PATIENTS

Acute care can also refer to care delivered in cases of sudden and frequently unanticipated deterioration in patients where an illness or injury has occurred creating an emergency scenario. Without rapid intervention there is high probability of disability or death (Hirshon et al., 2013). Therefore, an urgent assessment must be undertaken to determine the full extent of the presentation and the care needs of the patient (Clarke, 2016). The success rates of rapid intervention to improve health and well-being are mainly time sensitive and stress the importance of performing a rapid yet efficient assessment of the patient.

Successes in acute care are achieved when reversible factors are identified during assessment and interventions implemented as soon as possible within the realms of competency and capabilities (Nursing and Midwifery Council, 2015), treating the most significant threat to life or limb first and continuing in order of priority.

It is imperative to stress that while managing a patient during an acute presentation, technology is not always essential initially while stabilising a patient (Hirshon et al., 2013). This is especially significant in the community setting when a nurse may be a lone worker or visiting with limited equipment.

ACTIVITY 12.3

Discussion point
- What equipment does a community nurse have while undertaking visits?
- Considering the complexity of patients now being managed within the community is this sufficient?
- What do you consider to be essential items?
- If change is required how can you address or facilitate this?

NURSING ASSESSMENT IN ACUTE CARE

The importance of a holistic nursing assessment and decision making has been discussed in an earlier chapter. The significance of this should not be underplayed. Assessment is a complex process that requires knowledge and skills of the nurse to interpret findings and give meaning in relation to patient care. The nursing assessment has a direct impact on patient safety and well-being and when done ineffectively can lead to delivery of suboptimal care (National Institute for Health and Care Excellence, 2016).

It is also important that community nurses have expertise in managing care across the lifespan as discussed in Chapter 6 and are cognisant of the anatomical and physiological variances. Nurses require a good understanding of anatomy and physiology of the human body relevant to their specific role within the community team, and should have or be developing consultation, physical and psychological assessment and history-taking skills.

When presented with an acute situation and/or deteriorating patient a systematic approach to assessment is vital. A detailed approach initially is inappropriate for acutely unwell patients and indeed may be detrimental to their well-being. Lifesaving rapid assessment and intervention are required thus treating the patient before holistic assessment and diagnosis are complete (Douglas et al., 2013). It is acknowledged that this is in direct opposition to traditional theories of nursing assessment and can be initially challenging.

ACTIVITY 12.4

Discussion point
Identify assessment approaches that are conducive to apply within an acute assessment scenario.
• What are the advantages of this approach?
• What are the weaknesses of this approach?

The palliative/provoking, quality, radiation, severity, timing (PQRST) symptom analysis mnemonic outlines a framework by which to structure questioning during an acute situation (Macaluso and McNamara, 2012) (Table 12.2).

THE ABCDE APPROACH

A rapid and decisive approach must be utilised to determine the cause of a patient's deterioration and identify interventions that can be implemented in an attempt to stabilise their condition. Therefore, it is essential to think critically while undertaking assessment and diagnosing to deliver immediate management. Critical thinking relates to the ability to consider all possible options and outcomes within a scenario, including from other people's perspective (Standing, 2010). Coupled with clinical judgment, the application of information obtained from actual observation of a patient in conjunction with subjective and objective data leads to a conclusion (Mosby, 2008). This can be difficult to achieve during an acute episode when presented with a deteriorating patient. It is during such a scenario that reassurance can be obtained from utilising an assessment framework such as the ABCDE approach (Figure 12.2).

Table 12.2 Summary of the PQRST mnemonic

P	**Provocation/palliation** What initiates, starts or causes it? What helps, improves or makes it better? What does not help or makes it worse?
Q	**Quality and quantity** How does it feel, look or sound? How much is there?
R	**Radiation** Where is it? Does it spread?
S	**Severity** Does it interfere with activities? Rate the severity on a scale – mild, moderate, severe
T	**Timing** When does it begin? How often does this happen? Is it sudden or gradual?

ACTIVITY 12.5

Action point

During a visit to an individual you are nursing in the community utilise the PQRST mnemonic:

- How easy was it to utilise?
- Did it enhance the structure of your questioning?
- Did it impact on the information gleaned from the patient?
- Would you utilise this approach again?
- What were the strengths and weaknesses of this approach?

The Resuscitation Council's ABCDE approach provides a systematic and generic method of assessment utilised by all healthcare professionals (Resuscitation Council, 2015). It provides a logical system of assessment that allows the most significant threats to well-being to be identified first and interventions commenced immediately. The undoubted strength of the ABCDE approach is it remains the same regardless of patient presentation or suspected cause. It can be employed irrespective of grade or experience within clinical assessment and activation of interventions within the realms of competence (Nursing and Midwifery Council, 2015). During the ABCDE assessment establishing a diagnosis is not required. The whole ethos of the assessment is to intervene at any and every stage during the assessment when an abnormality has been detected in an attempt to reverse the situation.

Anticipating any medical emergency by recognising unsafe deviations out with safe parameters allows help to be summoned, thus improving quality of care. This approach relies on the healthcare professional utilising this system of assessment having a robust knowledge and understanding of anatomy, physiology and physiological parameters. Without this it would be unsafe to interpret findings and commence

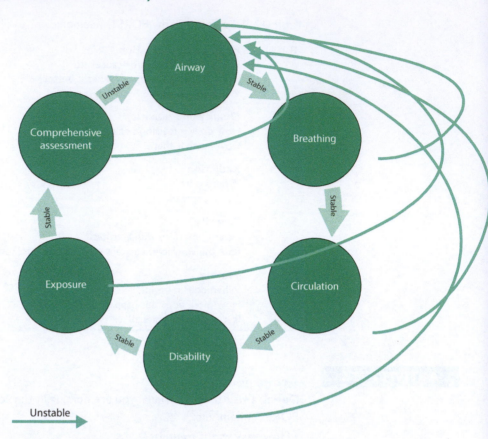

Figure 12.2 ABCDE assessment framework.

Action point
Is your current knowledge and understanding of anatomy and physiology adequate to enable you to safely undertake and interpret findings of an ABCDE assessment?

If not, what do you need to do to achieve this?

treatment. This approach is most apt allowing for rapid prioritising of treatment to stabilise patients (Impact, 2010).

Underlying principles of ABCDE approach

The approach to all deteriorating or critically ill patients is the same. The underlying principles are as follows:

1   Use the airway, breathing, circulation, disability, exposure (ABCDE) approach to assess and treat the patient.
2   Do a complete initial assessment and re-assess regularly.
3   Treat life-threatening problems before moving to the next part of assessment.
4   Assess the effects of treatment.

5   Recognise when you will need extra help. Call for appropriate help early.

6   Use all members of the team. This enables interventions (e.g. assessment, attaching monitors, intravenous access) to be undertaken simultaneously.

7   Communicate effectively – use the situation, background, assessment, recommendation (SBAR) or reason, story, vital signs, plan (RSVP) approach.

8   The aim of the initial treatment is to keep the patient alive, and achieve some clinical improvement. This will buy time for further treatment and making a diagnosis.

9   Remember – it can take a few minutes for treatments to work, so wait a short while before reassessing the patient after an intervention.

(Resuscitation Council, 2015)

The ABCDE approach should be utilised and continued until the patient is deemed stable. At this time, it would be appropriate to commence a comprehensive assessment to aid a differential diagnosis and construct a management plan. Should the patient begin to deteriorate again, then the ABCDE approach must be recommenced until such time as the patient stabilises again or help has arrived to support.

AIRWAY

Commencing with an assessment of the patient's airway, any obstruction of the airway is an emergency situation and expert help should be sought immediately. This is a life-threatening scenario as the patient is at high risk of cardiac arrest, hypoxia, acute kidney injury and death.

Signs of airway obstruction – The airway can be assessed using the look, listen and feel method:

Look

- Airway obstruction causes paradoxical chest and abdominal movements ('see-saw' respirations) and accessory muscles usage during respiration. A late sign of airway obstruction is the presence of central cyanosis.
- The mouth should be assessed for any physical obstruction such as foreign body, blood, vomit, swelling or secretions.
- Reduced level of consciousness often leads to airway obstruction in a critically ill patent due to depression for the central nervous system.

Listen

- In complete airway obstruction, there are no breath sounds at the mouth or nose.
- In a partial airway obstruction, air oasis:entry is diminished and frequently noisy.
- Although noisy breathing can be frightening to hear and distressing to observe, remember no sound at all is far more sinister. The airway is completely occluded, your patient has stopped breathing and has gone into respiratory arrest. When noisy breathing is evident, such as stridor then air is partially shifting and therefore the patient is experiencing a partial occlusion of the airway. This remains an emergency scenario and expert help is required immediately.

Feel

- To establish whether there is any movement of air place your cheek or hand next to the patient's nose and mouth.

(Resuscitation Council, 2011)

Any airway obstruction is a medical emergency and therefore expert help should be summoned immediately. An untreated airway obstruction has serious consequences: hypoxaemia with the risk of hypoxic injury, cardiac arrest and ultimately death.

Interventions

The majority of airway obstructions can be resolved with simple airway opening manoeuvres such as head tilt, chin lift. Suctioning should be considered and the insertion of an oropharyngeal or nasopharyngeal airway. Should these interventions be unsuccessful then intubation may be required (Resuscitation Council, 2015).

Oxygen therapy should be administered via an oxygen reservoir bag at 15 litres/minute aiming for oxygen saturations of 94%–98%. Oxygen can then be titrated down once the patient has stabilised, with a view to maintaining oxygen saturations between 94% and 98%. Critically ill patients at known risk of hypercapnia, due to established disease should also aim to be maintained with oxygen saturation of 94%–98% initially (Resuscitation Council, 2015).

Only when the airway is stable can the assessment progress to the next stage.

ACTIVITY 12.7

Discussion point

Mr Cameron is a known type 1 diabetic patient who is poorly controlled due to compliance issues. On arrival at his home to reassess his venous ulceration you find him in his bed and he has a reduced level of consciousness.

- How confident are you at assessing airway?
- What manoeuvres can you undertake to open an airway if compromised?
- What airway adjuncts would you have with you?
- Why does the airway become compromised in patients with reduced levels of consciousness?

BREATHING

Breathing can be assessed using the look, listen and feel method:

Look

- Is the patient showing signs of respiratory distress: use of accessory muscles, skin colour, distress, sweating, central cyanosis, abdominal breathing, patient position, nasal flaring, pursed lips, elevated jugular venous pressure (JVP)?
- Does the patient have a reduction in the level of consciousness?
- Check immediate surroundings for any aids or adjuncts: oxygen, inhalers, nebulisers.

- Does the patient have any chest deformity, scarring, signs of trauma or chest drains?

Listen

- Is the breathing pattern noisy, laboured, wheezy, rasping?
- Is the patient able to communicate in full sentences?

Feel

- Establish whether there is any movement of air by placing your cheek or hand next to the patient's nose and mouth.
- Is the patient hot and sweaty, cool and clammy?

(Resuscitation Council, 2011)

Assessing rate and depth of breathing is one of the easiest observations to record yet one that is frequently omitted. A patient who suddenly becomes tachypneic is alarming as breathing is frequently the first clinical observation to become impaired within a deteriorating patient. Breathing is therefore a good clinical indicator warning of an adverse event (NPSA, 2007; NICE, 2007).

Breathing must be measured for 1 minute, in addition to determining the number of breaths the depth and pattern of breathing should also be assessed. Any added sounds such as wheeze or stridor, presence of cough need to be considered (Woodrow, 2012). The percentage and rate of any supplementary oxygen in situ need to be factored into the assessment (SIGN, 2014).

When available a pulse oximeter should be utilised to measure SpO_2. Care should be taken when fitting the probe to ensure the area it is being attached to is warm and well perfused. Fingers and earlobes are commonly used sites; however, a deteriorating patient may have peripheral cyanosis which will impact on the accuracy of the result (Jackson, 2016). Percussion and auscultation of the chest should be undertaken, if within competencies and capabilities to assess for presence of fluid, consolidation, reduced or absent air oasis:entry (Resuscitation Council, 2015).

Interventions

Oxygen therapy should be administered via an oxygen reservoir bag at 15 litres/minute aiming for oxygen saturations of 94%–98%. The oxygen can be titrated down once the patient has stabilised with a view to maintaining oxygen saturations between 94% and 98% (British Thoracic Society, 2016). If the rate of breathing and/or depth is not stablised with this intervention, then bag-mask ventilation must be used to support the patient until expert help arrives or the patient stabilises (Resuscitation Council, 2011).

Patient positioning can also help to enhance oxygenation and whenever safe to do so patients should be nursed upright to optimise lung expansion. This may not be possible depending on their level of consciousness or intervention required (Jackson, 2016).

If the patient deteriorates then return to 'airway' and recommence the ABCDE assessment.

ACTIVITY 12.8

Discussion point

Having secured Mr Cameron's airway, you assess his breathing.

• How confident are you at assessing breathing?

• What position should patients be nursed in if breathing is compromised?

• What equipment would you have with you to help manage a breathing difficulty?

• How should individuals with COPD be managed in relation to oxygen therapy and target oxygen saturations?

CIRCULATION

Circulation can be assessed using the look, listen and feel method:

Look

• Note the colour at the patient's peripheries: pale, blue; pink.
• Assess their veins: are they collapsed or underfilled?
• Is there a reduction in the level of consciousness?
• If a urinary catheter is in situ look at urinary output.
• Are there signs of haemorrhage?

Listen

• Is the patient alert and orientated?
• Is the patient in pain?

Feel

• Assess the temperature of the patient's hands and feet; are they hot or cool?
• Assess the peripheral pulse, noting rate, rhythm and volume.
• Measure blood pressure.
• Measure capillary refill time.

Assessment

While measuring the peripheral pulses it is important to assess the rate, rhythm and volume of the pulse. A bounding pulse could be indicative of sepsis while a faint pulse could be due to reduced cardiac output (Resuscitation Council, 2015).

The systolic pressure measurement is the most significant while obtaining a blood pressure reading. It is used during the assessment phase as it is reputed to be the more reliable marker of well-being. It is important to recognise that blood pressure can appear normal in the presence of shock due to the body's compensatory mechanisms and be cognisant of this.

Discussion point
What are the main causes of hypotension?
• Considering preload, myocardial contractility and afterload

Capillary refill time (CRT) is ascertained by applying enough pressure to cause blanching of the skin using a fingertip for 5 seconds at approximately heart level. The length of time it takes for the skin to return to its normal colour after the release of pressure equates to the CRT. A normal value for CRT is less than 2 seconds, prolonged CRT is indicative of poor peripheral perfusion (Jevon and Ewens, 2012).

Urinary output is another crucial indicator, a urinary catheter should be inserted when there is concern regarding diminishing urinary output to allow for accurate monitoring. Consider whether the cause is pre-renal, renal or post-renal as highlighted below:

Pre-renal: Is there an adequate blood pressure or cardiac output?

Renal: Have the kidneys been poisoned?

Post-renal: Is there obstruction to the flow?

(Huether and McCance, 2016)

The main reason for a reduction in cardiac output occurs from a loss in circulating volume; therefore, it is imperative to assess for haemorrhage both externally and internally. Prolonged or severe diarrhoea and vomiting can also account for fluid loss leading to hypovolaemic shock if extensive enough (Huether and McCance, 2016). Hypovolaemia must be considered the primary cause of shock, within the vast majority of surgical and medical emergencies until proven otherwise (Resuscitation Council, 2015).

Interventions

Treatment specifics depend upon the cause of the reduction in cardiac output; however, initial interventions should be targeted at fluid replacement, control of any haemorrhage and tissue perfusion repair (Huether and McCance, 2016), intervening urgently with the most significant threats to life and well-being first.

A wide-bore cannulae(s) should be inserted if there is no venous access and routine blood scan should be drawn prior to the commencement of a fluid challenge(s). An initial bolus of 500 mL of warmed crystalloid solution (e.g. 0.9% sodium chloride) should be administered in the presence of hypotension, with an infusion rate of less than 15 minutes. If the patient is known or suspected to have cardiac failure, then a reduced volume of 250 mL is recommended. Close monitoring is essential to observe for fluid overload by auscultating the chest after each bolus.

Regular monitoring of the patient's pulse and blood pressure is required to determine whether the intervention(s) are effective. The goal is to restore blood pressure to normal or a systolic greater than 100 mm Hg. The fluid bolus should be repeated if there is no improvement in blood pressure and then reassessed. Intravenous fluids should be reduced in rate or discontinued if there are any concerns of cardiac failure (Resuscitation Council, 2015).

ACTIVITY 12.10

Discussion Point
• How would you measure the effectiveness of a fluid challenge (bolus)?

If the patient deteriorates then return to 'airway' and recommence the ABCDE assessment.

DISABILITY

Disability can be assessed using the look, listen and feel method:

Look

• Examine the size of the patient's pupils, checking for symmetry.
• Is there a reduction in the level of consciousness?
• Check immediate surroundings for any aids: blood glucose monitoring machine, insulin pens, alcohol, drugs – prescribed and illicit.
• Is there any asymmetry within the body, in particular the face and limbs?

Listen

• Is the patient orientated to time and place and coherent?

Feel

• Is the patient hot and sweaty, cool and clammy?

Assessment

An assessment of a patient's conscious level can be quickly and efficiently completed using the AVPU score:

    A – Alert

    V – Responsive to verbal stimuli

    P – Responsive to painful stimuli

    U – Unresponsive

If a patient is able to respond to you fully he or she is scored 'A' for alert. When the patient is able to respond after you verbally give him or her a command, for example, 'open your eyes for me' (always use the patient's name while doing so to maximise the chance of him or her responding), this would be a 'V' score. If a patient requires painful stimuli to respond this is scored 'P'; no response at all would score 'U'. Any patient achieving a 'P' or a 'U' score has an altered state of consciousness (Royal College of Physicians, 2015).

The Glasgow Coma Scale (GCS) is a more comprehensive system of assessment which can be utilised once the acute phase of assessment has been completed to provide further clarity of any deficits (Teasdale, 2014).

Check whether the patient has taken their prescribed drugs correctly – has there been any illicit drug use? Even when prescribed drugs have been taken correctly consideration should be given to drug toxicity and whether any are reversible (Resuscitation Council, 2015).

Intervention

Hypoglycaemia is a common cause of reduced conscious levels and must be discounted or treated during an ABCDE assessment. Local NHS policy should be followed to treat hypoglycaemia, initially 50 mL 10% glucose solution administered intravenously. Patients who are unconscious or have a reduced level of consciousness are unable to maintain their airway independently and therefore should be nursed in the lateral position. The main concern is the high risk of aspiration due to the loss of gag reflex (Resuscitation Council, 2015).

If the patient deteriorates then return to 'airway' and recommence the ABCDE assessment.

ACTIVITY 12.11

Discussion point

Mr Cameron is found to have a blood glucose level of 2.8 mmol/L on testing and although he has reduced levels of consciousness he is able to eat and drink:

- How confident are you at treating a hypoglycaemic episode?
- What resources do you have with you to enable you to manage this episode?
- Which food group snack should be given to patients after blood glucose increases initially to maintain blood glucose levels?
- If the patient had been unable to eat or drink how would you have managed this episode?

EXPOSURE

A full top to toe examination of the patient should be undertaken while maintaining dignity to assess for any clues or reversible causes to the patient presentation.

Exposure can be assessed using the look, listen and feel method:

Look

- The patient should be observed for any signs of a rash, discolouration, oedema, distension, injury, bleeding and abnormalities. Care needs to be taken to minimise heat loss during the assessment (Jevon and Ewens, 2012).

Listen

- Is the patient complaining of any pain, swelling, itch, discomfort, abnormality?

Feel

- Does the patient generally feel too hot or cold?
- Is there an area of localised heat, swelling, distension? Were both sides compared for symmetry?

Assessment

A patient's temperature needs to be obtained to determine the presence of a pyrexia or hypothermia. A pyrexia greater than 41°C can lead to convulsions and be fatal, whereas hypothermic temperatures of less than 32°C can lead to cardiac arrhythmia (Huether and McCance, 2016).

Intervention

Blood cultures should be obtained when pyrexia is present and greater than 38.3°C (NICE, 2016).

If the patient deteriorates then return to 'airway' and recommence the ABCDE assessment.

If the patient remains stable, then documentation can be completed and a comprehensive examination undertaken to establish a differential diagnosis and ongoing management plan.

ACTIVITY 12.12

Discussion point

During another visit Mr Cameron is found to have elevated blood glucose levels and is facially flushed and his skin is hot to touch. His temperature is 38.5°C:

- How confident are you at assessing exposure?
- What equipment would you have with you?

You discover that he has a pyrexia and on completion of a top to toe observation you notice an area of ulceration to his left shin which looks clinically infected:

- How would you manage this presentation?
- Are you able to take blood cultures? If not who can and how fast is this required?
- When should antipyrexials be administered?

Now that ABCDE has been described you may wish to explore this further and access:

(https://www.resus.org.uk/resuscitation-guidelines/)

Red flags

Good knowledge of pathology and clinical presentation allows for recognition of significant clinical findings more commonly referred to as *red flags*. The presence of such findings during history taking and/or clinical examination should trigger 'alarm bells' within the practitioner to the potential possibility of significant pathology. An urgent referral or escalation of care should be initiated as a matter of priority (Nuttal and Rutt-Howard, 2016).

Considering your patients and frequently seen presentations,
• Identify what you would consider red flags.
• What is the significance in terms of health and well-being?
• Who would you inform and/or refer the patient to?

COMMUNICATION STRATEGIES TO MANAGE ACUTE EPISODES OF CARE

Poor communication is frequently cited within NHS complaints, yet there are a small number of tools to support the delivery of effective verbal communication. Situation, background, assessment, recommendation (SBAR) is a communication tool to aid the effectiveness of conversations during a critical scenario. It provides a framework consisting of four sections to ensure that pivotal information is shared in a timely manner, thus fostering a culture of patient safety (NHS Institute for Innovation and Improvement, 2010) (Figure 12.3). This framework empowers staff to communicate assertively and effectively in a logical manner.

Pain assessment

However painful and unwanted a sensory experience pain is, it is essential to our well-being. The presence of pain indicates the occurrence of an injury or disease. Without this indicator of something being amiss irreversible and fatal damage

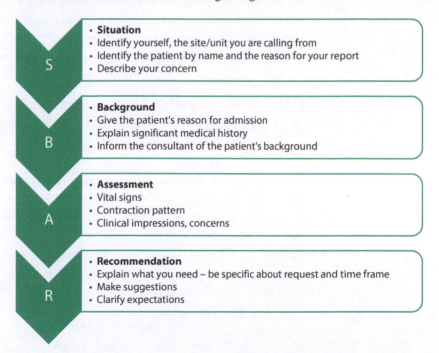

S
• **Situation**
• Identify yourself, the site/unit you are calling from
• Identify the patient by name and the reason for your report
• Describe your concern

B
• **Background**
• Give the patient's reason for admission
• Explain significant medical history
• Inform the consultant of the patient's background

A
• **Assessment**
• Vital signs
• Contraction pattern
• Clinical impressions, concerns

R
• **Recommendation**
• Explain what you need – be specific about request and time frame
• Make suggestions
• Clarify expectations

Figure 12.3 SBAR Communication Tool. (Adapted from NHS Institute for Innovation and Improvement, SBAR Situation-Background-Assessment-Recommendation. http://www.institute.nhs.uk/quality_and_service_improvement_tools/quality_and_service_improvement_tools/sbar_-_situation_-_background_-_assessment_-_recommendation.html, 2010.)

CASE STUDY

Miss Parker has had a history of COPD for 5 years; she has requested a visit as she has not been feeling well since last night. She states that she is struggling to breathe and feels hot.

Prior to arriving at the house to review Miss Parker what preparatory work could you complete in preparation for the visit?

On arrival at the house Miss Parker is clearly struggling to breathe.

- What visual clues would there be when a patient's breathing is compromised?
- What other clues can the immediate environment provide as to how she has been managing?

You undertake an ABCDE assessment to establish the extent of the presenting condition.

- What would you expect to find within each stage of the assessment?
- What interventions could you commence?
- Consider how you would communicate your assessment findings using the SBAR communication tool.

would occur. An episode of acute pain is indicative of an acute injury or disease compromising the body that requires acute intervention to resolve (Huether and McCance, 2016). It is imperative that a patient has their pain proficiently assessed and adequate analgesia prescribed and administered in a timely manner. Uncontrolled pain can contribute to a traumatic experience for patients that will impact and influence their ability to cope with future episodes of pain.

SOCRATES is a pain assessment framework (Table 12.3) which encompasses a variety of factors to establish a holistic pain assessment (Banicek, 2010). The

Table 12.3 Summary of SOCRATES mnemonic

S	**Site** – Where is the pain?
O	**Onset** – When/how did the pain start (e.g. sudden, gradual)?
C	**Character** – Describe the pain (e.g. dull ache, sharp stabbing).
R	**Radiation** – Does the pain move anywhere?
A	**Associations** – Any symptoms/signs associated with the pain?
T	**Timing** – How has the pain changed over time?
E	**Exacerbating/relieving factors** – Does anything worsen/relieve the pain?
S	**Severity** – How bad is the pain on a scale of 0–3 (no pain, mild, moderate, severe)?

ACTIVITY 12.14

Reflection point

Recall an episode or episodes of pain you have had either personally or related to a patient where the pain was difficult to control or was not controlled:

• What implications could this have about coping with a recurrence of pain in the future?

• How does it impact on a patient's coping mechanisms?

Physiological changes also manifest when pain is uncontrolled or poorly uncontrolled and have a detrimental effect on well-being and recovery.

Action point

• How many physiological changes can you identify that may occur due to poorly controlled pain?

• What is the relevance of this in relation to well-being?

• Review the symptoms that inadequate pain relief can cause.

All of the factors noted above can have a significant negative impact on the clinical outcome of an acutely unwell patient by placing the body under more stress.

Now utilise the SOCRATES mnemonic while undertaking a pain assessment with one of the individuals you nurse:

• Consider how well you could apply the mnemonic.

• Consider the information obtained from the patient and how this influenced management.

• Consider in relation to how you used to assess pain, if there is any difference.

• What are the strengths and weaknesses of using this in practice?

outcome of this assessment will provide the rationale for analgesic prescribing and can provide clues as to the nature of the ongoing presentation.

Pain control

The desire for patients to receive appropriate analgesics and effective pain control during an episode of pain is not a new phenomenon. As far back as 1996 the World Health Organization (WHO) recognised the importance of effective pain relief in cancer pain. The pain ladder was created in an attempt to guide and standardise prescribing practice and care received. Although devised within the field of cancer care, the principles of the pain ladder can be applied to any individual in pain. The ladder provides a stepwise approach to the level of analgesic required measured against the pain score (Figure 12.4).

PHARMACOLOGY KNOWLEDGE AND INTERVENTIONS

Medicine management is an integral element of nursing practice. It is imperative to have a comprehensive understanding of pharmacology to ensure safe management of medications (NMC, 2015). Patients within the community setting do not have the opportunity to remain under constant observation of a healthcare

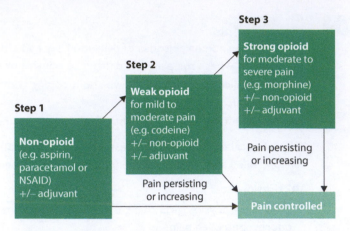

Figure 12.4 World Health Organization (1996) pain relief ladder.

ACTIVITY 12.15

Reflection point
Recall an episode or episodes of pain you have had either personally or related to a patient where the pain was difficult to control or was not controlled.
• What implications could this have about coping with a recurrence of pain in the future?
• How does it impact on a patient's coping mechanisms?

professional (Nuttall and Rutt-Howard, 2016). Therefore, it is essential that the community nurse is competent and can maintain safe medication practice, promoting and monitoring maintenance of adequate and safe drug levels in the body (NMC, 2015).

One of the most influential additions to the nurses' role in the community has been the introduction of nurse prescribing. The Cumberlege Report in 1986 identified ineffective ways of working and a significant wastage of hours by community staff to obtain a prescription for patients (Department of Health and Social Security, 1986). Initially prescribing was limited to safeguard patients, and the (Department of Health, 1989) Crown Report dictated how it could occur. A successful change of legislation in 1992 the Medicinal Products: Prescription by Nurses Act gave nurses the ability to prescribe in a wider context.

In 1999, the evolution of nurse prescribing continued with the publication of another Crown Report, Review of Prescribing, supply and administration of medicines which extended the prescribing responsibilities afforded to non-medical prescribers. In 2012, changes to the Misuse of Drug Regulations enabled a nurse prescriber to prescribe controlled drugs, except for prescribing in addiction unless within the prescriber's area of expertise (Department of Health, 2012).

Nurse prescribing can be undertaken within two different formats, independent and supplementary prescribing.

Independent prescribing

Independent prescribing enables a practitioner to independently assess patients with undiagnosed and diagnosed conditions to conclude a diagnosis and devise a management plan, which may or may not lead to the generation of a prescription within their area of practice and competence. This may be from a limited formulary according to the scope of your practice (NMC, 2015). Any form of prescribing should only be completed within the realms of capability and competence.

Supplementary prescribing

Supplementary prescribing enables a voluntary tripartite partnership between the patient, independent prescriber and supplementary prescriber working cohesively to agree to a clinical management plan. Within this partnership the independent prescriber retains accountability and responsibility for diagnosing and prescribing decisions (Nuttall and Rutt-Howard, 2016).

Gaining a non-medical prescribing qualification helps to facilitate nurses to extend their role and scope of practice. Furthermore, this can lead to a redesign of service and innovative ways of working. It is useful for all nurses working in evolving and developing roles and service to acknowledge and recognise skills and knowledge they bring. It is essential for all nurses to undertake continued professional development (CPD) in order to develop and maintain currency of their knowledge of recommended pharmacological regimes, development, manipulation and review of management plans and completion of a recognised prescribing course (NMC, 2015).

ACTIVITY 12.16

Reflection point
Reflect on and identify any personal knowledge deficits and develop an action plan to identify how you will access and achieve the knowledge and skills required to facilitate safe and competent patient management of medication in order to manage acute care in the community.
* Self-assess your current knowledge base of pharmacology.
* What is your understanding of pharmacokinetics and pharmacodynamics?
* Describe the processes of absorption, distribution, metabolism and excretion.
* What disease processes and factors affect how medications interact with the body's physiology?
* Reflect on how being a nurse prescriber can enhance your practice.

CONCLUSION

An acute episode can dramatically alter the whole dynamics of care needs. In summary, community nursing continues to evolve in responses to policy drivers, service provision and type and acuity of the patients cared for in the community. Improving practice is an essential component of practice, and as a practitioner the individual has a responsibility to remain up to date and continue to strive to push the boundaries to enhance the patient experience and outcomes (Department of Health, 2010). It is imperative that practitioners deliver evidence-based practice, while acting as a positive role model to others (Royal College of Nursing, 2014). The role of the community nurse is dynamic, challenging and rewarding; however, it is vital that the practitioner adheres to the requirements as dictated within the governing code of conduct, is a lifelong learner and is always aware of their limitations (Nursing and Midwifery Council, 2015).

REFERENCES

Baker A, Leak P, Ritchie LD et al. (2012) Anticipatory care planning and integration. *British Journal of General Practice* 62:e113–20.

Banicek J (2010) How to ensure acute pain in older people is appropriately assessed and managed. *Nursing Times* 106(29):14–7.

British Thoracic Society (2016) *Guideline for Emergency Use Oxygen in Adult Patients*, 2nd edn. London: British Thoracic Society.

Clarke D (2016) The importance of nursing assessment in acute care. In Clarke D and Maleccki-Ketchell A (eds) *Nursing the Acutely Ill Patient: Priorities in Assessment and Management*. London: Palgrave.

Crumbie A (2008) Professional role. In Hincliff S and Rogers R (eds) *Competencies for Advanced Nursing Practice*. London: Edward Arnold.

Department of Health (DH) (1989) *Report of the Advisory Group on Nurse Prescribing (Crown Report)*. London: Department of Health.

Department of Health (2010) Advanced level nursing: A position statement. London. http://www.dh.gov.uk/prodconsum dh/groups/dh digitalassets/@dh/@en/@ps/documents/digitalasset/dh 121738.pdf.

Department of Health (2012) The misuse of drugs act 1971 (Amendment) order 2012. http://www.legislation.gov.uk/ukdsi/2012/9780111520857/pdfs/ukdsi_9780111520857_en.pdf.

Department of Health (2014) *Five Year Forward View*. London: Department of Health.

Department of Health England (2013) *Care in Local Communities: A New Vision and Model for District Nursing*. London: Department of Health.

Department of Health and Social Security (DHSS) (1986) *Neighbourhood Nursing—A Focus for Care (Cumberlege Report)*. London: HMSO.

Department of Health, Social Services and Public Safety (2011) *Transforming Your Care: A Review of Health and Social Care in Northern Ireland*. Belfast: DHSSPS.

Douglas G, Nicol F and Robertson C (2013) *MacLeod's Clinical Examination*, 13th edn. London: Churchill Livingstone.

Edwards N (2014) *Community Services: How They Can Transform Care*. London: King's Fund.

Health Foundation (2013) *Improving Patient Flow: How Two Trusts Focussed on Flow To Improve the Quality of Care and Use of Capacity Effectively*. London: Health Foundation.

Hewison A (2009) UK health policy and health service reform. In McGee P (ed) *Advanced Practice in Nursing and Allied Health Professions*. Chichester: Wiley-Blackwell.

Hirshon JM, Risko N, Calvello, EJB et al. (2013) Health systems and services: The role of acute care. *Bulletin of the World Health Organization* 91:386–8.

Huether SE and McCance KL (2016) *Understanding Pathophysiology*, 6th edn. Missouri: Elsevier.

Impact (2010) Impact (III medical patients' acute care and treatment). Impact medical. http://www.impactmedical.org/index.html.

Information Service Division Scotland (2016) Information service division. http://www.isdscotland.org/index.asp.

Jackson J (2016) Principles of assessment. In Clarke D and Maleccki-Ketchell A (eds) *Nursing the Acutely III Patient: Priorities in Assessment and Management*. London: Palgrave.

Jevon P and Ewens B (2012) *Monitoring the Critically III Patient (Essential Clinical Skills for Nurses)*. Chichester: Blackwell Publishing.

Macaluso CR and McNamara RM (2012) Evaluation and management of acute abdominal pain in the emergency department. *International Journal of General Medicine* 5:789–97.

Maybin J, Charles A and Honeyman M (2016) *Understanding Quality in District Nursing Services*. London: King's Fund.

Mosby (2008) *Mosby's Medical Dictionary*, 8th edn. St Louis: Mosby.

Naidoo J and Wills J (2016) *Foundations for Health Promotion*, 4th edn. London: Elsevier.

National Institute for Health and Care Excellence (2016) Sepsis: Recognition, diagnosis and early management (NG51). https://www.nice.org.uk/guidance/ng51.

National Institute for Health and Care Excellence (2007) Acutely III adults in hospital: Recognising and responding to deterioration. https://www.nice.org.uk/Guidance/CG50.

National Patient Safety Agency (2007) Recognising and responding appropriately to early signs of deterioration in hospitalised patients. (Accessed 28 September 2016) http://www.nrls.npsa.nhs.uk/resources/?EntryId45=59834.

Naylor C, Alderwick H and Honeyman M (2015) *Acute Hospitals and Integrated Care: From Hospitals to Health Systems*. London: King's Fund.

NHS Education for Scotland (2016) Community hospitals and intermediate care networks. http://www.knowledge.scot.nhs.uk/chin/intermediate-care/hospital-at-home-services.aspx.

NHS Institute for Innovation and Improvement (2010) SBAR Situation-Background-Assessment-Recommendation. http://www.institute.nhs.uk/quality_and_service_improvement_tools/quality_and_service_improvement_tools/sbar_-_situation_-_background_-_assessment_-_recommendation.html.

Nursing and Midwifery Council (2015) *The Code: Professional Standards of Practice and Behaviour for Nurses and Midwives*. London: NMC.

Nuttall D and Rutt-Howard J (2016) *The Textbook of Non Medical Prescribing*, 2nd edn. Chichester: John Wiley & Sons.

Queen's Nursing Institute/Queen's Nursing Institute Scotland (2015). *The QNI/QNIS Voluntary Standards for District Nurse Education and Practice*. London: QNI.

Purdy S (2010) *Avoiding Hospital Admissions: What Does the Research Evidence Say?* London: King's Fund.

Resuscitation Council (UK) (2011) *Advanced Life Support*, 6th edn. London: Resuscitation Council.

Resuscitation Council (UK) (2015) *A Systematic Approach to the Acutely III Patient: The ABCDE Approach*. London: Resuscitation Council.

Royal College of Nursing (2013) *District Nursing: Harnessing the Potential. The RCN's UK Position on District Nursing.* London: Royal College of Nursing.

Royal College of Nursing (2014) *Moving Care to the Community: An International Perspective.* London: Royal College of Nursing.

Royal College of Physicians (2015) *National Early Warning Score (NEWS). Standardising the Assessment of Acute-Illness Severity within the NHS.* London: Royal College of Physicians. (Accessed 5 July 2016) https://www.rcplondon.ac.uk/projects/outputs/national-early-warning-score-news.

Scottish Government (2011) *Achieving Sustainable Quality in Scotland's Healthcare. A '20:20' Vision.* Edinburgh: Scottish Government.

Scottish Government (2013) *A Route Map to the 2020 Vision for Health and Social Care.* Edinburgh: Scottish Government.

Scottish Government (2015) *Pulling Together: Transforming Urgent Care for the People of Scotland. The Report of the Independent Review of Primary Care Out of Hours Services.* Edinburgh: Scottish Government.

Scottish Government (2016) *Pulling Together: Transforming Urgent Care for the People of Scotland.* Edinburgh: Scottish Government.

Scottish Intercollegiate Guidelines Network (2014) *SIGN 139 Care of Deteriorating Patients.* Edinburgh: Scottish Intercollegiate Guidelines Network.

Standing M (2010) *Clinical Judgement and Decision Making.* Milton Keynes: Open University Press.

Teasdale G (2014) The glasgow structured approach to assessment of the glasgow comma scale. (Accessed 16 September 2016) www.glasgowcommascale.org.

Welsh Assembly Government (2010) *Setting the Direction: Primary and Community Service Strategic Delivery Programme.* Cardiff: Welsh Assembly Government.

Woodrow P (2012) *Intensive Care Nursing,* 3rd edn. Abingdon: Routledge.

World Health Organization (1996) WHO's cancer pain ladder for adults. http://www.who.int/cancer/palliative/painladder/en/.

CHAPTER 13

Emerging issues in long-term conditions

Lois Seddon

LEARNING OUTCOMES

- Critically analyse relevant current government policy and how this influences the management of long-term conditions (LTCs) within the current health agenda.
- Discuss the ways in which LTCs can be proactively managed using ideas and techniques to solve problems.
- Appraise the potential impact of LTCs on individuals and their families and carers.
- Review information to enable you to make judgements about the values of different models that empower professionals to support people with LTCs including the principles of case management and the concept self-care/self-management.
- Reflect on your developing essential skills for successful decision making and delivering care in complex cases.

INTRODUCTION

The purpose of this chapter is to highlight the key considerations for the community nurse when working with people with long-term conditions (LTCs), their carers and their families. The themes raised in this chapter focus specifically on the delivery of person-centred and needs-based care, and include performing assessment, handling case management, supporting self-care, promoting behaviour change, and addressing issues of vulnerability.

Other important topics related to LTCs such as assessing mental health, the use of telehealth in managing LTCs, the important role of carers and the integration of health and social care are explored in other chapters in this edition.

LONG-TERM CONDITIONS

An LTC is one that generally lasts a year or longer and impacts on a person's life (National Institute for Health and Care Excellence [NICE], 2015). Examples include arthritis, asthma, cancer, dementia, diabetes, heart disease, mental health conditions, respiratory disorders, gastroenterological conditions and stroke. Long-term conditions have also traditionally been known as 'chronic' conditions.

In the past there has been a tendency to define LTCs as chronic conditions without cure, but more recently there has been a different approach, for example, describing LTCs as

> [T]he irreversible presence, accumulation, or latency of disease states or impairments that involve the total human environment for supportive care and self-care, maintenance of function and prevention of further disability.
>
> *(Curtin and Lubkin, cited in Larsen and Lubkin, 2009: 5)*

As you can see from this definition, latterly the emphasis is on a more holistic approach and a more comprehensive understanding of what can be done to alleviate the impact of having a LTC. This means that care for people with LTCs should be more about supporting the person to manage rather than trying to treat the condition. It is generally agreed that this approach calls for a model of care that sits more easily within a nursing rather than a medical domain (Larsen and Lubkin, 2009)

A longer life expectancy, due to improved technical and medical advances, means that more people are surviving into old age. It is also known that contemporary lifestyle choices can lead to more people suffering from long-term illnesses (Nuffield Trust, 2013). So despite living longer, our UK populations are not necessarily living much healthier and many people reach their later years with multiple or complex LTCs. Additionally, because most people prefer to be cared for in their own homes, wishing to avoid hospital admissions, there is an increasing need for a range of community services, particularly community nursing. In order to understand why and how community nursing services play such a major role in delivery of care, it is important to consider how key drivers and government policy translate into strategies for the management of LTCs.

POLICY DRIVERS AND GOVERNMENT STRATEGY

Understandably, the management of LTCs has a major impact on health and social care resources across the United Kingdom. It is estimated that 70% of the money spent in England on health and social care is for caring for people who have LTCs. This is because there is an estimated 17.5 million people living with at least one LTC in England. It is thought there are many more that are undiagnosed and the number of people with multiple (more than one) LTCs in England is projected to rise to 2.9 million by 2018 (Department of Health [DH], 2012).

In other parts of the United Kingdom, the picture is much the same. According to Audit Scotland, the number of people aged 75 and over will rise by 60% between 2004 and 2031. By the age of 65, nearly two-thirds of people will have developed a LTC. Around 2 million people, 40% of the Scottish population, have at least one LTC (NHS Scotland, 2010).

It is also estimated that there are 500,000 people living with at least one LTC in Northern Ireland, and it is expected that there will be a significant increase in these numbers over the next 20 years (Department of Health, Social Service and Public Safety [DHSSPS], 2012).

The impact of LTCs is also growing in Wales. One-third of the adult population, an estimated 800,000 people, report having at least one LTC, such as diabetes, chronic obstructive pulmonary disease (COPD) or coronary heart disease (CHD). Two-thirds of the population of Wales aged 65 or older report having at least one chronic condition, while one-third have multiple LTCs, and the burden will increase as the population ages. The number of those aged 65 and over in Wales is projected to increase by around 32% between 2010 and 2026 (Wales Audit Office, 2014).

Policy papers

It has been acknowledged for some time that if people with LTCs are supported and cared for effectively in the community, their health status is likely to remain relatively stable, with less health crises, avoided hospital visits and an overall improved quality of life (Ross et al., 2011). So, community-based care is not only better for the health outcomes of people receiving care, but is also seen to be more effective in terms of healthcare costs. The most recent health strategy documents and policies associated with LTCs therefore incorporate a noticeable emphasis on developing models of cost-effective community-based care, and central to the success of community-based care is of course the contribution of community nursing services.

Over recent years, there has been a steady increase in UK policies with a focus on supporting a more effective approach to the management of LTCs. In 2010, the UK government launched the White Paper, *Liberating the NHS – Legislative Frame-work and Next Steps* (DH, 2010a). This set out the NHS Outcomes Framework which incorporates five domains, one of which is 'Enhancing Quality of Life for People with Long Term Conditions' emphasising the responsibility of health service providers to develop local strategies to help address the needs of those with LTCs.

In 2012, the coalition government published the first NHS Mandate, and within this it allocates the responsibility to NHS England for coming up with plans to help make life better for people with LTCs by

- *Helping them to get the skills to manage their own health*
- *Agreeing with them on a care plan that is based on their personal needs*
- *Making sure their care is better co-ordinated*

The focus on managing LTCs is also reflected in policies and strategies in other countries of the United Kingdom. For example in Scotland, a 'National Action Plan' was developed in 2009, outlining seven high-impact changes that are needed to improve the care of those with LTCs. These are partnership, mutuality, self-management, workforce development, integrated care, quality improvement and clinical information systems (Scottish Government, 2009). In Wales, meeting the needs of people with LTCs has been a priority for the NHS since 2005 when the Welsh Government outlined its intention to develop an integrated framework for LTCs. The plan was to change services from an overreliance on acute hospitals and towards greater use of primary and community services, and in 2012, the Welsh Government reaffirmed its commit-ment to community-based care with a plan to provide a greater range of services available at all times. Their achievements so far with this vision have recently been evaluated by the Welsh Audit Office and results can be accessed in their report, *The Management of Chronic Conditions in Wales – An Update* (Wales Audit Office, 2014). In Northern Ireland, the Primary Care Development Unit has been developing a policy framework specifically focused on supporting people with LTCs. The framework is based on six underpinning principles: working in partnership, supporting self-management, information to service users and carers, managing medicines, carers as partners and anticipatory care (DHSSPS, 2012).

This focus on LTCs, user involvement, personal choice and self-care for LTC management is however not new. There are a number of helpful archived documents developed that are worth a look and include *Our Health Our Care Our Say* (DH, 2006a), *Supporting People with Long-Term Conditions* (DH, 2005b) and *Supporting People with Long-Term Conditions to Self Care* (DH, 2006b).

The National Institute for Health and Care Excellence (NICE) has recently published a guideline which although developed to guide practitioners in specifically supporting older people with LTCs, provides a useful model for managing LTCs generally (NICE, 2015). The focus in this new guideline is clearly on pulling together health and social care services in supporting people with complex care needs and multiple LTCs. This integration agenda is discussed and explored in more depth in Chapter 11 of this text.

A PERSON-CENTRED PERSPECTIVE AND PSYCHOLOGICAL RESPONSES TO DIAGNOSES

It is important to remember that behind all these figures and policies are individuals experiencing life-affecting disorders. The diagnosis of a LTC can be devastating. When the individual has been experiencing symptoms for some time and is anxiously awaiting results, he or she may feel an initial period of relief of knowing at last what is wrong. However, depending on personal perspectives and circumstances, together with the nature of the condition, the diagnosis normally means that the person's life will never be the same again (NHS, 2008). Learning to live with the pressures of the condition can pose major challenges: disability, pain, anxiety, fear and lack of knowledge and understanding are just some. There may be many personal losses, for example, independence, social status, financial stability and social connections, particularly if employment is affected. Body image may be affected and personal relationships may suffer (NHS, 2008).

There can be a number of responses following diagnosis, including shock, denial, distress with symptoms and interventions, exaggerated independence alternating with collapse and into dependency. In particular, the NHS Positive Practice Guide (NHS, 2008) outlines the impact of co-morbidity of chronic disease and mental ill health and illustrates the impact of specific chronic diseases on mental health and vice versa. Individual coping mechanisms will vary and a range of emotions is likely to occur – there may be feelings of stress, guilt and resentment (Nichols, 2003).

Nichols suggests three levels of intervention for the health professional in helping a person through these early stages of diagnosis:

Level 1 includes health professionals' awareness and understanding and ability to communicate with patients.

Level 2 involves monitoring, providing support, counselling, advocacy and referral.

Level 3 refers to specialist therapeutic interventions.

ACTIVITY 13.1

Reflection point

This first activity invites reflection on what may be needed to guide you as a health professional, but starting from the patient's perspective.

Scenario

You have recently been diagnosed with type 2 diabetes. Please access the Diabetes UK website www.diabetesuk.org and reflect on how helpful this could be for you. Do you discover more about the condition and what to expect in terms of care and support? Do you feel that it gives you some more confidence in discussing your condition with healthcare professionals? Navigate through the various sections of the site and consider the presentation and content. You may wish to look at specific aspects that interest you, for example, if you have visual impairment or perhaps you want to know more about healthy eating.

Reflection

Is the site useful for you as a health professional?

How might this resource complement the management provided by the healthcare team?

How can you make this information available to patients who do not have access to the Internet?

In terms of the interventions outlined by Nichols (above), what would you as a person diagnosed with diabetes expect from the community nurse?

DEVELOPING A PERSON-CENTRED APPROACH: SELF-CARE AND SELF-MANAGEMENT AND THE ROLE OF THE COMMUNITY NURSE

Self-care refers to those activities that we might perform for ourselves that keep us well. The Self Care Forum (www.selfcareforum.org) presents a very useful model that illustrates how the level of self-care varies along a continuum. For example, a person might self-care for a minor ailment he or she is suffering by purchasing an over-the-counter treatment, but following a major trauma a person would require a high level of medical intervention and in this case self-care is only likely to 'kick in' once recovery is well underway. The notion of self-care is considered a key element of LTC management in each of the countries of the United Kingdom. It is an underpinning principle of the Health and Social Care Model (Figure 13.1) which is widely adopted in respect of LTC management across Scotland, England, and in Wales a similar model is followed. The model shows the proposed different levels of intervention by health and social care services. The base level and the middle level of the pyramid in Figure 13.1 account for more than 80% of the population who are affected by LTCs, and this is where support for self-care is mostly targeted. However, even for the top 20% who suffer from multiple or complex conditions, there is still potential for some degree of self-care, for example, individuals will be able to monitor and report changes in their health status to the case manager/responsible health professional.

Promoting self-care is generally regarded as a positive approach to healthcare. Empowering people with the confidence to look after themselves and independently manage their LTC when they can will give people greater control of their own health and is known to encourage healthy behaviour and improve overall well-being. As mentioned previously, the management of long-term conditions accounts for 70% of total health spending in the United Kingdom, but it has been shown that encouraging self-management of LTCs can reduce the extent of nursing or medical interventions and consequently can help reduce overall healthcare costs (Health Foundation, 2014). However, there must be adequate support within the health and social care systems to underpin this approach and to ensure that people are properly prepared to take on self-care so that their health and well-being remain optimal.

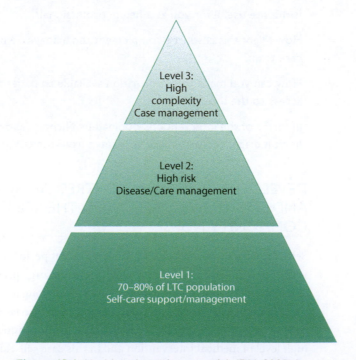

Figure 13.1 Health and social care model. (DH, 2005b.)

Community nurses play a key role in preparing and supporting those with LTCs to self-care while also ensuring that people stay safe. Joint decision making is a central facet of self-care, where the practitioner, the person with the LTCs and their family and carers work together to set out a personalised care plan. This can only be achieved by making sure people are informed and guided not just about their condition(s), but also about the skills needed to self-manage. All professionals, including community nurses working with people who have LTCs, have an important educational and coaching role and so sound communication skills are essential (DH, 2010b). The document 'Improving the Health and Well Being of People with Long Term Conditions' (DH, 2010b) clearly spells out the attitudes, approaches, skills, knowledge and competences that are expected of the workforce supporting people with LTCs. This includes helping people monitor their own symptoms and teaching them when they need to take appropriate action and who and how to access further support when it is needed. When people are encouraged to take on 'ownership' of their condition they will also need to be taught risk management and problem-solving skills (DH, 2010b). The provision of high-quality tailored information is therefore crucial. Checking and ensuring understanding is a key skill when imparting information, and community nurses will need to consider that the ability of people to process information can be highly variable, especially when they are contending with the pressures of the LTCs. Other factors may include age, gender, culture, religion and social class and the level of health literacy (levels of literacy and numeracy combined with beliefs about health) (Royal College of General Practitioners, 2014). In addition to calling on their knowledge of disease processes, the community nurse will need to use skills in counselling to help guide people through managing the social and emotional impacts of their condition as well as the physical changes associated with the illness (NHS, 2008).

HELPING PEOPLE TO CHANGE BEHAVIOUR

The focus of government strategy across the United Kingdom includes not only the management and care of individuals with LTCs, but also prevention, early diagnosis and engagement with individuals to achieve better health outcomes. There are currently a number of broad and encompassing public health and health promotion strategies relevant to the role of the community nurse and these are discussed in more depth in Chapter 2. In this section, we focus principally on behaviour change in relation to LTCs and how the community nurse might use different models and skills to help people more actively engage in the self-management agenda.

The Health Belief Model, modified by Becker (1974), cited in Naidoo and Wills (2016), describes a set of functions that impacts on a person's decision making. (You can access further discussion regarding the Health Belief Model in Chapter 2 of this text.) A person's perceptions in terms of their susceptibility to a condition and severity of a disease can be modified by demographic and sociopsychological variables. This means that a person's knowledge base regarding their health action and perceived threat of disease are combined with external triggers such as familial attitudes and media influence. These can determine whether a person will take a specific action in relation to their health behaviour. The person's confidence is also a factor and is related to their 'locus of control' (Morrison and Bennett, 2012). This means do they believe that the events that govern their lives are initiated from within or outside themselves? And consequently, do they feel they have the ability to make desired change? An appropriate level of support from the health professional, in this case the community nurse, can make all the difference. The community nurse will also need to assess the person's 'readiness to change' in relation to 'The Stages of Change Model'. The four stages of change were originally identified by Prochasta and Di Clemente (1984, cited by Naidoo and Wills, 2016). The first stage is pre-contemplation, where the individual is not yet ready to make the change; second is contemplation, where the person is open to considering altering their behaviour. The remaining stages involve planning for and maintaining change. Each stage is led by the individual who may not be able to move readily from one stage to the next. However, a skilled professional senses the stage which a person reaches and offers the appropriate support and encouragement to move on when the person is ready.

Motivational interviewing

Often, when faced with the notion of making lifestyle or health behaviour changes, a person will feel a degree of conflict about whether to take action. It is in this area of ambivalence that another tool, motivational interviewing (MI), can help. MI is also referred to in Chapters 2 and 8. MI was developed in the 1980s by William Miller and his fellow psychologists working in the area of substance misuse. More recently, it has been found to be useful in many situations where health behaviour change would be advisable. A partnership between the individual and health professional is developed. In this way they together explore this ambivalence to identify a way of moving forward by appraising the 'change talk' expressed by the patient. This includes such statements as 'I wish I could…' 'It would be better if ….' Careful listening and clarification, combined with a non-judgemental, empathetic and encouraging attitude, will lead the individual to discover and believe in their own motivation and abilities and make plans for taking action. Rollnick et al. (2008) set out the four guiding principles for professionals which are resisting the righting reflex, understanding the person's motivation, listening to and empowering the patient. In addition, three fundamental core skills are crucial if professionals are to achieve this: asking, listening and informing. This approach is underpinned by the spirit of MI, which has three components: collaboration, evocation and patient autonomy. Developing skills in these techniques will enable community nurses to more confidently support those who are grappling with the challenges of behaviour change associated with taking more self-management of their illness and their lives. There are a number of resources available, for example, the website www.motivationalinterviewing.org/ where information on formal and online training is available.

CASE MANAGEMENT IN LONG-TERM CONDITIONS

Owing to global demographics the challenge of managing LTCs is not confined to the United Kingdom, and health and social care strategists across the globe have sought ways to address this increasing health need. In the United States, for example, models of management have been developed by companies such as Evercare and Kaiser Permanente. It is from their models of care that the UK models for managing LTCs have been developed. The evidence from the United States has shown how the concept of case management of patients with LTCs can have significant potential to deliver both better care for patients and cost savings. Although there is a marked difference in the configuration of healthcare provision in the United States, especially in terms of funding, it was felt that much could be gained by adopting similar approaches in the United Kingdom (Snodden, 2010).

The case management model is community based and incorporates a targeted, proactive approach to care. The process involves case-finding, care assessment, care planning and care co-ordination, and where implemented effectively it has been shown to improve the experiences of individuals and their carers. This has meant better health outcomes for both and so reduced the need for hospital-based care, thus enabling a more cost-effective use of health resources (Ross et al., 2011). However, any model of case management must be well designed and be co-ordinated by appropriately trained and prepared professionals. Also, it is imperative that whichever model of case management is applied, it is soundly embedded in a wider system based on the integration of health and social care (Ross et al., 2011). This is an underpinning principle for the model of LTC management across the United Kingdom (DH, 2005a; Scottish Government, 2009; DHSSPS, 2012).

Essentially, case management is based on one crucial underpinning principle of practice which is care co-ordination. This role is usually undertaken by an individual case manager. In some areas this will be an advanced nursing practitioner, who may have the title of community matron, or it may be an allied health professional such as an occupational therapist or a physiotherapist. In other localities the responsibility of case management may be allocated to a small team of health and social care practitioners. However, increasingly case management is seen as a district nursing role. The responsibilities of the case manager will include, but are not limited to, a full holistic assessment, medication management (and prescribing of medicines if a community matron or a health practitioner with an appropriate non-medical prescribing qualification), self-care support, advocacy and negotiation, psychosocial support, monitoring of health status and review of the care planning. The role of the community nurse will be to support the case manager in the process of case management, collecting information to inform the assessment and monitoring change and response to care plans, and reporting back to the case manager.

ACTIVITY 13.2

This activity is designed for you to consider how the needs of a person with multiple or complex conditions might be assessed and to consider how the resources available to provide support in the community might be set in place to address these needs.

Scenario

Mr A recently registered with the general practitioner (GP) practice. He is 70 years old with chronic obstructive pulmonary disease (COPD) having been referred to the practice nurse because he is experiencing difficulty in using his inhaled medication. He has had several hospital admissions and also suffers from Parkinson's disease; he has high blood pressure and rheumatoid arthritis. He has recently moved to the area to live closer to his daughter. What skills are required to undertake a full assessment? What specific areas would need an in-depth assessment? What resources will be required to provide ongoing care, including input from other nurses, health professionals and agencies, and who will co-ordinate his care? What will be the referral process? Which policy documents underpin and support relevant standards of care?

Mr A would be in the population located in the top third of the LTC pyramid; he has highly complex needs. His assessment and ongoing care will require a high level of expertise and support from various professionals and agencies. In terms of direct management and care, the case manager's skills and depth of knowledge will ensure that Mr A's condition is closely monitored. For example, the case manager will have a major role in medicines management. Mr A will potentially be taking several medicines for each of his conditions, including pain relief. In accordance with the regulations set down in the NMC Code (Nursing and Midwifery Council [NMC], 2015), the case manager will work closely with Mr A, developing a concordant relationship to promote adherence to the therapeutic regime and so effective use of medication. If the case manager is an independent prescriber he or she can make prescribing decisions according to their specific area of competence as per the NMC Code (NMC, 2015). An example of this is the management of COPD where the case manager can help avoid unnecessary hospital admission. People with COPD often suffer from exacerbations of their condition which require hospital admission. The case manager can encourage self-care not only by teaching and providing information and if a non-medical prescriber could prescribe a 'rescue pack' for Mr A to use when he feels his condition is deteriorating. The pack will consist of antibiotics and steroids, thus a hospital admission is avoided.

Mr A will also require input from several other professionals. Depending upon his needs, a mental health professional, allied health professional, social worker or district nurse may fulfil the role of case manager or may be involved in providing separate elements of his care. Consider what specialist input each of these may contribute to the care of Mr A.

Referral to other health departments and wider agencies may be required and the skills needed for this include developing effective networking and fostering collaborative relationships with others.

The virtual ward

People such as Mr A who have multiple LTCs are frequently at risk of admission and readmission to acute care due to exacerbations or other complications associated with their conditions (King's Fund, 2013). Clearly, this is a disruptive experience for the person and that person's family and carers, and will often incur substantial costs to the wider health services. In order to address this, some community trusts have developed *virtual* ward environments for those who have a high risk of readmission. This model is based on the principle of collaborative working and the community nurse is often at the centre of the model, specifically taking on a role of monitoring and supporting the individual. The 'ward' mirrors an actual hospital setting but the person remains in their own home, with ward rounds including involvement of the relevant professionals who network 'electronically' making decisions and plans for ongoing care. In the United Kingdom, there are currently a number of different models to guide the provision of virtual wards (Nuffield Trust, 2013). A typical model will be based on the following points:

- The primary care provider will co-ordinate the infrastructure for virtual wards, employing the virtual ward staff and establishing a contract with each GP practice participating in the virtual wards programme.
- The local council provides a named social worker for each virtual ward.
- The local NHS acute hospital establishes honorary contracts to all virtual ward staff so they can visit patients on the wards, obtain laboratory results, and perform other functions.
- The out of hours primary care service will take over the ward clerk telephone number at night and has access to the virtual ward electronic patient records.
- Voluntary organizations assign a named representative to each virtual ward as the link to voluntary services, such as befriending services, advice helplines, and cultural groups.
- When a patient is admitted to a virtual ward, the case manager visits the patient at home and conducts an initial detailed assessment, often accompanied by the ward physician. The assessment includes screening for certain conditions.
- Working with the patient, the case manager drafts an initial action plan, which is entered into a set of electronic notes that all ward staff can access.
- The virtual ward staff conduct an office-based ward round each working day, with teleconference facilities available for staff who wish to join remotely. Newly admitted patients are discussed, changes to current patients' care plans are proposed and tasks allocated. Frequency of the patient's review depends on the patient's circumstances and clinical stability. (In the Croydon virtual ward model, of the 100 patients on each ward, typically about five patients would be

reviewed daily, 35 patients would be reviewed weekly, and the remaining 60 would be reviewed monthly.) So on any given ward round, around 15 current patients are discussed in addition to any new admissions or soon to be discharged patients.

- The GP practice is informed of all significant changes to a patient's condition or management.
- Every night a list of each virtual ward's current patients is e-mailed securely to local hospitals and out of hours services, who upload the information to their own clinical computer systems.
- The emergency room (ER) sets up a system so that the arrival of a virtual ward patient at the ER triggers an alert to prompt the ER receptionist to contact the patient's virtual ward clerk. The local ambulance service may set up a similar alert system and will dispatch an Emergency Care Practitioner or ambulance crew to virtual ward patients.
- Secondary care staff contact the virtual ward clerk to obtain current details of the patient's care and work in partnership with the virtual ward staff to try to avoid a hospital admission; if a patient must be hospitalized, hospital staff will arrange early discharge back to the care of the virtual ward team.
- If a patient has been cared for uneventfully for several months, following assessment by all relevant virtual ward staff the team will decide when the patient is ready to be discharged back to the care of the primary care practice. The length of time that a patient is cared for on a virtual ward can range from a few weeks to over a year.
- When a patient is discharged from a virtual ward back to the sole care of his or her GP, the virtual ward clerk sends the practice a discharge summary and sends a discharge letter (using lay terminology) to the patient.

An informal evaluation of virtual ward patients in Croydon has shown that their satisfaction with the service was very high (Commonwealth Fund, 2010).

ACTIVITY 13.3

You might consider how this model could be used in supporting Mr A. What do you see are the main differences between the usual model of care and the virtual ward model? What would be the benefits for Mr A and the health and social care professionals? Who would be the key staff needed in the virtual ward for Mr A and what would be their role?

YOUNGER PEOPLE AND LONG-TERM CONDITIONS

It is important to remember that although the picture of our national demographics shows that we have an ageing population who are subject to increasing and multiple LTCs, a diagnosis of a chronic illness can, and does, happen at any age. The challenges for the community nurse in supporting younger people often are often quite specific and they may be quite complex.

THE IMPACT OF A LONG-TERM CONDITION ON THE FAMILY UNIT

ACTIVITY 13.4

The purpose of this exercise is to explore, reflect upon and address potential risks for the family when a parent is dealing with a LTC.

Scenario

Mrs B (41 years old) has been referred to you for assessment. She has just been diagnosed with multiple sclerosis, having had distressing neurological symptoms for some months. She is having problems going out as she tends to lose her balance and she is very concerned about difficulties she has with continence. Mrs B is married and lives with her husband in the family home (for which they pay a mortgage) with their two children aged 13 and 9 years. Prior to her diagnosis, Mrs B had been the main wage earner in the household, being employed as an administrator in a local government department.

Consider your assessment of Mrs B and identify potential risks there may be in terms of her physical and psychosocial well-being. What are the risks for her husband and children? How can these risks be addressed by community nursing, the wider health and social care agencies and non-statutory sector? You may wish to revisit Chapter 9 for further suggestions on how to support carers. It may help to create a mind map or spider diagram of the various teams who need to be involved.

In the complex situation in Activity 13.4, there are numerous aspects to consider and the exercise emphasises the importance of a fully comprehensive and holistic assessment. The physical aspects alone present profound implications for life change. They include disability in a young woman, risk of falls; perhaps difficulties in getting to the toilet and as immobility increases there may be problems with tissue viability. There will be increasing loss of sensation, pain and fatigue.

Psychological considerations are at least as challenging. Will Mrs B be able to continue working? If not, there may be an economic risk to the family. What about her status within the family, the local community and the workplace? Will her relationship with her husband be threatened? Will a sexual relationship still be possible? What is Mrs B's understanding of and what are her concerns for her future health? How will she deal with the unpredictable nature of her condition? What are Mr B's needs? Is he prepared for potential caring responsibilities?

There are a number of potential risks in this situation and addressing them will need sensitive and informed enquiry and support. It is important to consider potential negative effects such as relationship or family breakdown, substance misuse or even domestic abuse. The children's schooling may be disrupted; they may be called on to provide care for their mother, which will raise enquiry around their well-being as young carers. Family carers are an integral part of LTC management and their needs and concerns should be included in all plans of care and in this scenario the carers' role(s) may be quite complex. (Here you may like to refer to Chapter 9 for further information regarding the key role of carers.)

There may, however, be very positive responses and outcomes, and high levels of support and care are frequently developed within families who are dealing with the challenge of LTCs as indicated in the anecdotal evidence gathered by the organisation Healthtalk.org (see www.healthtalk.org/peoples-experiences/long-term-conditions/chronic-pain/impact-family). However, even when there is a positive family approach, the community nurse should be fully aware of the local availability of both statutory and voluntary sources of support and local pathways of care. It is also essential to be fully confident in implementing safeguarding procedures including those associated with domestic abuse. Sensitive ongoing monitoring of the situation will be a key responsibility of the lead health professional.

SUPPORTING YOUNG PEOPLE WITH LONG-TERM CONDITIONS

ACTIVITY 13.5

Owing to medical advances and developments in neonatal and early childhood health care, more infants and children with life-threatening disorders or congenital conditions are now surviving into adolescence and adulthood, and this is of course to be celebrated. It is however important to also consider that these young people may be growing and developing with the challenge of ongoing LTCs and associated vulnerabilities. In addition, the conditions that they have to contend with can follow varying courses of progression. They might be lifelong (for example, deafness), slowly deteriorating (for example, muscular dystrophy), potentially curable (for example, cancer) or of a variable course (for example, cystic fibrosis) (www.healthtalk.org 2016). It is also essential that health professionals supporting young people with LTCs recognise that the needs of the child or young person will be very different to those of adults and that their needs and those of their families will change over time as the young person grows and develops. This can present major challenges for health service professionals and others involved in providing age-appropriate treatment, care and support. The following exercise will help you explore the specific needs of children and young people who are suffering from LTCs and consider how these might be addressed.

Scenario

Annie, who is 17 years old, was diagnosed 2 years ago with chronic renal disease. She had not really felt unwell but her legs frequently became swollen and blood tests suggested some issues with renal function. A renal biopsy confirmed the diagnosis. Annie was prescribed steroid therapy, and was for a while very stable, so the dose was gradually reduced.

Two months ago, unexpectedly, further tests showed that Annie's kidneys were deteriorating rapidly. She was retaining a lot of extra fluid and was unable to walk around and was in a great deal of pain. Annie was admitted to hospital is now having to have dialysis although she had been told at the time of her diagnosis that it would be a long time before that would be the case.

ACTIVITY 13.5

Annie lives at home with her mum and dad and you have been asked to assess her needs while she is currently recovering from a recent hospital admission.

Consider her physical needs, who should be involved in ensuring Annie has the optimal physical care, who might be the lead professional in this aspect of her care?

Consider her psychological and emotional needs, what/who might help her cope with these?

Up to now, Annie's mum and dad have helped her make decisions about her care, but Annie is now a young woman. What are the specific considerations as Annie is on the verge of entering adult services rather than accessing child and young person services?

What information and support can you offer Annie?

Physical needs

Following your initial assessment advice can be sought from the specialist renal team, many nephrology teams have outreach services that can dialyse at home and help individuals manage their own dialysis either at home or in hospital. There may be a specialist nurse who can offer Annie and her family, and you, support and information.

Chronic tiredness/fatigue is a common feature of many long-term illnesses, so it is important to assess how this is affecting Annie in her day-to-day activities and whether there is any advice you can give her in managing this fatigue. Pain is an issue to consider for Annie – is it being managed sufficiently for Annie to be pain free? Pain and tiredness often go together because pain makes it hard to sleep, or even rest or sit still. Annie may have periods of relapse or remission and so it might be difficult for her to know exactly how she will feel at any time. It is important to liaise with the GP and specialist team to ensure that pain relief for Annie is appropriate and effective.

Emotional needs

Understandably, it can be particularly difficult for teenagers to be diagnosed with a chronic condition that requires long-term treatment and medical supervision. Annie will have found the decision to have dialysis a big shock and may be feeling upset and let down as she was not expecting this so early in the progression of her illness. She may feel very vulnerable in respect of her own mortality and the need to depend on a machine and/or a transplant, and she may be feeling angry and depressed. Some young people may react to a diagnosis with suicidal thoughts (www.healthtalk.org – see the list of resources) so it is essential to explore her feelings sensitively but thoroughly so that specialist support for her mental health is arranged if required.

Like any other young person, Annie will have plans and goals to achieve, including the desire to have a 'normal' life. During the teenage years and into young adulthood individuals are likely to be going through a number of life changes. Those with LTCs will have more to contend with and consequently will have specific emotional and social needs. Many will be entering relationships or starting work. They may be leaving home for the first time, or planning to move away to university (Mathews, 2012). Annie may be studying and busy preparing for exams and coursework at college or at school working, or looking for work, or working and studying at the same time. How will she also cope with the demands and treatment regime of this illness? How debilitating are the relapses or periods of treatment and how do they interfere with her mobility and engagement with life generally? The community nurse is well placed to recognise and acknowledge Annie's individual emotional and/or psychological needs, to reassure Annie that they are taken seriously and signpost Annie to specialist support services or peer support groups. The website 'Healthtalk' at http://www.healthtalk.org/young-peoples-experiences/long-term-health-conditions/topics provides insight and advice for professionals supporting young people with LTCs.

Information and support

When young people are diagnosed with a disease that may affect them for years to come they will have many questions. What information has Annie already accessed, are there any information gaps or misinformation? Annie will doubtless already have undertaken her own 'research' and it is appropriate to sensitively caution about accessing trustworthy Internet sites and being aware that some information can be alarming. There are a number of national voluntary organisations associated with this condition that can offer facts and figures and give insight to other people's experiences; they might also link to chat rooms, e-mail and other social media. However, some young people do not always want a lot of health information – they may prefer to concentrate on other things and not feel that they are being defined by their condition.

In recognition of the specific needs of young people with ongoing health conditions the Department of Health published, in 2007, guidance for commissioners of local health services in the 'You're Welcome Quality Criteria for Young People Friendly Health Services'. This was updated in May 2011. The criteria set out principles that will help primary and secondary care health services (including non-NHS provision) become young people friendly (DH, 2011). In addition, the government strategy for young people 'Positive for Youth: A New Approach to Cross-Government Policy for Young People Aged 13–19' was published in 2011 and updated in 2013. It provides comprehensive detail on all the government's policies for young people aged 13–19 covering a wide range of issues – from education and youth services, to health, crime, housing and more.

In Scotland – 'Getting it Right for Every Child' is a focused project on bringing information to parents and their children. This has a number of very useful resources and includes a summary of advice to doctors and nurses who work with children and young people. This is accessible at www.alliance-scotland.org.uk/what-we-do/our-work/children-and-young-people/getting-to-know-girfec/.

Transition to adult services

For many young people this can be a difficult time as they experience greater independence and young people may find adult services very different from paediatric care. Annie will be expected to take much greater responsibility and to actively participate in the management of her condition. How will she embrace this change? Will she find it threatening or welcome the chance to have more control over her condition and treatment? Her parents have been very supportive, what will be their role now? Has there been a proactive plan established for the transition of Annie to adult services, because this will be key to a smooth transition.

There is plenty of guidance on what makes for good transition planning and good commissioning of care (see below); however, a Care Quality Commission (CQC) review in 2014 found a significant shortfall between policy and practice (CQC, 2014). The report found that some families are confused and distressed by the lack of information and support given to them, that certain children's services stop before their equivalent adult services start, and that there is a general variation in people's experience across the localities and countries of the United Kingdom. The recommendations that evolved from this review offer helpful advice to the community nurse in supporting young people like Annie.

The CQC advise that every young person with complex physical health needs, from age 14 should have

- A key accountable individual responsible for supporting their move to adult health services
- A documented transition plan that includes their health needs
- A communication or 'health passport' to ensure relevant professionals have access to essential information about the young person
- Health services provided in an appropriate environment that takes account of their needs without gaps in provision between children's and adult services
- Training and advice to prepare them and their parents for the transition to adult care, including consent and advocacy
- Respite and short break facilities available to meet their needs and those of their families

In addition, as a consequence of the CQC Report and acknowledging that the period of transition is a vulnerable time for young people and their families, the National Institute for Health and Care Excellence has recently issued a guideline that covers the period before, during and after a young person moves from children's to adult services. It aims to help young people and their carers have a better experience of transition by improving the way it is planned and carried out. It covers both health and social care and provides a comprehensive guide to all health and social care professionals supporting young people such as Annie (NICE, 2016).

DEVELOPING COMPETENCE IN LONG-TERM CONDITIONS MANAGEMENT

This chapter has been designed to encourage reflection on how care can be provided for people with LTCs by nurses working in the community. The contemporary vision is to promote a person-centred approach and increase a person's involvement in a model of self-care. This chapter has shown how helping people manage their LTCs is currently, and will continue to be, a key role for community nurses. The potential contribution of the community nurse is immense and will encompass many of the topics covered elsewhere in this text. Subsequently, you will undoubtedly find, in many of the other chapters, guidance in developing competences that apply to this particular area of community nursing practice. For example, in Chapter 8 you will find information about supporting mental health, Chapter 9 illustrates how carers and families might be supported, and Chapter 17 outlines the skills needed when using eHealth as a means of supporting people in the community.

This list is not exhaustive, and reflecting on practice experiences includes learning from those in our care as well as our colleagues to enhance shared learning,

ACTIVITY 13.6

In order to be well prepared to practice effectively in the community it is useful to reflect on your current skills and identify any gaps. Nurses working in the community will practice with a number of key skills and attributes. Reflect on how the following skills, specifically related to supporting people in the community with LTCs, feature in your practice. What are your strengths and what skills do you need to develop or refresh?

- Contributing to comprehensive and holistic assessment
- Highlighting specific needs of individuals
- Supporting senior colleagues in leading and co-ordinating care
- Being non-judgemental
- Helping people become creative in managing their LTC
- Understanding and building on a person's strengths
- Helping people keep safe
- Motivational interviewing
- Offering health promotion advice
- Working in partnership with individuals and their families
- Collaboratively working with other agencies and other professionals
- Being informed of local and national support networks
- Showing sensitivity and response to the emotional aspects of suffering from LTCs
- Being aware of disease processes and applying that knowledge to helping people manage their symptoms
- Being aware of agencies that can advise on financial support/benefits for people being nursed in the community

desired health outcomes and improved quality of life for people living with LTCs and those close to them.

In addition, there are a range of community nursing disciplines involved in the delivery of primary care and many roles continue to be developed. Some of these roles are designed to actively prevent LTCs and reduce the effects. Consider, for example, the work of the school nurse in addressing childhood obesity or the general practice nurse offering help with the management of asthma. Other essential roles include community mental health nurses and community children's nurses and teams of practitioners who provide end-of-life care. Liaison and co-ordinating care with other nurses such as these is an essential element of successful management of LTCs.

CONCLUSION

This chapter has provided an introduction to a number of emerging issues associated with the current LTCs agenda and explored why it is important to consider this in the context of community nursing. If the challenges posed are to be successfully tackled, the new generation of community nurses will need to acquire, maintain and update specific skills and apply new models of intervention. Care and support for people with LTCs must take account of individual needs and preferences and people must be given the opportunity to make properly informed decisions about managing their own care, in partnership with health and social care practitioners (NICE, 2015). The main contemporary policy drivers have been identified and it is clear that these will continue to focus on home-based collaborative and co-ordinated care, where the community nurse role will remain pivotal.

FURTHER READING

Margereson C and Trenoweth S (2010) (eds) *Developing Holistic Care for Long-Term Conditions*. Oxford: Routledge.

McVeigh H (2009) *Fundamental Aspects of Long-Term Conditions*. London: Quay Books.

Nicol J (2011) *Nursing Adults with Long Term Conditions*. Exeter: Learning Matters. (Transforming nursing practice series).

Presho M (2008) *Managing Long Term Conditions: A Social Model for Community Practice*. Chichester: John Wiley and Sons.

Randall S and Ford H (eds) (2011) *Long Term Conditions: A Guide for Nurses and Health Care Professionals*. Chichester: John Wiley and Sons.

Walker R and Rodgers J (2011) *Implementing Personalised Care Planning In Long Term Conditions*. Northampton: SD Publications.

FURTHER RESOURCES

There are an infinite number of relevant materials available via textbooks and websites. In addition to the websites mentioned below, it is worth noting that almost all conditions will have at least one dedicated website.

www.qni.org.uk/transition The Queen's Nursing Institute provides information about the transition to community nursing and includes a section about LTCs

www.nmc-uk.org/nurses-and-midwives Provides professional standards

Self-care and self-management:

http://selfmanagementuk.org/ Provides advice for individuals and professionals

http://smns.alliance-scotland.org.uk/ Self Management Network Scotland

Most consumer-led sites are involved in advocacy and campaigning. Good examples are

www.mind.org.uk

www.ageuk.org.uk

Patient- and carer-focused sites include

www.carersuk.org

NHS Choices at

www.nhs.uk/pages/home.aspx

Clinical information can be accessed in the evidence section of NICE:

www.nice.org.uk/

www.selfcareforum.org

Enhancing co-ordinated care:

www.england.nhs.uk/wp-content/uploads/2013/05/nv-narrative-cc.pdf

Living with LTCs:

www.dhsspsni.gov.uk/sites/default/files/publications/dhssps/living-longterm-conditions.pdf

Motivational interviewing:

www.motivationalinterviewing.org/

Information to help support young people can be accessed at the following:

www.alliance-scotland.org.uk/what-we-do/policy-and-campaigns/current-work/children-and-young-people/

Children and Young People's Health Outcomes Forum – Report of the Long-Term Conditions, Disability and Palliative Care Sub-Group

www.gov.uk/government/uploads/system/uploads/attachment_data/file/216856/CYP-Long-Term-Conditions.pdf

Association for Young People's Health:

www.ayph.org.uk/publications/242_Final%20Summary%20RU9%20Long-term%20Conditions%20Feb%202012.pdf

POLICY: 2010–2015 Government Policy: Long-term Health Conditions:

www.gov.uk/government/publications/2010-to-2015-government-policy-long-term-health-conditions/2010-to-2015-government-policy-long-term-health-conditions

REFERENCES

Becker MH (ed) (1974) *The Health Belief Model and Personal Health Behaviour.* Thorofare, NJ: Slack.

Care Quality Commission (2014) From the Pond to the Sea. (Accessed July 2016) https://www.cqc.org.uk/sites/default/files/CQC_Transition%20Report.pdf.

The Commonwealth Fund (2010) Predictive modelling in action: How 'virtual wards' help high risk patients receive hospital care at home. (Accessed July 2016) http://www.commonwealthfund.org/Publications/Issue-Briefs/2010/Aug/Predictive-Modeling-in-Action.aspx.

Department of Health (DH) (2005a) *The National Service Framework for Long Term Conditions*. London: The Stationery Office.

DH (2005b) *Supporting People with Long-Term Conditions: Liberating the Talents of Nurses Who Care for People with Long-Term Conditions*. London: DH.

DH (2006a) *Our Health Our Care Our Say*. London: DH.

DH (2006b) *Supporting People with Long-Term Conditions to Self Care*. London: DH.

DH (2010a) *Liberating the NHS: Legislative Framework and Next Steps*. London: The Stationery Office.

DH (2010b) Improving the health and wellbeing of people with long term conditions. (Accessed July 2016) http://www.yearofcare.co.uk/sites/default/files/pdfs/dh_improving%20the%20h%26wb%20of%20people%20with%20LTCs.pdf.

DH (2011) You're welcome – quality criteria for young people friendly health services. (Accessed January 2016) https://www.gov.uk/government/publications/quality-criteria-for-young-people-friendly-health-services.

DH (2012) Long term conditions compendium of information, 3rd edn (Accessed January 2016) https://www.gov.uk/government/uploads/system/uploads/attachment_data/file/216528/dh_134486.pdf

Department of Health, Social Service and Public Safety (DHSSPS) (2012) *Living with Long Term Conditions—A Policy Framework*. Northern Ireland: Primary Care Development Unit. (Accessed January 2016) http://www.dhsspsni.gov.uk/living-longterm-conditions.pdf.

Health Foundation (2014). The self care NHS Trust—The future for NHS Choices. (Accessed January 2016) http://www.health.org.uk/blog/self-care-nhs-trust-%E2%80%93-future-nhs-choices.

King's Fund (2013) *South Devon and Torbay Proactive Case Management Using the Community Virtual Ward and the Devon Predictive Model*. London: King's Fund. (Accessed July 2016) http://www.kingsfund.org.uk/sites/files/kf/field/field_publication_file/south-devon-and-torbay-coordinated-care-case-study-king'sfund13.pdf.

Larsen PD and Lubkin I (2009) *Chronic Illness: Impact and Intervention*, 7th edn. London: Jones & Bartlett.

Mathews (2012) Supporting young adults with long term conditions. (Accessed January 2016) http://www.nursinginpractice.com/article/supporting-young-adults-long-term-conditions.

Morrison V and Bennett P (2012) *An Introduction to Health Psychology*, 3rd edn. Oxford: Pearson Higher Education.

National Institute for Health and Care Excellence (NICE) (2015) Older people with social care needs and multiple long term conditions. (Accessed January 2016) http://nice.org.uk/guidance/ng22.

NICE (2016) Transition from children's to adults' services for young people using health or social care services. (Accessed July 2016) https://www.nice.org.uk/guidance/ng43.

NHS (2008) Improving access to psychological therapies. *Long Term Conditions Positive Practice Guide*. (Accessed January 2016) http://www.iapt.nhs.uk/silo/files/longterm-conditions-positive-practice-guide.pdf.

NHS Scotland (2010) Quality Strategy—Putting people at the heart of our NHS. (Accessed January 2016) http://www.gov.scot/Publications/2010/05/10102307/0.

Naidoo J and Wills J (2016) *Foundations for Health Promotion*, 4th edn. London: Elsevier.

Nichols K (2003) *Psychological Care for Ill and Injured People—A Clinical Guide*. Maidenhead: Open University Press.

Nuffield Trust (2013) Examining the effectiveness of virtual wards. (Accessed January 2016) http://www.nuffieldtrust.org.uk/our-work/projects/examining-effectiveness-virtual-wards.

Nursing and Midwifery Council (NMC) 2015 *The Code*. London: NMC.

Prochasta JO and DiClemente C (1984) The transtheoretical approach: Crossing traditional foundations of change Don Jones/Irwin. In Naidoo J and Wills J (Eds.) *Foundations for Health Promotion*, 4th edn. London: Elsevier.

Rollnick S, Miller WR and Butler C (2008) *Motivational Interviewing in Health Care: Helping Patients to Change Behaviour*. New York, NY: The Guilford Press.

Ross S, Curry N and Goodwin N (2011) *Case Management—What it is and How it Can Best be Implemented*. London: King's Fund. (Accessed January 2016) http://www.kingsfund.org.uk/sites/files/kf/Case-Management-paper-The-Kings-Fund-Paper-November-2011_0.pdf.

Royal College of General Practitioners (2014) Health literacy report from an RCGP-led health literacy workshop. (Accessed July 2016) http://www.rcgp.org.uk/news/2014/june/~/media/Files/Policy/RCGP-Health-Literacy-2014.ashx.

Scottish Government (2009) Improving the health & wellbeing of people with long-term conditions in Scotland: A national action plan 2009. (Accessed January 2016) http://www.sehd.scot.nhs.uk/mels/CEL2009_23.pdf.

Snodden J (2010) *Case Management of Long Term Conditions: Principles and Practices for Nurses*. Oxford: Wiley Blackwell.

Wales Audit Office (2014). The management of chronic conditions in wales—An update. (Accessed January 2016) http://www.audit.wales/system/files/publications/The%20Management%20of%20Chronic%20Conditions%20in%20Wales%20-%20An%20Update.pdf.

Providing quality care at the end of life

Gina King

INTRODUCTION

The term 'end-of-life care' (EoLC) is still a relatively new phenomenon, and it encompasses all aspects of care at the end of an individual's life. Rather than describing care as palliative, supportive or terminal, EoLC is now the preferred term when identifying a person who is in the final stages of life, which may last years, months, weeks or days. The importance of this term is that it helps professionals acknowledge and more actively plan ahead for the care that may be needed to optimise quality of life and focus on living rather than dying. The six steps of the EoL pathway outlined in the *End of Life Care Strategy* (DH, 2008) have been used to structure this chapter and each one will be discussed in turn with a cross-reference to the national *Ambitions for Palliative and End of Life Care* (2015).

Each year in England around half a million people die, of which two-thirds are aged over 75 years. This is predicted to increase to 550,000 by 2035 (The Choice in End of Life Care Programme Board, 2015). Most deaths (58%) occur in National Health System (NHS) hospitals, with around 18% occurring at home, 17% in care homes, 4% in hospices and 3% elsewhere (ONS, 2014). Although the number of people dying in their 'usual place of residence', that is, at home or in care homes has risen from under 38% in 2008 to 44.5% (NEoLCIN, 2015). However, the evidence still suggests over 60% would prefer to die at home (NHS England, 2014), demonstrating a vast difference in preferences and actual place of death. There are several contributing factors that can influence this outcome. The older the population, the more likely it is that they have complex needs and require integrated care packages (Ellershaw and Murphy, 2005). In addition, the need for hospital admissions increases due to disease progression and carer crises, all of which reduce the patient's and family's confidence and ability to cope with dying at home (Munday et al., 2007). The number of deaths is set to increase by 17% between 2012 and 2030 in England and Wales, and for those over 85 years from 32% to 44% (DH, 2014), which will have a significant impact on community service provision (Age UK, 2014) and nurses will need to be equipped with the appropriate knowledge and skills so they can offer high-quality care (DH, 2009a).

The aim of high-quality EoLC is to support all individuals with advanced, progressive and incurable illnesses regardless of diagnosis, stage or setting, to live as well as possible until they die, therefore to be able to live with a quality of life and have mechanisms in place to enable discussions and make informed decisions about their preferences and choices so they die where and how they choose (DH, 2008). The National Council for Palliative Care (NCPC) stresses the importance of identifying the supportive and palliative needs of both patients and family throughout the last phase of life and into bereavement, which includes the management of pain and other symptoms and provision of psychological, social, spiritual and practical support (NCHSPCS, 2002; National Institute of Clinical Excellence [NICE], 2011; The Choice in End of Life Care Programme Board, 2015). Although the United Kingdom was ranked top of the league table (93.4 out of 100) for providing the best in EoLC in the world which praised the quality and availability of services (BBC News, 2015), there is still evident need for improvement in providing equity in all care settings.

Over the past century the demographics of dying in relation to age profile, cause and place of death have changed fundamentally, as previously a greater number of deaths occurred either in childhood or young adulthood. As a result, the public's social contact with dying has been reduced and an experience of someone dying who is close to them does not tend to occur until later in their own lives (Hanks et al., 2010). The stigma associated with dying in society today means that we do not tend to discuss death and dying openly, causing difficulties in communication when end of life approaches either for the individual concerned or someone close to them (Seymour et al., 2010).

Each individual has their own perspective in terms of what constitutes a 'good death', and the majority agree that it is about being

- Treated as an individual, with dignity and respect
- Without pain and other symptoms
- In familiar surroundings
- In the company of close family and/or friends (DH, 2008)

These elements of high-quality EoLC are important to achieve for the individual concerned and especially for the family if we respect the words of Dame Cecily Saunders, the founder of the Hospice movement, when she stated 'How people die remains in the memory of those who live on' (Saunders, 1989).

ACTIVITY 14.1

Reflection point

Reflect on a patient you have cared for who has died. Consider what you felt about their quality of life and the care received.

END-OF-LIFE CARE STRATEGY

The end-of-life care strategy was produced in July 2008 by the Department of Health and was the first ever paper to identify that there was a need for equitable and standardised care for all individuals regardless of their diagnosis, setting or stage (Gray, 2011).

Historically, those with a cancer diagnosis had easier access to care, resources and services (NAO, 2008). Other reports and white papers, such as the National Institute for Health and Care Excellence guidance for improving palliative and supportive care (NICE, 2004), *Our Health, Our Care, Our Say* (DH, 2006), *Living and Dying Well* (NHS Scotland, 2008), *Transforming Community Services* (DH, 2009b), *Dementia Strategy* (DH, 2009c), *Palliative and End of Life Care Strategy for Northern Ireland* (DHSSPSNI, 2009; House of Commons Health Committee, 2015), Better Endings Right Care, Right Place, Right Time (NIHR, 2015), *NICE Guideline for the Care of Dying Adults in the Last Days of Life* (2015) and DH (2016) have reinforced the call for all health, social and voluntary care professionals and organisations to examine their service provision in order to provide good-quality EoLC.

The *End of Life Care Strategy* (DH, 2008) provides processes and themes for organisations and individual professionals involved in the provision of EoLC to use in developing practice and improving the delivery of care over a 10-year plan (Gray, 2011). Its overall aim is to provide high-quality care for all at the end of life, not just within hospices and specialist palliative care services but in other care settings as well (Gray, 2011). The paper is based on the following 12 principles:

1. Raising the profile on death and dying
2. Strategically commissioning services to provide the best quality care
3. Identifying people approaching the end of life
4. Planning care
5. Co-ordinating care
6. Permitting rapid access to care
7. Delivering high-quality services in all locations
8. Providing care in the last days of life and care after death
9. Involving and supporting carers
10. Educating and training and continuing professional development
11. Performing measurement and research
12. Obtaining funding to support these principles

(DH, 2008)

The *Ambitions for Palliative and End of Life Care* that was released in 2015 built on the national EoLC strategy and the associated 12 key principles, highlighting the need for leadership from commissioning and health and social care provider organisations, in particular Health and Well-Being Boards. The ambitions include six goals based on learning from papers such as the Francis Report (2013), *More Care, Less Pathway* (Neuberger, 2013), *One Chance to Get It Right* (Leadership Alliance for the Care of Dying People [LACDP] 2014) and the Ombudsman Report (PHSO, 2015). The ambitions are underpinned by 'building blocks' that provide foundations for providing high-quality care (Figure 14.1) The six ambitions are as shown in Figure 14.1.

As the six ambitions are built on the previous goals set by the National EoLC Strategy (2008), in community nursing practice, the six steps of the EoL pathway outlined in the strategy still provide a useful tool to help apply theory to practice (Figure 14.2).

Step 1: Discussions as EoLC approaches: Identification of people approaching the end of life and initiating discussions about preferences for EoLC

The key aspect of the EoL pathway is to identify those patients who are approaching the end of their life. Historically, this has presented a challenge not only in relation to prognostic tools that can be complex to use, but also in acknowledging the time when care becomes palliative as opposed to curative. However, unless all members of the multidisciplinary team (MDT) work together to identify patients regardless of their diagnosis, discussions around preferences and options will not take place, families and friends will not be appropriately supported and patients will not achieve a good death (Hubbard, 2011). Early identification of the EoL stage is one of the most important processes to take place to allow sufficient time for the individual to discuss their preferences and wishes (NICE, 2011). The *Dying without Dignity* investigations led by the Parliamentary and Health Service Ombudsman into complaints about EoL care (PHSO, 2015) highlighted several key themes such as the lack of recognition that people are dying leaving insufficient time for care to be planned and discussed as well as open and honest conversations with the person and those important to them.

The Gold Standards Framework advocated by the *End of Life Care Strategy* (DH, 2008) has produced a 'Prognostic Indicator Guidance' which outlines the Karnofsky Performance Status Score, the three main disease trajectories (cancer, neurological conditions and dementia/frailty) and, most importantly, recommended the adoption of the 'surprise question', Would you be surprised if this patient were to die in the

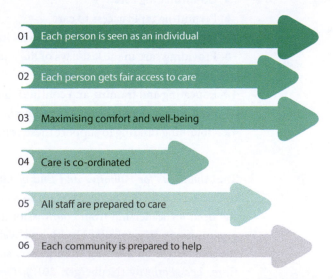

01 Each person is seen as an individual

02 Each person gets fair access to care

03 Maximising comfort and well-being

04 Care is co-ordinated

05 All staff are prepared to care

06 Each community is prepared to help

Figure 14.1 The six ambitions for palliative and end of life care. (Taken from *Ambitions for Palliative and End of Life Care*, 2015.)

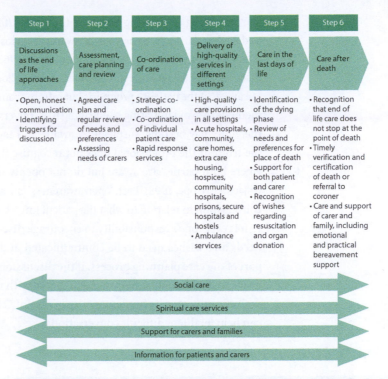

Figure 14.2 The six steps of the EoL Pathway outlined in the EoLC Strategy. (See Department of Health, *End of Life Care Strategy: Promoting High Quality Care for All Adults at the End of Life,* The Stationery Office, London, 2008. With kind permission from the National End of Life Care Programme.)

next 6–12 months? (GSF, 2011). This question has been regarded as one of the most effective instruments in identifying EoLC because of its simplicity and application to any diagnosis or just old age (Boyd and Murray, 2010). This is now supported with further questions: Do they have general indicators of decline? followed by: Do they display specific clinical indicators? (GSF, 2011). The Supportive and Palliative Care Indicator Tool (SPCIT) produced by NHS Lothian offers a similar model that breaks down the process into four steps (NHS Lothian, 2016). This also includes the 'surprise question' in its first step titled 'Ask', followed by 'Look for two or more general clinical indicators', 'Now look for two or more disease related indicators', and finally 'Assess patient and family for supportive and palliative care needs. Review treatment/ medication. Plan care. Consider patient for general practice palliative care register'.

Good communication skills are essential not only to initiate conversations and discussions with patients and their families as EoLC approaches but also to provide support, help and advice to them along their journey and to help them feel valued (Munday et al., 2007). It is the professional's responsibility to recognise that it is a two-way process and that the individual's information needs will vary over time and circumstances (responsive communication) (NICE, 2011). This can be a challenging prospect for many health professionals as it may provoke professional discomfort based on many influencing factors, such as the professional's accountability and responsibility; knowledge, skills, attitude and expertise; workload pressures; and the fear of getting or creating upset for the patient/family (Watson et al., 2009; Barclay and Maher, 2010). Four aspects of awareness (closed, suspicion, mutual pretense and open) were identified by Glaser and Strauss in 1965 (Cope, 1998) which may influence discussions between professionals and patients. Closed awareness is where professionals are aware of the patient's prognosis but refrain from disclosing the information and use methods to avoid initiating or engaging in a conversation (Seale et al., 1997). The patient therefore may become 'suspiciously aware' and try to use tactics such as cues to find the truth. If the professional does not recognise it, this can lead to 'mutual pretense', where both parties are aware but do not openly discuss and acknowledge the dying trajectory (Cope, 1998). Last, 'open awareness' is when both parties are able to engage in conversation in relation to what the patient knows and understands (Seale et al., 1997).

It is everyone's responsibility to encourage discussions, and the patient's identified needs and wishes need to be communicated and co-ordinated within the MDT as part of the care planning process. If the discussion has not taken place then the MDT needs to decide who will open the dialogue with the patient (Hanks et al., 2010).

Communication is fundamental to good EoLC (Watson et al., 2009) and Table 14.1 can help facilitate difficult conversations.

Table 14.1 How to promote good communication

Factors to consider	Guidelines	Example
The environment	Privacy, no interruptions	Quiet room, arranged time
Body language	Understanding how your posture may reflect barriers in communication Observing the patient's body language	Barriers: arms and legs crossed, tapping of a foot, clenching of hands
Non-verbal communication	Personal space, posture, gestures	Relaxed facial expressions, eye contact
Verbal communication	Use of simple language and open-focused questions	'How have you been feeling since your last visit to the doctor?'
Listening	Use of silence and use of body language to acknowledge that you have 'heard'. Also what is being said. What is the meaning behind the words and the non-verbal communication to identify triggers and cues for further exploration	Gentle nodding of head: 'You sound very angry about what has been happening to you'
Demonstrating empathy	Acknowledge feelings	'I understand how difficult this must be for you'
Reflection	Assess level of understanding and document/share with MDT for further discussion – seamless care	'So from what you were saying I understand that ...'
Barriers	The patient may have internal and external factors that are affecting the communication process	Disease progression, tiredness, lack of understanding, language, environment, feelings of loss

Sources: Heyse-Moore, L., *Speaking of Dying*, Jessica Kingsley, London, 2009; Watson, M., Lucas, C., Hoy, A., and Wells, J., *Oxford Handbook of Palliative Care*, 2nd edn., Oxford University Press, Oxford, 2009; NHS National End of Life Care Programme (NEOLCP), *Support Sheet 2: Principles of Good Communication*, National End of Life Care Programme, Leicester, 2010a; Fallowfield, L., In *Oxford Textbook of Palliative Medicine*, 4th edn., Oxford University Press, Oxford, 2010; Barclay, S. and Maher, J., *British Medical Journal*, 341, c4862, 2010.

Sensitivity and respect should be displayed around the discussion as some individuals may not feel ready to have the dialogue at that particular point in time (Barclay and Maher, 2010). Everyone should have the opportunity to be offered honest and well-informed conversations about their future, that may include discussions around death and dying, and everyone must be seen as individual (NPELCP, 2015). There is no particular point on the EoL pathway that is the optimum time to initiate a discussion around EoLC; however, the 'earlier the better' is advocated to allow the patient the opportunity to make an informed choice and support the process of advance care planning (ACP) (Barclay and Maher, 2010).

ACP is a process of discussion between an individual and their care provider irrespective of discipline. If desired by the patient, family and friends are included. With the individual's agreement, this discussion should be documented, regularly reviewed and communicated to key people involved in their care (Henry and Seymour, 2007). The difference between ACP and general care planning is that the purpose of ACP is to clarify a patient's wishes and decisions (e.g. preferred place of death) and for these to be incorporated into a general care plan so the MDT can provide appropriate care and support on their EoL pathway (NEOLCP, 2010d).

The two key terms used in ACP are an advance statement and an advance decision (Table 14.2).

A statement can be either verbal or written and identifies the individual's wishes, preferences, beliefs and values. It is not legally binding but must be taken into account when the person loses capacity to advocate their wishes and preferences in their best interests. An advance decision states that specific medical treatment is to be refused in the circumstances that are stated and is written by the individual with support from professionals, relatives or carers. It becomes effective once the individual has lost capacity by giving consent or refusing treatment even if it puts

Table 14.2 Advance decisions to refuse treatment

Patient considerations	Family/carers and professionals
It is a voluntary process and may be initiated by the patient	Family members, carers, partners may be involved if requested by the patient
Must be aged 18 and over and have capacity to discuss the options available and be able to agree to them	Professionals supporting the patient must follow the appropriate guidance 'Advance decisions to refuse treatment – A guide for health and social care staff'
The individual's responsibility is to keep the ADRT up to date and to keep professionals involved in their care informed and up to date	To establish whether an advance decision is valid and applicable, healthcare professionals must try to find out if the person: – Has done anything that clearly goes against their advance decision – Has withdrawn their decision – Has subsequently conferred the power to make that decision on an attorney – Would have changed their decision if they had known more about the current circumstances

Source: Taken from *Advance Decisions to Refuse Treatment (ADRT) – A Guide for Health and Social Care Professionals* (NEOLCP, 2008) with permission from the National End of Life Care Programme.

their life at risk. However, it cannot be prepared if the individual has lost capacity and therefore must meet all the requirements of the Mental Capacity Act and will be legally binding for social and healthcare professionals (NEOLCP, 2008).

ACTIVITY 14.2

Consider who you feel is the most appropriate member of the MDT to initiate discussions for a patient approaching EoLC and why.

Step 2: Assessment, care planning and review: Assessing needs and preferences, agreeing on a care plan to reflect these and reviewing these regularly

A holistic common assessment (psychological, spiritual, physical and social) of the patient and family needs is essential to ensure that all the individual's wishes are taken into account and helps to identify any unmet areas of care (King's Fund, 2007). The MDT can then co-ordinate and communicate the best possible care dependent on the level and availability of the services (Hanks et al., 2010), as supported by the NICE Quality Standard for EoLC (2011). This is a joint assessment with the individual that involves their consent. It should be based on the principles of person-centred care and is a continuous process, as information cannot always be gathered at one visit (NEOLCP, 2010b).

The most important aspect of the holistic assessment is verifying the individual's and their family's levels of understanding of their diagnosis, treatment options and prognosis (National Cancer Action Team, 2010). This knowledge then enables discussions in relation to their preferences and choices at the end of life, development of a proactive and personalised plan of care and anticipation of crises supported by contingency plans to prevent readmission to hospital (NEOLCP, 2010d; NICE, 2011). There are five domains of the assessment, which are background information and assessment preferences, physical needs, social and occupational needs, physical well-being, and spiritual well-being and life goals (NEOLCP, 2010c). The NICE guidance for EoLC (2011) recommends that an assessment for the person and their families approaching EoLC should involve

- Provision of written and other forms of information
- Face-to-face communication
- Individual involvement in decision making
- Control of physical symptoms
- Provision of psychological support
- Social support
- Spiritual support
- Organ and tissue donation

The House of Care Model (NHS England, 2014) provides a whole system approach to long-term care management. It focuses on goal setting, action planning, sharing of information, support, long-term decision making and putting the person central to their care.

Figure 14.3 highlights how the person is at the centre of their care.

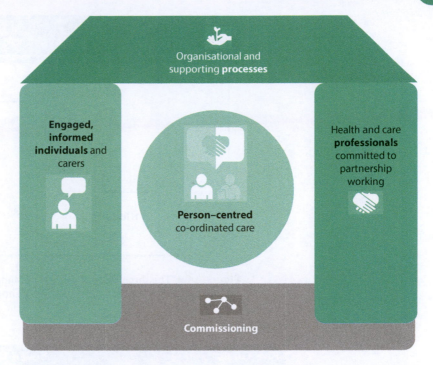

Figure 14.3 The house of care model. (Taken from NHS England, *Actions for End of Life Care: 2014–16*, 2014.)

A holistic assessment forms an essential part of the Gold Standards Framework (GSF).

The Gold Standards Framework

The Gold Standards Framework (GSF) is a system-focused approach formalising best practice for individuals in their last year of life (Gray, 2011). It provides tools and resources to identify, assess and plan care in a more co-ordinated and communicated way so that all professionals feel empowered to give the best possible care (Thomas, 2003; GSF, 2009). It originated initially in general practices in 2001 and is now being adopted in care homes, community and acute hospitals across the United Kingdom (Munday and Dale, 2007; GSF, 2015). The key aspect of the GSF is that it enables the MDT, at regular meetings, to proactively plan ahead, anticipate possible crises, assess carers' needs and manage bereavement concerns of the family/relatives and those important to them (NPELCP, 2015). It involves the holistic assessment of the individual and their family, advance care planning and care of the dying (Thomas, 2003; GSF, 2009). The GSF in the community setting has been paramount in changing how professionals plan care and involve other members of the MDT (for example, specialist palliative care, allied health professionals, social care, receptionist) who are involved in the patient's pathway (Munday and Dale, 2007).

The GSF comprises one aim, three steps, five goals and seven Cs (Table 14.3).

• *One aim* – To deliver a 'gold' standard of care for all patients nearing the end of life.

• *Three steps (see Figure 14.4)*

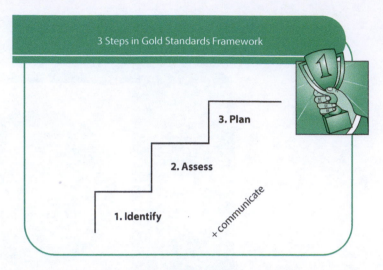

Figure 14.4 The three steps of the Gold Standards Framework. (With kind permission from Professor Keri Thomas.)

Table 14.3

Five Goals	Seven Cs
1. Consistent high-quality care	Communication
2. Alignment with patients' preferences	Co-ordination
3. Pre-planning and anticipation of needs	Control of symptoms
4. Improved staff confidence and teamwork	Continuity of care
5. More home-based, less hospital-based care	Continued learning Care support Care of the dying

Source: Gold Standards Framework (GSF), *Community Nurses GSF,* Factsheet 1, National Gold Standards Framework Centre, London, 2009. With kind permission from Professor Keri Thomas.

The first step is to identify the last year of life (6–12 months) and list those identified patients on a GSF Register for the MDT to proactively plan care. Their disease trajectory is predicted by using the Needs-Based Coding (Figure 14.5) to estimate their stage to plan their care needs.

Support in line with needs – GSF helps identify people earlier and meet their needs

• Months
• Weeks
• Days

| A - Blue 'All' from diagnosis Stable Year plus prognosis | B - Green 'Benefits' - DS1500 Unstable / Advanced disease Months prognosis | C - Yellow 'Continuing Care' Deteriorating Weeks prognosis | D - Red 'Days' Final days / Terminal care Days prognosis | Navy 'After Care' |

Figure 14.5 Needs-based coding – using the 'surprise question' to predict main areas of need and support required. (With kind permission from Professor Keri Thomas.)

The second step is to assess through a holistic common assessment including their benefits – patients may be entitled to claim for non-means-tested benefits, for example, DS1500 to support a Personal Independence Allowance if aged between 16 and 64 years or if over 65 years, an Attendance allowance. Assess the patient's possible needs such as anticipatory care and prescribing including ACP. Most of all, early assessment of carers' needs is advocated (formal assessment) along with provision of written information.

The third step is to plan general care generated from the holistic common and carers' assessment, the ACP discussions and any recorded wishes/choices. It is about thinking proactively and anticipating possible crises, by ordering medication and equipment and co-ordinating and communicating with the MDT especially out-of-hours (OOH) services. Identification and allocation of a key worker can support the patient and family in the EoL Pathway and guide the MDT discussions (GSF, 2009).

ACTIVITY 14.3

Consider how you would implement and/or evaluate the GSF into your GP and what resources you would need to achieve this.

Step 3: Co-ordination of care

Co-ordinating an individual's care and fair access are one of the key aspects at the end of life (Ambitions, 2015). Organisations also need to work together and be effective, providing realistic outcomes for the individual to ensure care is delivered in the right way and time (NICE, 2011). If their wishes and preferences are not respected, the individual and their family may feel devalued and experience unnecessary anxiety. The GSF is one tool that can ensure that the MDT is communicating and co-ordinating care (Munday and Dale, 2007). The importance of every health and social care professional being involved in an integrated personalised care plan that is regularly reviewed is essential to ensure the patient's needs are supported (NEOLCP, 2010c). Communication links with the OOH services such as medical 'hubs' and evening and night community nursing services are paramount as there is more likelihood of a crisis happening at that time (NICE, 2011). The patient and family feel more vulnerable and isolated at home when carers' or professionals' visits and contact are less frequent (Munday et al., 2007). By using the tools within the GSF such as the OOH communication tool or special notes on electronic systems, community nurses can inform these services that the patient is now end of life and outline any possible predicament. In some areas of the United Kingdom, the MDT use an End of Life Locality register alternatively known as an Electronic Palliative Care Co-ordination System, which is a template comprising a "checklist" that is communicated to OOH services and other care providers. This lists all the key information surrounding decisions and actions in the last 6–12 months of life in a tick-box format (Social Research Institute, 2011).

As a community nurse, it is necessary to involve and include the MDT resourcefully such as specialist palliative care dependent on how much the patient and family require or want their involvement (Boyd and Murray, 2010). The key component is that every person is an individual with changing needs and feelings. It is important to remember that although patients may decline support or refuse equipment at certain points along the pathway, their needs still exist, and it is the nurse's role to encourage and support the individual regardless and enable them to maintain independence, choice and control (Barclay and Maher, 2010). As outlined in the communication section, just listening and encouraging the patient to express their feelings and anxieties can initiate discussions about dying and alleviate their feelings of isolation and loneliness. However, it is important to respect the person's privacy as it is their home, their environment and their space. Family members and carers, friends and neighbours play an essential part in a person's pathway and need to be included in joint discussions and decisions (NEOLCP, 2010d).

ACTIVITY 14.4

Reflect on how you can assess whether all the services are communicating and co-ordinating care.

Support for carers, both during a person's illness and after their death – Many family members become unpaid carers and there are now around half a million people who provide care for a terminally ill relative or friend in the United Kingdom (Payne, 2010). This figure is set to increase due to the rising demographics of the older population (NHS England, 2014). The role is an intricate one as although they are still the individual's relative they are dealing with an unpredictable journey, providing intimate care that they would never have envisaged and experiencing the emotional strain that they will eventually be bereaved. Also, they are often 'thrown' into this role without any previous knowledge or experience (Payne, 2010). The ongoing pressure of the caring role is one of the key reasons why patients are admitted to hospital during their pathway and at the end of life (Jack and O'Brien, 2010). Therefore, many carers need respite, support, guidance and information to help them cope with their daily lives (NAO, 2008). Although for some it may be a temporary role, it can still affect the carer's work and impact on the rest of their life with regard to their future role in life (for further information refer to Chapter 9). It is important that the community nurse assesses, co-ordinates and supports the care in a proactive way to ensure that the carer is involved and able to cope with the ever-changing circumstances at the end of life (Jack and O' Brien, 2010; Milne et al., 2007; NICE, 2011). Additionally, it is important to explore what community networks are available for the carer and what support is around locally that might be prepared to help with ongoing tasks (Abel et al., 2016), and also to recognise that if support is declined initially by the carer that there is opportunity to change their minds later on, if so desired, with timely intervention (NICE, 2011).

ACTIVITY 14.5

Joan is 78 years old and has been married to Harold for 60 years. She has had dementia for 3 years, with a history of arthritis in her hands. Harold is her main carer and has been finding it increasingly difficult to cope recently as Joan is unable to communicate her needs and has begun wandering at night. The GP has referred Joan to an Alzheimer Adviser/Admiral Nurse for further support and information for Harold. How can you as a community nurse assess Joan and Harold's needs in co-ordination with the Alzheimer Adviser/Admiral Nurse to identify the cause of Joan's change in condition? What other support is available to Harold to ensure he feels he is able to manage?

Step 4: Delivery of high-quality services

Patients and families may need to use a combination and range of services from across different organisations and settings, and it is imperative that they should receive high-quality and equitable care regardless of its origin (NEOLCP, 2010d). The role of the community nurse is to make certain that all information is documented and shared with all the professionals involved in the patient's care. It is an essential part of the community nurse's role to recognise their accountability for the delivery of care and to ensure all documentation is an accurate record of events (LACDP, 2014).

Diversity, equality and language

People approaching the end of life and their families and carers should have access to the high-quality care (NPELCP, 2015) described in this quality standard on the basis of need and that takes into account their preferences, regardless of their individual circumstances, including the following:

- Gender
- Ethnicity
- Disability
- Cognitive impairment
- Age
- Sexual orientation
- Gender reassignment
- Religion and belief
- Culture or lifestyle
- Marriage and civil partnership
- Pregnancy and maternity
- Socio-economic status
- Mental capacity
- Diagnosis
- Choices they make about their care
- Location and setting in which they are receiving care

(Taken from NICE 2011 Quality Standard in EoLC)

The key aim of this chapter is to ensure that the community nurse is aware of EoLC tools and the EoL Pathway in order to provide a high standard of care. It is, however, an individual practitioner's responsibility to be aware of their own and the team's training needs, to meet these learning needs and to develop their practice (Skills for Care and for Health, 2017) and be prepared to care (NPELCP, 2015).

ACTIVITY 14.6

Reflection point
Reflect on a patient you have recently cared for and for whom you felt the care could have been better managed. What personal and professional development needs can you identify that would help you feel more effective in the future?

Step 5: Care in the last days of life

The dying process

Supporting the family through the dying process is a sensitive and emotional experience. Being aware of the general issues that an individual may experience will enable the community nurse to prepare the family to deal with the changes (NEOLCP, 2010b). For further guidance, refer to the five priorities of care outlined in the *One Chance to Get It Right* by the LACDP (2014).

The Liverpool Care Pathway – Neuberger Report

The Liverpool Care Pathway (LCP) was introduced in the late 1990s and was used to standardise and improve care in the last hours and days of life (Dee and Endacott, 2011). The model originated from the Hospital Specialist Palliative Care Team at the Royal Liverpool and Broadgreen University Hospital NHS Trust and staff from the Marie Curie Hospice in Liverpool who identified that the majority of patients died in hospital (60%). As a result, they wanted to transfer best practice from a hospice setting to a hospital setting (Taylor, 2009). It had been previously criticised in some literature for supporting euthanasia, for not effectively meeting spiritual and religious needs and for not adequately preparing or training staff to use the tool (Taylor, 2009). However, despite the supporting evidence that found it helped to improve the care of dying patients and provide positive outcomes for the MDT in changing attitudes and methods of working (Paterson et al., 2009), it was recommended in the independent "Review of the Liverpool Care Pathway" (Neuberger, 2013) to phase out the LCP within 6–12 months and change this approach to be more focused on individualised and personalised care planning. This was the result of an in-depth investigation triggered by complaints of poor care, unnecessary withholding of hydration and nutrition, lack of communication and consent (Liddament, 2015) and built on the findings of the Francis Report (2013).

One Chance to Get It Right

The *One Chance to Get It Right* – Improving people's experience of care in the last few days and hours of life (LACDP, 2014) was produced in response to the Neuberger Report (2013) and identified five key priorities that would instead replace a national care plan. This is also highlighted in the *Ambitions for Palliative and End of Life Care* (2015) (Figure 14.6).

Priorities for Care of the Dying Person

The Priorities for Care are that, when it is thought that a person may die within the next few days or hours.

1. This possibility is recognised and communicated clearly, decisions are made and actions taken in accordance with the person's needs and wishes, and these are regularly reviewed and decisions revised accordingly.

2. Sensitive communication takes place between staff and the dying person, and those identified as important to them.

3. The dying person, and those identified as important to them, are involved in decisions about treatment and care to the extent that the dying person wants.

4. The needs of families and others identified as important to the dying person are actively explored, respected and met as far as possible.

5. An individual plan of care, which includes food and drink, symptom control and psychological, social and spiritual support, is agreed, co-ordinated and delivered with compassion.

Figure 14.6 The five priorities for Care of the Dying Person. (Taken from Leadership Alliance for the Care of Dying People, *One Chance to Get It Right*, Leadership Alliance for the Care of Dying People, London, 2014.)

The *One Chance to Get It Right* (LACDP, 2014) Report highlights the key aspects of communicating with the individual and family/carers throughout their journey to ensure all their needs are met. The decision to identify 'recognition of dying' that the person is in their last days and hours of life will usually be assessed by the GP, district nurse and other members of the MDT (DH, 2013) and an identified "lead" should be nominated. The patient and/or the family should also be involved in these discussions with sensitive communication and supportive information available (NICE, 2011; LACDP, 2014). Information that is offered to people approaching the end of life, and their families and carers, should include the following:

- Treatment and care options, medication
- What to expect at each stage of the journey towards the end of life
- Who they can contact at any time of day or night to obtain advice, support or services
- Practical advice and details of other relevant services such as benefits support
- Details of relevant local and national self-help and support groups

(NICE, 2011)

Conversations around the diminished need for food and drink should be included and for professionals to recognise that provision, that may in some cases provide risks, can often provide comfort to the patient and family/carers (LACDP, 2014). It is essential that clear and understandable communication regularly occurs to support ongoing concerns and uncertainties with all those involved in their care (Liddament, 2015). The main priority is maximising comfort and well-being (NPELCP, 2015). This will in cases, include discussions around limits of treatment including Do Not Attempt Cardiopulmonary Resuscitation (DNACPR) – withholding and withdrawing treatment and preferred place of care and death (LACDP, 2014). It is important to consider that these difficult conversations for the person and their family need to be communicated with empathy and the recognition of emotional stress and distress that have been caused (LACDP, 2014). Being fully informed about the process related to decisions around DNACPR including the Mental Capacity Act (2005) will support individuals and those important to them in making informed choices about their future care.

The NICE Guidance of the Care of dying adults in the last days of life (2015) was produced in response to the removal of the Liverpool Care Pathway and the recommendations set out by the *One Chance to Get It Right* Report (LACDP, 2014). It covers the clinical care of adults (18 years and over) identified as dying in the last 2–3 days of life. It includes all the key points highlighted in the report, such as clear and sensitive communication with the person and those important to them and discussions around maintaining hydration. It also provides a repository of information around comfort and dignity, anticipatory prescribing, the management of symptoms and the side effects of medications to support care in the last days of life and maximising comfort and well-being (NPELCP, 2015). For further reading, see https://www.nice.org.uk/guidance/ng31/chapter/context (Figure 14.7).

The community nurse needs to recognise that when caring for a person in the last days of life, it includes being prepared to support individual and unique relationships of the related friends, family, carers and peers in their community. This will mean also helping those loved ones to be prepared for their loss, grief and bereavement (NPELCP, 2015).

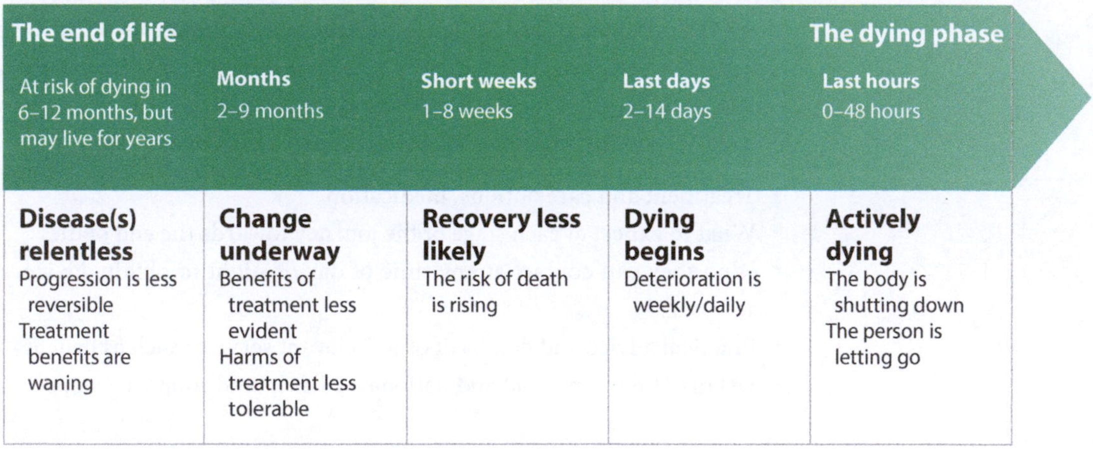

The end of life				The dying phase
At risk of dying in 6–12 months, but may live for years	**Months** 2–9 months	**Short weeks** 1–8 weeks	**Last days** 2–14 days	**Last hours** 0–48 hours
Disease(s) relentless Progression is less reversible Treatment benefits are waning	**Change underway** Benefits of treatment less evident Harms of treatment less tolerable	**Recovery less likely** The risk of death is rising	**Dying begins** Deterioration is weekly/daily	**Actively dying** The body is shutting down The person is letting go

Figure 14.7 Time frames in the dying process.

Step 6: Care after death – Bereavement

What to do when someone dies

When a patient dies, even though it is expected, it can be a difficult, emotional and stressful time for the bereaved relatives and for the community nurse. Each individual's family situation is different and sometimes complex due to previous psychosocial issues within the family's matrix (Watson et al., 2009). Table 14.4

Table 14.4 'What to do after a death in England or Wales' (2014) Department for Work and Pensions

Process	Example
Provide information to the family on what to do next	'What to do after a death in England or Wales' and a localised bereavement leaflet
Inform services of the death	GP practice, out of hours service
Verify the death	The death can be verified (if certified competent) or refer to the doctor who will verify and certify the death
Inform the coroner	Unexpected death or patient not seen by the GP for 14 days (GP and police to be informed first)
Request for a post-mortem	An unexpected death that the coroner decides needs further investigation
Contact the funeral director	Once the death certificate is issued
Register the death	Within 5 days and then a burial or cremation certificate will be issued by the registrar

ACTIVITY 14.7

Consider what you might need to include in a personalised care plan as part of your holistic common assessment for an individual's last days of life.

provides an aide-memoire for this time based on information provided in 'What to do after a death in England or Wales' (DWP, 2014).

The most vital component is to reassure, support and offer comfort to those present and allow privacy if desired and, if no one is present, to notify the family as quickly as possible. An individualised personalised care plan is a useful tool based on the *One Chance to Get It Right* (LACDP, 2014) five priorities of care to support the community nurse through the care after death and ensures that families are supported. Careful consideration must be included to the individual's and families' spiritual and religious needs with referrals to spiritual care providers for guidance and involvement as appropriate which can be of great support at this time (NICE, 2011). For further information, see Chapter 10 on spirituality.

A stepped approach to emotional and bereavement support may be appropriate, which could include but is not limited to

- Information about local support services
- Practical support such as advice on arranging a funeral, information on whom to inform of a death, help with contacting other family members and information on what to do with equipment and medication
- General emotional and bereavement support, such as supportive conversations with generalist health and social care workers or support from the voluntary, community and faith sectors
- Referral to more specialist support from trained bereavement counsellors or mental health workers

(Taken from NICE Quality Standard EoLC, 2011)

The bereavement process

There are some well-known theories that explore and explain grief which may help community nurses understand the process and support the bereaved person. However, as each bereavement is individual and unique it is often difficult to theorise. It is sometimes difficult to make sense of the emotions involved that may pose challenges for health and social care professionals (Alpack, 2010). This section will not explore the grief process in detail but will provide further guidance.

The grieving process does not always begin when the person dies; for many it begins when the prognosis is given or when it becomes apparent the person is dying. This is why it is important to identify the EoLC phase earlier in the pathway to allow time for the patient and family to go through the process of grieving and have opportunities to discuss their feelings and to identify any 'unfinished business' (Heyse-Moore, 2009). Grief is a normal response to bereavement or a significant loss in a person's life and their experience varies dependent on the relationship or the impact of the loss (Watson et al., 2009). Individuals need to process their loss at their own pace. Although each journey is unique, Kubler-Ross (1969) cited by Kissane and Zaider (2010) was recognised for her work on identifying the five stages (denial, anger, bargaining, depression, acceptance) that people might enter. However, since then this work has been criticised by other researchers who state that there is no particular sequence that the bereaved may experience, and that some people may experience several emotions at one time (Freidman and James, 2008). However, not all emotions in bereavement are negative, as some individuals have a positive response when they feel they have done as much as they possibly could in the dying phase (Davies et al., 1998; Koop and Strang, 2003). Over a period of time, individuals should be able to recover from the loss and return to the daily functions of life and establish a new way of living without their loved one. The role of the community nurse is to identify those who are less likely to cope and are at risk of complicated grief and signpost the bereaved to appropriate care such as their own GP or bereavement services. For further reading please refer to Chapter 15.6 in Hanks et al. (2010).

ACTIVITY 14.8

Reflect on a family that has been bereaved. What emotions were displayed and how did you feel they coped with them? What strategies did you use to manage the situation?

CONCLUSION

This chapter has outlined the importance of the provision of good quality EoLC in the community setting by using the six steps from the EoL Pathway as a framework for best practice. It has highlighted the need for earlier discussions in the pathway, even for the public to start thinking about having conversations before identification of EoLC occurs. It has also identified the essential need for ongoing communication and ACP throughout the pathway around the patient's identified wishes and preferences. Ongoing assessment, care planning and review of the patient and family, with involvement of the MDT across different services, can ensure co-ordinated care. Finally, EoLC tools, policies and NICE guidance that have been discussed can guide, reinforce and document care but cannot dictate the delivery as only the community nurse can determine the level of care they provide.

In striving for optimum standards of care, it is important to reflect on the statement made by the National End of Life Care Strategy (2008) which indicates that 'How we care for the dying is an indicator of how we care for all sick and vulnerable people' (National End of Life Care Strategy 2008, Executive Summary: 10).

FURTHER RESOURCES

www.goldstandardsframework.org.uk/

www.terminalillness.co.uk/understanding-grieving-process.html

www.dyingmatters.org

www.nhs.uk/carersdirect

http://www.ageuk.org.uk/

www.hospiceuk.org.uk

endoflifecareambitions.org.uk/

www.macmillan.org.uk

www.ncpc.org.uk/

www.endoflifecare-intelligence.org.uk/home

www.mariecurie.org.uk/help

https://www.gov.uk/government/organisations/office-of-the-public-guardian

www.resus.org.uk/dnacpr/decisions-relating-to-cpr/

http://www.cqc.org.uk/sites/default/files/20160505%20CQC_EOLC_OVERVIEW_
    FINAL_3.pdf

www.ons.gov.uk/peoplepopulationandcommunity/healthandsocialcare/
    healthcaresystem/datasets/nationalsurveyofbereavedpeoplevoices

www.england.nhs.uk/wp-content/uploads/2016/05/identifying-assessing-carer-hlth-
    wellbeing.pdf

www.gov.uk/government/uploads/system/uploads/attachment_data/file/496231/Faith_
    at_end_of_life_-_a_resource.pdf

www.fpm.ac.uk/faculty-of-pain-medicine/opioids-aware

www.e-lfh.org.uk/programmes/end-of-life-care/

REFERENCES

Abel J, Kerrin M, Murray S and Sallnow L (2016) *Each Community is Prepared to Help: Community Development in End of Life Care – Guidance on Ambition Six*. London: NCPC.

Age UK (2014) *Care in Crisis – What Next for Social Care*. London: Age UK.

Alpack J (2010) *Sorrow Profiles: Death Grief and Crisis in the Family*. London: Karnac Books.

Barclay S and Maher J (2010) Having difficult conversations about end of life care. *British Medical Journal* 341:c4862.

BBC News (2015) (Accessed 6 October 2015) http://www.bbc.co.uk/news/health-34415362.

Boyd K and Murray SA (2010) Recognising and managing key transitions in end of life care. *British Medical Journal* 341:c4863.

Cope G (1998) A review of current theories of death and dying. *Journal of Advanced Nursing* 28:382–90.

Davies B, Deveau E, De Veber B et al. (1998) Experiences of mothers in five countries whose child died of cancer. *Cancer Nursing* 21:301.

Dee JF and Endacott R (2011) Doing the right thing at the right time. *Journal of Nursing Management* 19(2):186–92.

Department for Work and Pensions (2014) *What to Do After a Death in England or Wales*. London: Department for Work and Pensions.

Department of Health (DH) (2006) *Our Health, Our Care, Our Say: A New Direction for Community Services*. London: The Stationery Office.

DH (2008) *End of Life Care Strategy: Promoting High Quality Care for All Adults at the End of Life*. London: The Stationery Office.

DH (2009a) *Transforming Community Services*. London: The Stationery Office.

DH (2009b) *Dementia Strategy*. London: The Stationery Office.

DH (2009c) *End of Life Care Strategy Quality Markers and Measures for the End of Life*. London: The Stationery Office.

DH (2016) *Our Commitment to You for End of Life Care*. London: The Stationery Office.

Department of Health, Social Services and Public Safety (2010) *Living Matters, Dying Matters. A Palliative and End of Life Care Strategy for Adults in Northern Ireland*. Department of Health, Social Services and Public Safety, Castle Buildings, Belfast.

DHSSPSNI (2009) *Palliative and End of Life Care Strategy for Northern Ireland – Consultation Document*. Belfast: DHSSPSNI.

Ellershaw J and Murphy D (2005) The Liverpool Care Pathway (LCP) influencing the UK national agenda on care of the dying. *International Journal of Palliative Nursing* 11:132–4.

Fallowfield L (2010) Communication and palliative medicine. In Watson M, Lucas C, Hoy A, and Wells J (Eds.), *Oxford Handbook of Palliative Care*, 2nd edn. Oxford: Oxford University Press.

Francis R (2013) *Report of the Mid Staffordshire NHS Foundation Trust Public Inquiry. Executive Summary*. London: The Stationery Office.

Freidman R and James JW (2008) The myth of the stages of death, dying and grief. *Skeptic* 14:37–42.

Gold Standards Framework (GSF) (2009) *Community Nurses GSF*. Factsheet 1. London: National Gold Standards Framework Centre.

GSF (2011) *Prognostic Indicator Guidance*, 4th edn. London: National Gold Standards Framework.

GSF (2015) (Accessed 23 July 2015) http://www.goldstandardsframework.org.uk/.

Gray B (2011) *England's Approach to Improving End-of-Life Care: A Strategy for Honoring Patients' Choices. Issues in International Health Policy*. London: The Commonwealth Fund.

Hanks G, Cherny N, Christakis NA et al. (2010) *Oxford Textbook of Palliative Medicine*, 4th edn. Oxford: Oxford University Press.

Henry C and Seymour J (2007) *Advance Care Planning: A Guide for Health and Social Care Staff*. London: The Stationery Office.

Heyse-Moore L (2009) *Speaking of Dying*. London: Jessica Kingsley Publishers.

House of Commons Health Committee (2015) *End of Life Care Fifth Report of Session 2014–15*. London: The Stationery Office Limited.

Hubbard G (2011) The surprise question in end of life care. *British Journal of Community Nursing* 16:109.

Jack B and O'Brien M (2010) Dying at home: Community nurses' views of the impact of informal carers on cancer patient's place of death. *European Journal of Cancer Care* 19:636–42.

King's Fund (2007) *Holistic Common Assessment of Supportive and Palliative Care Needs for Adults with Cancer.* London: Department of Health.

Kissane DW and Zaider T (2010) Bereavement. In GW Hanks GW, NI Cherny, NA Christakis (eds.), *Oxford Textbook of Palliative Medicine.* 4th edn. Oxford: Oxford University Press.

Koop PM and Strang VR (2003) The bereavement experience following home-based family care giving for persons with advanced cancer. *Clinical Nursing Research* 12:127.

Kubler-Ross E (1969) *On Death and Dying.* New York: The Macmillan Company.

Leadership Alliance for the Care of Dying People (2014) *One Chance to Get It Right.* London: Leadership Alliance for the Care of Dying People.

Liddament A (2015) The community matron's role in providing end-of-life care. *Journal of Community Nursing* 29(3): 34–38.

Milne A, Hatzidimitriadou E, Chryssanthopoulou C and Owen T (2007) *Caring in Later Life: Reviewing the Role of Older Carers* (Executive summary). London: Help the Aged.

Munday D and Dale J (2007) Palliative care in the community (Editorial). *British Medical Journal* 334:809.

Munday D, Dale J and Murray S (2007) Choice and place of death, individual preferences uncertainty and the availability of care. *Journal of Social Medicine* 100:211–5.

National Audit Office (NAO) (2008) *Patient and Carer Experiences Regarding End of Life Care in England.* Leeds: OVE ARUP and Porters.

National Cancer Action Team (2010) *Holistic Common Assessment of Supportive and Palliative Care Needs for Adults Requiring End of Life Care.* London: National Cancer Action Team.

National Council for Hospice and Specialist Palliative Care Services (NCHSPCS) (2002) *Definitions of Supportive and Palliative Care.* London: NCHSPCS.

National Institute of Clinical Excellence (NICE) (2004) *Guidance on Cancer Services: Improving Supportive and Palliative Care for Adults with Cancer.* London: NICE.

National Institute of Clinical Excellence (NICE) (2011) *End of Life Care for Adults.* London: NICE.

National Institute of Clinical Excellence (NICE) (2015) *Care of Dying Adults in the last days of life.* London: NICE.

National Intelligence End of Life Care Network (NEoLCIN) (2015) (Accessed 23 July 2015) http://www.endoflifecare-intelligence.org.uk/data_sources/place_of_death.

National Palliative and End of Life Care Partnership (NPELCP) (2015) *Ambitions for Palliative and End of Life Care: A National Framework for Local Action 2015-2020.* NPELCP.

NEOLCP (2008) *Advance Decisions to Refuse Treatment (ADRT) – A Guide for Health and Social Care Professionals.* Leicester: National End of Life Care Programme.

NEOLCP (2010a) *Support Sheet 2: Principles of Good Communication.* Leicester: National End of Life Care Programme.

NEOLCP (2010b) *Support Sheet 8: The Dying Process.* Leicester: National End of Life Care Programme.

NEOLCP (2010c) *Differences Between General Care Planning and Decisions Made in Advance.* Leicester: National End of Life Care Programme.

NEOLCP (2010d) *Route to Success in Care Homes*. Leicester: National End of Life Care Programme.

Neuberger J (2013) *More Care, Less Pathway: A Review of the Liverpool Care Pathway*. London: The Stationary Office.

NHS England (2014) *Actions for End of Life Care: 2014–16*. London: NHS England.

NHS Lothian (2016) *Supportive & Palliative Care Indicators Tool*. Scotland: NHS Lothian and University of Edinburgh.

NHS Scotland (2008) *Living and Dying Well a National Action Plan for Palliative and End of Life Care in Scotland*. Edinburgh: The Scottish Government.

NHS Wales Health Board (2013) *Together for Health –Delivering End of Life Care: A Delivery Plan up to 2016 for NHS Wales and its Partners*. NHS Wales Health Board

NIHR (2015) *Better Endings Right Care, Right Place, Right Time*. Cardiff: NIHR Dissemination Centre.

Office for National Statistics (2014) *National Survey of Bereaved People (VOICES)*. London: ONS.

Parliamentary and Health Service Ombudsman (PHSO) (2015) *Dying Without Dignity Investigations by the Parliamentary and Health Service Ombudsman into Complaints About End of Life Care*. London: PHHSO.

Paterson BC, Duncan R, Conway R et al. (2009) Introduction of the Liverpool Care Pathway for end of life care to emergency medicine. *Emergency Medicine Journal* 26:777–9.

Payne S (2010) Following bereavement, poor health is more likely in carers who perceived that their support from health services was insufficient or whose family member did not die in the carer's preferred place of death. *Evidence Based Nursing* 13:94–5.

Saunders C (1989) Pain and impending death. In Wall PD and Melzak R (eds) *Textbook of Pain*, 2nd edn. Oxford: Churchill Livingstone, pp. 624–31.

Seale C, Addington-Hall J and McCarthy M (1997) Awareness of dying: Prevalence, causes and consequences. *Social Science Medicine* 45:477–84.

Seymour J, French J and Richardson E (2010) Dying matters: Let's talk about it. *British Medical Journal* 341:c4860.

Skills for Care and for Health (2017) *End of Life Care Core Skills Education and Training Framework*. London: Health Education England.

Social Research Institute (2011) *End of Life Locality Registers Evaluation Interim Report*. London: Ipsos MORI.

Taylor H (2009) Liverpool Care Pathway. Bevan Britan: This article was previously published in the February 2010 edition of *Health Care Risk Report*.

The Choice in End of Life Care Programme Board (TCEoLCP) (2015) *What's Important to Me: A Review of Choice in End of Life Care*. London: The Stationery Office.

Thomas K (2003) *Caring for the Dying at Home: Companions on the Journey*. Abingdon: Radcliffe Medical Press.

Watson M, Lucas C, Hoy A and Wells J (2009) *Oxford Handbook of Palliative Care*, 2nd edn. Oxford: Oxford University Press.

Organisation and management of care

Jill Y. Gould

INTRODUCTION

Community services in the United Kingdom undertake approximately 100 million contacts each year (Addicott et al., 2015). As these range widely from universal public health (health visiting and school nursing) to targeted clinical interventions, it is no wonder that nursing in the community setting is seen as varied, complicated and challenging (Drennan et al., 2005; Barrett et al., 2007). Community nurses work in a dynamic and constantly changing care environment with potentially limitless demands (Bowers and Durrant, 2014). On this 'ward without walls' it is difficult to apply restrictions to the number or complexity of patients with little control over increased workload or new referrals (RCN, 2010; Ball et al., 2014). Evidence suggests there is a growing gap between demand and capacity, alongside the increasingly complex care being delivered (Maybin et al., 2016). Practitioners need to be responsive to routinely fluctuating workload demands as well as less predictable wide-scale crises such as flu epidemics. In addition to managing the risks associated with a continually shifting caseload, community nurses are responsible for safeguarding vulnerable groups, seeking health needs and actively identifying potential patients, employing a patient-centred, proactive, pre-emptive approach to service provision (Kane, 2008; NMC, 2009; DH, 2013).

Some community nurses such as practice nurses, who work in general practice (GP) surgeries, or community matrons, who provide 'advanced nursing and clinical care, as well as effective case management' (DH, 2006), have a more clearly defined patient population or can 'close' when their lists are full. This is not normally an option for those providing universal services or caring for the more vulnerable or housebound population, so these practitioners need to prioritise and organise care, as well as make difficult daily decisions about what gets left undone. Professional accountability encompasses clinical decision making, delegation and raising concerns if care delivery could be viewed as 'unsafe or harmful' (NMC, 2010a, 2015a). With the constantly changing work environment, community nurses are routinely responsible for individual care decisions but must also seek out, appraise, communicate and respond to the needs of their wider populations. The management of care, prioritisation and directing resources towards areas of greatest need are a professional obligation as well as being vital to the cost-effectiveness and high quality of care provided (DH, 2011a; NMC, 2015a).

As illustrated in Table 15.1, there is a great range of community nurses with new services, roles and job titles emerging in response to localised identified need and the progression towards commissioning based, outcomes-focused services (DH, 2010a, 2011b). While the diversity of services is vital, this chapter focuses on district nurses, health visitors and school nurses who have responsibility for the population's health through the lifespan and are expected to have higher levels of judgement in clinical practice, leadership, management, quality assurance, care organisation and service development (NMC, 2001, 2004; DH, 2010c; QNI and

Table 15.1 Example of nursing services in primary care

Population	'Core' services	Supplementary or 'Specialist' services	
Child and family	Midwifery health visiting school nursing	Family–nurse partnerships; Sure Start Centres	
		Youth Offending Services	
		Children not in mainstream education (i.e. pupil referral units [PRUs])	
		Family planning/sexual health services	
		'Specialist' nurses:	Safeguarding leads
			Continence/bowel care
			Children's community nurses
			Learning disability nurses
Adult	District nurses Practice nurses	Community matrons/case managers Occupational health nurses	
		Nurse consultants/advanced practitioners; out-of-hours, primary care centres or minor injuries clinics	
		'Intermediate care'/step-down units	
		'Specialist' nurses:	Chronic disease: e.g. diabetes, congestive heart failure (CHF)/coronary heart disease (CHD), chronic obstructive pulmonary disease (COPD)/respiratory, neurological, continence
			Tissue viability, etc.
Mental health	Community mental health	Alcohol and drug dependency services, outreach teams, Child and Adolescent Mental Health Services (CAHMS), etc.	
ALL	Public health department(s), NHS Direct; smoking cessation services; community hospitals/minor injuries, community outpatients, maternity units, etc.		

QNIS, 2015). District nurses provide one of the few 7-day (and in some instances, 24-hour) services in the community setting, managing the acute, long-term, complex and palliative care needs for a diverse and often vulnerable, housebound population. Health visitors and school nurses are responsible for 'universal services' throughout the lifespan, also providing intensive support for higher-risk individuals and families.

This chapter explores the practical application of care organisation and considers the wider context of practitioners' need to minimise risk, be responsive to changes, influence service provision and act as leaders to enhance the quality of care provision in the community. Topics relating to the organisation and management of care covered in this chapter include work organisation in the community setting, service design and referral criteria; skill mix, educating for competence; and caseload/workload management.

WORK ORGANISATION AND CARE DELIVERY IN THE COMMUNITY SETTING

The practicalities of work organisation and prioritisation differ between discrete disciplines in the community setting. These distinct roles have been affected to a varying extent by the emergence of new funding streams, quality outcomes and the commissioning agenda (DH, 2009a,b, 2011b, 2014). Changes to healthcare policy have resulted in a growing need to quantify, categorise and record clinical activity and to meet defined health outcomes. Research by Haycock-Stuart et al. (2008) suggests that district nurses routinely prioritise direct patient care over administrative duties, although this expanding need to measure activity and increased data input has an impact on the amount of time spent on patient care. Similarly, there is pressure on health visitors and school nurses to meet commissioned targets (immunisation rates, for example) and generate more thorough and precise documentation, particularly in relation to safeguarding, also influencing the amount of time spent on direct contact. The impact of increasing paperwork was illustrated poignantly in the Laming Report (2009: 23) with one teenager stating: 'It seems like they have to do all this form filling… it makes them forget about us.'

While the growing need for quality metrics, robust documentation and computer-generated records is common to most community nurses, as is the need to prioritise interventions, the disciplines have discrete foci for their routine work organisation. The emphasis for district nurses is on clinical need such as acute, long-term ill-health and end-of-life care can be seen as more aligned with these types of transforming community services 'streams' (DH, 2009a, 2011b). Conversely, health visitors and school nurses are encouraged to take a more pre-emptive public health, population-wide approach, relating to public health funding streams now within the remit of local authorities in some regions of the United Kingdom, such as England (NMC, 2004; DH, 2011c, 2015a).

Despite the less pronounced clinical role, public health nurses are also required to meet commissioned targets for specified contact points (e.g. the 6-week baby check) and respond to acute situations such as safeguarding. There is little in the literature to detail how clinical work is prioritised and delegated in these aspects of care, although numerous attempts have been made to measure and quantify workload (Kerr, 2004; Hurst, 2005, 2006; Baldwin, 2006; Kane, 2008; Reid et al., 2008; Kirby and Hurst, 2014; Chapman et al, 2017).

ACTIVITY 15.1

Reflection point

Jo is a staff nurse who is the acting team leader of a busy district nursing team. It is 9 AM and she has received a sick call from Dee, who was going to do two of the daily insulin injections on her way in to the office. There is a message that one patient has a blocked urethral catheter and another message that a palliative care patient has deteriorated overnight and needs an urgent visit. There are another 30 visits of varying complexity to be delegated between Jo, two staff nurses and a nursing auxiliary.

• What would be the priorities?
• What would influence the decision making?

Care organisation, prioritisation and delegation for a district nursing caseload of patients involve the scrutiny of diverse factors with varying degrees of importance (Luker and Kenrick, 1992). Theoretical models are widely applied to nursing, but Kennedy (2002: 710) found that they are not as applicable to the complex and varied nature of community nurses' knowledge. Community nurses need to be able to swiftly grasp and weigh the significance of the many variables that add to the complexity of decision making in primary care (Kennedy, 2004). As a general starting point, prioritisation is based on determining the most significant or urgent of the identified clinical needs.

However, even within the simple illustration in Activity 15.1, other factors such as 'knowing the patient' (Speed and Luker, 2004; Kennedy, 2004; Bain, 2015) could influence decision making. For example, if the patient referred for a 'blocked' urethral catheter was known to bypass urine regularly, that patient would not be considered as urgent unless he or she had expressed a symptom atypical for them. Conversely, some patients may be known as having more pressing psychosocial needs, so in this example, the visit could be deemed more urgent if the patient was isolated and had anxieties relating to the fear of a 'blocked' catheter. Maybin et al. (2016) found that patients considered 'psychosocial support' to be of equal importance as 'clinical expertise', with a number of respondents commenting that clinical expertise is of secondary importance. Other factors influencing care priorities and delegation include available skill mix, clinical expertise, experience, various crises, geographical location and sometimes factors such as traffic or weather conditions (Haycock-Stuart et al., 2008). In addition to prioritisation, the district nurse needs to consider if the referral is appropriate (Audit Commission, 1999). Some of the many influences on prioritisation and delegation are outlined in Table 15.2.

Work organisation can be seen to start with the services' referral criteria, which can be complicated due to the evolving commissioning agenda where organisations

Table 15.2 Prioritisation/delegation – Example of influencing factors

Variables	District nurse	Health visitor	Specialist nurse	Other
Clinical need	'Urgent' (requiring rapid intervention but not deemed to be a 'medical emergency') or higher priority: e.g. pain, discomfort, trauma, distress, potential harm if untreated; end-of-life care: Prevention of hospital admission Non-urgent (but still requiring a visit within 24 hours) Many examples: some wound care, medication/injection, etc. Routine: anything that can be safely deferred	'Urgent' or higher priority: Safeguarding emotional/ post-natal health issues, emerging PH crises Non-urgent (but planned for a specific time) Clinics/screening, etc. Surveillance: prevention of acute issues Routine: anything that can be safely deferred	'Urgent' or higher priority: Safeguarding emotional or sexual health issues, emerging PH crises Non-urgent (but planned for a specific time) Drop-in clinics/ teaching sessions/ screening, etc. Surveillance: prevention of acute issues Routine: anything that can be safely deferred	Specialists/community matrons: prevention of hospital admission Routine/ support visits Practice nurses: non-routine/ urgent situations Patient clinics Community mental health team: urgent or routine
	OTHER: Higher priority: refusal of referral to other services or hospital admission identified as being necessary for well-being/safety			
Skill mix and service configuration	Working arrangements: Referral criteria; service specification/commissioned services; team or individual practitioners; corporate caseload/geographical working or GP attached Delegation based on: Staff competence: skills, experience, knowledge, training; NMC standards; employment contracts/ policies, staff availability Liaison with other services/referral processes			
Geographic location	Visits organised to optimise efficiency within the confines of skill mix – may be GP attached or working geographically			
Traffic/weather, etc.	May need to request assistance for travel; reorganise planned care/visits			
Public health 'crises'/ disasters	For example, flu epidemic/immunisation programmes/natural disasters: organisations have contingency plans which should include policies and protocols to guide the prioritisation of care services, some use dependency scoring tools for this			

are in a process of change or merger and the fact that services are often commissioned using block contracts. Bridging a vast range of conditions from acute to long term, district nurses can be seen as 'the only professionals with no limit to their workload' (QNI, 2009a: 22). The varied and 'invisible' nature of the work is not helped by a lack of clearly defined referral criteria (Audit Commission, 1999; RCN, 2003; QNI, 2006, 2009a, 2016a; Jarvis et al., 2006; DH, 2013). Maybin et al., (2016) suggest a possible response to the demand-capacity gap as the rejection of incomplete referrals, but note this poses risks of damaging or delaying patient care. The development of referral criteria is recommended to reduce the number of inappropriate referrals, to clarify and add legitimacy to the district nursing role and to help ensure the best use of their skills and judgement (RCN, 2003; Jarvis et al., 2006). The establishment and implementation of referral processes can thus be seen as a fundamental step in organising and managing nursing care in the community setting, particularly for district nurses, who have little control over their workload (Kane, 2015; Maybin et al., 2016).

Provider organisations should have documented referral criteria as a basis by which district nurses can monitor and direct the number and types of patients on their active caseload. Referrals can be received from a range of sources including general practice (GP), hospitals, residential homes, day centres, social services, family, carers and the patients themselves. However, there are variations in the use of referral criteria for a number of reasons, including

- *Detail/specifics* – Inconsistency between care organisations/providers; poor quality information within referrals
- *Implementation* – A lack of awareness or patchy support for their use
- *The commissioning agenda* – The need for services to be more 'marketable' and efficient, and thus more flexible. Referral criteria based on 'block contracts' comprise only a general outline of the types of care provided by district nursing services

While there are variations in relation to referral criteria, the Royal College of Nursing (RCN, 2003: 26) recommends that referrals are categorised in a way that aids prioritisation:

- *Urgent* – Contact necessary within 4 hours
- *Non-urgent* – Contact within 24 hours and visiting date agreed
- *Routine* – Contact within 48 hours and visiting date agreed

The Audit Commission Report (1999) into district nursing services found great variations between different geographical areas/community nursing teams of the number and types of patients on district nurse caseloads. Although there have been no subsequent large-scale studies and a recognised absence of data on community health services at a national level, indications are that these variations have worsened (QNI, 2009b; Maybin et al., 2016). Given widespread health service changes, for example, the diversification of roles (e.g. 'case managers', 'community matrons' and 'intervention teams'), it can be implied there is growing variation between district nursing teams. Further to considering the appropriateness of new referrals, district nurses need to evaluate each of the scheduled visits on the basis of their clinical need, identifying those of higher priority. As suggested in Table 15.2, from that starting point a range of influences on prioritisation and delegation is examined before decision making occurs.

Health visitors and school nurses also provide a range of services and show wide differences in this provision. However, health visitors have worked hard to establish clear service aims (DH, 2009c) and are broadly viewed as leaders in public health and within the Darzi stream of 'children's services' (DH, 2009a). There is a recognised decline in the number of specialist qualified district nurses (Cook et al., 2009; QNI, 2009a, 2010, 2015; HSCIC, 2016; Maybin et al., 2016). Policy in England aimed to redress a shortfall in health visitors by denoting a target number to be educated and employed, although despite achieving the targets (DH, 2015b), it has been reported that caseload sizes have not reduced (Turnball, 2015). The policy was likely in response to concerns over increased workload, with one survey finding that nearly 70% of health visitors reported they no longer had the capacity to support the most vulnerable children (Unite/CPHVA Omnibus Survey, 2008). The remit to provide universal services for the health visitor (Figure 15.1) populations and additionally target those with greater needs may be more clearly delineated than the equivalent for district nursing services, but remains highly challenging.

This model suggests health visitors work in partnership with other services to provide universal care for all, as well as support the most vulnerable families, particularly those where there are safeguarding concerns (DH, 2011c). While there is potential for flexibility in how outcomes are achieved and services are delivered, the exigency of safeguarding can be a barrier to practice innovation (Wakefield et al., 2010). Some public health or population-based health issues have an insubstantial evidence base potentially leading to variations. As with specialist district nursing practice, it is difficult to establish an evidence base to make explicit the need to 'employ health visitors rather than other workers to deliver their traditional role' (DH, 2009c: 3).

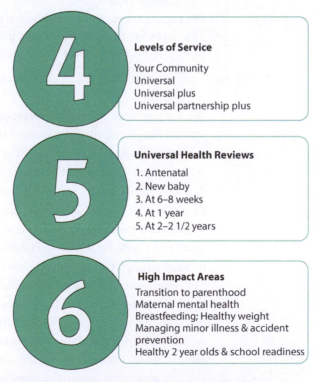

Levels of Service

Your Community
Universal
Universal plus
Universal partnership plus

Universal Health Reviews

1. Antenatal
2. New baby
3. At 6–8 weeks
4. At 1 year
5. At 2–2 1/2 years

High Impact Areas

Transition to parenthood
Maternal mental health
Breastfeeding; Healthy weight
Managing minor illness & accident prevention
Healthy 2 year olds & school readiness

Figure 15.1 Bennett (2015) 4-5-6 Model for Health Visiting. (Based on the NHS England National Core Health Visiting Service Specification for 2015–16. https:// vivbennett.blog.gov.uk/wp-content/uploads/sites/ 90/2015/03/4-5-6-Model.pdf.)

Care organisation has myriad influences, some of which arise from the key contrasts between hospital-based and community care (Box 15.1). While pre-registration nursing standards (NMC, 2010b, 2014) have since aimed to redress the imbalance between hospital and community-based education, this analysis helpfully identified some of the key differences between these settings. Despite the fact that current pre-registration nurse training is aimed at equipping nurses to work in any care setting on registration, Health Education England (HEE, 2015: 15) suggest that 'the majority of newly qualified nurses need support to develop the skills and competence required to work in community and/or primary care'.

Box 15.1 Nursing in community settings (Drennan et al., 2005)

Prior to the revised pre-registration nursing standards in response to the policy drive for services 'closer to home', a study commissioned by the Department of Health found that nurses new to the community 'become novice practitioners again' for these four main reasons:

1. The patient is in control of all decisions affecting their health and well-being, including their home environment.
2. The patients and their carers undertake most of their own health maintenance, treatment and care activities.
3. The multiple systems and infrastructures that support the delivery of health and social care vary between local areas.
4. The nurse has to make clinical and professional decisions, sometimes rapidly in less than ideal circumstances, at a physical distance from professional colleagues.

---

1 The centrality of the patient perspective: care organisation must take into account the clients' interpretation of their needs. This fundamental premise of the patient being at the centre of their own care has since been reflected in the '6 C's' and the updated NMC Code (2015a). Community nurses must recognise that patients at home are much more in control of their decisions (NHS Employers, 2006) and take into account their personal preferences. For instance, if a patient is relatively active and requires daily wound packing, he or she may prefer to be visited at a specified time. However, as with the constraints of institutional settings, this consideration has to be balanced with other influences on care organisation such as urgent unplanned visits, staff absence or higher priority needs. The centrality of the patient perspective can also be seen in a recent report by Maybin et al., (2016: 16) where 'good care' is described in their findings as 'staff caring for the whole person and providing holistic, person-centred care rather than taking a task-focused approach'.

2 Patients and carers undertake most of the care activities: unlike the hospital setting, much community-based work involves ongoing identification and analysis of need, promotion of self-care or co-ordination of services. Integral to this is ensuring support is available to those providing the bulk of the care. It

has been calculated that the economic value of the contribution made by informal carers is 'more than the annual cost of all aspects of the NHS' (Carers UK, 2007: 2). It is recognised that carers have distinct needs with the introduction of recent strategies, including support for greater personalisation and improved quality of care (HM Government, 2010), and revisions to the Care Act (2014), where carers now have the legal right to their own assessment. Maybin et al. (2016: 16) found that 'good care' is seen to include the involvement of informal carers and family members through offering practical support, including them in decision making, valuing their contributions and expertise and addressing carers' own needs and personal well-being.

3 The multiple systems and infrastructures: care organisation is highly dependent on the accessibility of services and resources. With a vast array of systems and structures (such as statutory and voluntary organisations), community nurses need to have excellent communications skills and sustain an extensive working knowledge of these resources. The people most likely to be affected by resource constraints (such as cuts to social care services) are often very vulnerable, requiring community nurses to advocate for services where gaps are identified.

4 Clinical and professional decision making in isolation: the need to make care decisions at a physical distance from colleagues can be daunting for practitioners new to nursing or to the community setting. The ranging skills within a community nursing team demand that more experienced practitioners delegating tasks need to be assured of the skill level of each team member and must aim to minimise the risk of less experienced or skilled staff performing visits which may be, or prove to be, outside their scope of practice. Decisions made by community nurses, as lone workers, may encompass elements of risk, particularly when patients are new to the service.

Care organisation in primary care is dependent on a variety of factors that are constantly fluctuating. The requisite skills of community nurses are wide-ranging and are seen to include 'proactively targeting services where most needed, addressing the wider causes of ill health, managing risks associated with patients and carers making their own decisions and understanding and influencing practice-based commissioning' (NHS Employers, 2006: 2). Practitioners are responsible for maintaining a continued currency of knowledge and skills, not only in relation to assessment and prioritisation, but also in the local knowledge of available services and structures, the needs of carers and an awareness of risk factors requiring a strong skill mix within teams. The next section looks more closely at this topic of skill mix, roles, responsibilities and delegation.

SKILL MIX, ROLES AND RESPONSIBILITIES

A series of policy documents has proposed that care is moved away from the hospital setting and closer to the patients' homes (DH, 2009a, 2013; Scottish Government, 2016; NHS England, 2014, 2017; NHS Wales, 2015). Despite the resulting pressures on the community-based workforce, findings indicate a decrease in the supply of skilled nurses (QNI, 2010: 2), with a loss of nearly 50% of specialist qualified district nurses since 2005 and an overall reduction in the number of community nurses over the past 5 years (Maybin et al., 2016; NHS Digital, 2017). This has developed through a combination of not recruiting when posts become vacant, dilution of the workforce with practitioners who are lesser trained and the ageing workforce. Maybin et al. (2016: 4) suggest the 'dissonance between the frequently stated policy ambition to offer "more care close to home" and the apparent neglect of community health services over recent years is striking'. The impact has not been fully examined although it has led to 'serious concerns about workforce pressures' (Foot et al., 2014: 28) and there are distinct implications for skill mix, roles, responsibility and accountability. The leadership role is recognised as 'pivotal' with the DH (2011a: 8) stating that, 'the strength of that leadership has an unambiguous link to the quality of care and the reputation of the profession'. While all community staff have professional accountability, larger and more fragmented teams coupled with ambiguous lines of leadership can present challenges for less experienced community nursing staff and impact upon the safe delegation of care by team leaders.

Most employment contracts and the Nursing and Midwifery Council (NMC) standards (NMC, 2001, 2015a) indicate that specialist practitioners (district nurses) remain accountable for their own practice and for the safe and conscientious delegation of work. However, with teams rapidly expanding and moving from GP attachment to larger corporate caseloads, it is challenging for team leaders to sustain a working knowledge of the patient caseload or the competence level of individual practitioners. In some areas, caseloads of active patients (requiring regular visits) have grown substantially, with one study identifying an average of 15 staff members per team (Ball et al., 2014). The scale of these teams and potential complexity of the caseload implies district nurses may have difficulty in maintaining the NMC standards for specialist practice (NMC, 2001) or working within the professional Code (NMC, 2015a) in relation to delegation. A survey of community nurses (Ball et al., 2014) found that 75% of respondents reported insufficient district nurses on their team, 81% reported they had worked additional hours on their last shift, and many were concerned about the quality of care they were able to provide.

Delegation, with its intrinsic accountability, has been viewed as 'subjective... based on custom and practice' (QNI, 2014a), with a suggestion that community nursing teams are moving towards the more objective, computer-aided practice of 'patient allocation'. A review of literature on workforce planning (QNI, 2014a) suggests that manual, labour-intensive processes of patient allocation are being replaced by electronic, automated processes (Dean, 2013). Where a team leader district nurse takes responsibility for their defined caseload population and is accountable for the prioritisation and delegation of work (NMC, 2001, 2015a), this presupposes authority over patient allocation, a knowledge of the patients and sufficient awareness of individual practitioners' knowledge and skills.

Both the traditional processes and new models where 'tasks' are allocated electronically, rely on team members articulating if they consider a visit or task to be beyond their scope of practice (NMC, 2015a). This can be tricky for new members of staff who are unaware of their lack of expertise until they are in the situation or in circumstances where the visit has an element of complication. The district nurse team leader can be seen as reducing risks for less experienced staff as well as safeguarding their vulnerable populations through expert team and caseload management. Recognised community qualifications help employers identify people with the right skills to lead teams and the policy objective of delivering care closer to or in the home requires the expertise and leadership of specialist qualified district nurses (QNI, 2015; NHS England, 2015; RCN, 2016).

ACTIVITY 15.2

Reflection point

Jo is a staff nurse in a semi-rural district nursing team. It is becoming an increasingly busy caseload, especially the daily insulin injections. She is 'in charge' most days as the team leader is now based at a different geographical location. The Band 3 nursing auxiliary (Cee) has expressed an interest in learning to administer insulin injections, but Jo is unsure of Trust policy. She also has some concerns over Cee's general knowledge and understanding of diabetes.

• How might she approach these challenges?

• What are the implications in relation to professional accountability?

The DH Commissioned Report by Drennan et al. (2005) found that the requisite knowledge and skills for primary care were often 'covert' and needed to be made explicit in order to create clear guidelines for employers to prepare nurses for community practice. An outline of the preparation needed for this transition would be of benefit to any practitioner embarking on a career in community care and it has been suggested that this should begin with pre-registration nursing programmes (QNI, 2010; NMC, 2010b; Willis, 2013). A number of tools to assist in knowledge, skills and competence development are available, including the 'Transition to community nursing practice' resource (Aldridge-Bent et al., 2013) and the Skills for Health (SFH, 2010) resources website. SFH resources include standards and an educational framework for 'unregulated' staff as well as registered nurses, with tools and competencies cross-referenced to the Knowledge and Skills Framework (KSF) (DH, 2004). While there are clear advantages to applying frameworks, it has been suggested that KSFs could be used more effectively as there is currently variation and a non-standardised approach (Bentley and Dandy-Hughes, 2010).

NHS Education for Scotland (2011) produced a career and development framework for community nursing and more recently Health Education England (2015) has published an education and career framework for district nurses and general practice nurses. Both these frameworks identify core knowledge, skills and educational attainment at various points in the career trajectory of community nurses, with an expectation of continued development. With greater accountability and a need for more stringent methods of professional regulation (NMC, 2015a,b; TSO, 2007), it is beneficial for practitioners to find clear and effective ways to assess, verify and record their competence and continuing professional development.

In line with NMC (2001, 2004) specialist standards and the broader health policy agenda, community practitioners need to address the immediate prioritisation of daily work but also look beyond to ensure the right balance of skills and knowledge to meet the needs of their population. The next section looks at methods of service evaluation, caseload, workload and workforce management to help this process of matching skills to service need.

CASELOAD, WORKLOAD AND WORKFORCE MANAGEMENT

Care organisation and caseload management vary according to geographical area, employer and professional discipline but can be seen broadly as focusing on the identification of need and efficient use of resources to meet this need. While community nurses in the United Kingdom have little authority over budget management (in contrast, see Box 15.2 for The Buurtzorg Model), other factors such as time and caseload management can be influenced to make potentially significant improvements to efficiency and client care. For example, efficient caseload management includes appropriate and timely discharge to avoid inappropriate visits and the potential erosion of patient autonomy. It is notable that these proactive initiatives, such as patient/carer education or patient reassessment and discharge, are often compromised when there are pressures on the service and staff feel they don't have time for these activities (Maybin et al., 2016).

BOX 15.2 The Buurtzorg Model

Started in 2007 with the aim of providing a more efficient care delivery model, it has a non-hierarchical structure with independent teams of a maximum of 12 nurses. These teams provide co-ordinated care for a specific catchment area, typically consisting of between 40 and 60 patients. The teams organise and are responsible for the complete process:

• Clients, nurses, planning, education and finance
• Assessment and care of all types of clients: generalists
• 70% registered nurses
• Their own education budget
• Informal networks in the neighbourhood and close collaboration with GPs (RCN, 2015)

The Buurtzorg model comprises six key services:

1. Conduct holistic assessment of the client's needs which includes medical, long-term conditions and personal/social care needs. Care plans are drafted from this assessment.
2. Map networks of informal care and assess ways to involve these carers in the client's treatment plan.
3. Identify any other formal carers and help to co-ordinate care between providers.
4. Provide care delivery.
5. Support the client in his or her social environment.
6. Promote self-care and independence.

(Buurtzorg Nederland, 2011)

Health visiting has traditionally been arranged around a 'caseload' of patients, but there is very little research literature relating to this topic (Cowley and Bidmead, 2009; DH, 2009c). Brewerton (2015) reports that a simple weighting tool to suggest ratios of health visits per population was developed by Cowley in 2009 and has since been adapted and used widely throughout the United Kingdom. While this tool helpfully takes deprivation indices into account, Cowley (Brewerton, 2015a) suggests other factors such as local variations need to be taken into consideration. When evaluating one health visiting workload tool, Pollock et al. (2002) concluded that it produced such inaccurate data it would be unsafe to use unless significant improvements were made. Problems with interpretation centred on the need for a more rigorous process for weighting elements of 'health visiting need' and scoring more accurately the wide variation in need among families (Pollock et al., 2002).

This illustrates the inherent difficulties of workload assessment and dependency scoring, also substantiated by a systematic review of caseload management tools and models that found there was 'a poor evidence base' (Kolehmainen et al., 2010: 47). This extensive review reported that despite 'considerable literature on caseload management' it was not possible to draw conclusions aside from a need to critically appraise methods and tools. Another literature review (Newland, 2014) found approaches to be inconsistent or subjective, but suggested computer based tools were improving this, while Roberson's (2016) review was unable to achieving its aim of identifying the most effective validated tool. Maybin et al. (2016: 4) recommends that 'robust mechanisms for monitoring resources, activity and workforce must be developed' while acknowledging the difficulties in achieving this. Notwithstanding the inherent challenges, service review is recognised as an important element of care organisation (Ervin, 2008; Kane, 2008; Bain and Baguley, 2012; Macdonald et al., 2013; Newland, 2014; Brewerton, 2015a). Research by Bramwell et al. (2014: 6) concluded that the 'lack of data about community service activity is a significant problem… (it) prevents the development of clear guidance about the staffing levels required to provide services for a given population'. Supporting this conclusion, Maybin et al. (2016: 73) suggest the absence of 'robust national data on activity levels in district nursing services… makes it very difficult to demonstrate, understand and monitor the demand-capacity gap'.

ACTIVITY 15.3

Reflection point
Reflect on the scenario below and consider the following:
• How might organisational structures affect service review findings?
• How could service review be used to influence/improve service delivery and care organisation?

Scenario
Organisation A has a 'traditional' pattern of employing their district nursing services in that the teams are relatively small (three to eight members) and

they are attached to a single GP practice. While the GP practices range in size, the caseloads of each of the district nursing teams are proportionate, with an average of 60 patients per whole time equivalent (WTE). The team leader doesn't visit every patient on the caseload but as a co-ordinator and provider of care is familiar with most patients and acts as a mentor/educational resource for the team, particularly for those who are less experienced. There is a community matron who is also GP attached who has a caseload of high-intensity patients with long-term conditions (LTCs).

Organisation B has moved away from the 'traditional' model, and the much larger district nursing teams work with 'corporate caseloads'. They communicate with a number of GP surgeries over the geographical patch. The staff nurses need to be more self-directed as the caseload size is so large that the team leader wouldn't necessarily be able to identify individual clients. The team leader acts as a manager in directing and delegating care, identifying educational needs and sometimes undertaking patient visits. The community matrons also work geographically and have a separate caseload of high-intensity patients with LTCs.

Organisation C has moved away from the job title of 'district nursing'. The practitioners who had been district nurses in the past are now 'case managers' whose client group are housebound patients with chronic diseases. They mainly work geographically although some are GP attached. Staff nurses constitute the 'intervention teams' and are geographically based. These teams are quite large, focus on 'episodic care' and are managed by an intervention team leader who covers what would have previously been three or four district nursing teams.

Caseload management skills are recognised as important for community practitioners and it is argued that continuing education and staff development programmes need to include these competencies 'to improve the efficiency and quality of nursing care' (Ervin, 2008: 127). Caseload management, the measurement and comparison of caseload information can be used to improve the quality of care (Kane, 2008). While the process of caseload and workload assessment (profiling) can be viewed as onerous, in one evaluative study (Gould, 2010) district nurse practice teachers described service review positively in terms of its usefulness and contribution to service organisation and development. Benefits identified included the ability to uncover unmet need, match skills to demands and introduce changes to practice to address gaps and the development of 'business skills' in advocating for improving services.

Service review can be seen as a combination of caseload profiling (the types and needs of the client group) and workload assessment that aims to measure and quantify the work or dependency of the client group. It has long been recognised that there is a need to quantify the work of community nursing teams in order to effectively meet service requirements and to manage the needs of populations efficiently (Audit Commission, 1999). More recently, the commissioning of services from provider organisations has prompted the need to quantify the work undertaken by community nursing teams and to demonstrate the achievement of measurable outcomes (DH, 2014). For example, the 'Service Spec' for health visitors (NHS England, 2014) requires health visitors to undertake and record data on new birth visits, 6–8 week checks, and so on, which is then published monthly by NHS Digital (2017).

These metrics exemplify the move towards outcome-driven service provision and while it's useful to have clearly defined objectives, this may impact on professional autonomy and judgment when prioritising care. Given the often unpredictable and sometimes immeasurable aspects of community-based care, it is imperative that practitioners have a degree of control over their caseload and work. This can be aided by the use of profiling and caseload management systems that enable practitioners to access the information they collect in a user-friendly way (Kane, 2014). Rigorous data collection methods can also be seen as a way to support safe staffing levels, skill mix and develop effective community services (Jackson et al., 2015a).

Basic caseload profiling tools normally involve providing a 'snapshot' of the types and numbers of clients, families or patients on the caseload and may include the following:

- Number of patients/families on the caseload
- Referral rates (including one-off referrals)/referral source
- Discharge rates
- Types of patients ('case mix')
- Patient profile (ages/sex) (Audit Commission, 1999; Kane, 2008)

To estimate the work associated with a caseload, it also includes the following:

- Frequency of visits for each patient on the caseload
- Duration of visits

Table 15.3 illustrates some of the recognised caseload, workload and workforce management tools.

While there is some overlap of terminology, workload tools are normally more concerned with quantifying the work associated with a caseload population or measuring the dependency levels of the clients. It may also encompass the emerging issues of 'capacity and demand' and safe staffing (Fields and Brett, 2015; Jackson et al., 2016). The difficulties in measuring workload have been well documented with a variety of tools and methods tried over a period of time that aim to go beyond counting contacts to provide better quality information (Bentley and Tite, 2000; Hurst, 2006; Jones and Russell, 2007; Kane, 2008; Lewis and Pontin, 2008; Kolehmainen et al., 2010; Grafen and MacKenzie, 2015). Workload tools can be 'prospective' or 'retrospective'. Prospective tools such as the 'Warrington' provide a numerical estimate of the amount of time certain procedures take (Baldwin, 2006). Retrospective tools aim to record the numbers of visits and time spent by practitioners on care-related and administrative tasks. All methods are reliant on the accuracy of the practitioner in recording activity and the complexity associated with

Table 15.3 Overview of caseload, workload and workforce management tools

Name of Tool	Key Features/Aims	Number of Visits	Type (Activity/Task or Diagnosis)	Duration; or Dependency	Other: e.g. The Number of Referrals, Admissions and Discharges; Non-Contact Time
Warrington Workload Tool (Frame and O'Donnell, 1996; Baldwin, 2006)	Prospective: Uses a point-based system to predict (and subsequently record) task time and patient dependency; staff are given a number of points; aims to measure workload and staffing	Daily visits recorded	Yes; Agreed units assigned per identified care/task	Patient tasks assigned a score along a finite continuum; standardised per task, e.g. weighting: 15 minutes = 1 point	Some versions include: travel; documentation; multidisciplinary team liaison/ arranging equipment; carer advice and support

Notes: One of the original weighting systems for community nursing care, Frame and O'Donnell (1996) based dependency scores on frequency of patient visits multiplied by the length of each visit, converting estimated task time into units. This still forms the basis of other workload systems, with recent research finding benefits and challenges: 'The Warrington tool can provide an accurate picture of time spent providing direct patient care', but this is dependent on it being completed accurately and consistently across teams (Baldwin, 2006). It can be combined with a caseload profiling tool to provide richer data. Originally 'paper based' (but transferrable to spreadsheets).

Name of Tool	Key Features/Aims	Number of Visits	Type (Activity/Task or Diagnosis)	Duration; or Dependency	Other
The West Hertfordshire Activity and Time Dependency Tool (WHATT) (Thomas et al., 2006)	Patient allocation system that measures actual time used by the DN service, by requiring verification after care delivery	Daily visits recorded	Yes Agreed units assigned per identified care/ task	Standardised as per task; activity is in 15-minute units	May also include: As above

The development of this and similar systems is dependent on the creation of well-informed software design and requires significant engagement of district nurses with the skills, knowledge and experience to articulate and justify the specification (Thomas et al., 2006).

Name of Tool	Key Features/Aims	Number of Visits	Type (Activity/Task or Diagnosis)	Duration; or Dependency	Other: e.g. The Number of Referrals, Admissions and Discharges; Non-Contact Time
Community Client Need Classification System (CCNCS) (Byrne et al., 2007; Brady et al., 2007, 2008)	A workload measurement system designed to capture the direct and indirect elements of community nursing work; enables prediction to be made about client need (dependency); retrospective data oasis:entry produces a report outlining team members' time over a defined period	Time per task	Seven assessment criteria; 1. Assessment 2. Physical Care 3. Psychosocial 4. Child and Family Support 5. Teaching and Health Promotion 6. Case Management 7. Environment	Based on level of need: dependency scoring; Need classification via scores between 1 and 5 based on level of need	Includes all care groups in the community including maternity, older persons, adults and children of all ages The seven assessment criteria used are nursing assessment; physical care needs; psychosocial needs; teaching and health promotion needs; case management; carer and family support; environmental needs; and travel time

With a 'combined' public health and community nursing role in some areas (such as Ireland), this tool captures the multi-dimensional aspects of the health needs for all clients of 'Public Health Nurses', rather than recording and measuring specific tasks.

Name of Tool	Key Features/Aims	Number of Visits	Type (Activity/Task or Diagnosis)	Duration; or Dependency	Other
Electronic Caseload Assessment Tool 'eCat' (Reid et al., 2008; Kane, 2014, 2015)	A knowledge-based tool that aims to provide effective caseload management; developed over a period of years as a bespoke electronic tool that gives access to contemporaneous, comparative data at each level of district nursing, from caseload holders to commissioners	Number of patients on the working caseload (with visits more often than monthly) and frequency	Reason for visit (24 variables to define primary need); reviews (8 variables)	Dependency: A bespoke measure developed for the tool on two levels: Activities of daily living (ADL dependency) and dependency on the nursing team (team dependency)	Records information on: Demography (e.g. staffing, population, GP attached or geographical; or mixed) Caseload size (number of patients) Visiting patterns (eight variables to describe the visiting frequency) Caseload throughput (e.g. admissions, discharges, etc.)

Name of Tool	Key Features/Aims	Number of Visits	Type (Activity/Task or Diagnosis)	Duration; or Dependency	Other: e.g. The Number of Referrals, Admissions and Discharges; Non-Contact Time
Scottish Community Workload Measurement Tool (SCWMT) (Grafen and MacKenzie, 2015)	Part of a suite of tools aiming to ensure a consistent approach to measuring nursing workload across NHS Scotland and to support evidence-based decision making on staffing and workforce needs; enables community nurses to record and report their actual workload by collecting information on six categories of activity	Counts face-to-face contacts (and associated workload)	Not specific tasks but four levels of intervention are defined, ranging from Level 1: 'straightforward' to Level 4: 'complex'	A workload tool as opposed to a caseload-profiling tool, so the level of complexity relates to the workload demands of each patient during each contact rather than the overall complexity of the patient; also records daily working hours	Used in tandem with a professional judgment tool and quality data appropriate to specific areas to triangulate the findings Records: Face-to-face contacts and non-face-to-face contact; visits and associated workload (such as management, administrative, meetings and development activity); travel and exception reporting; tool is generally used on an occasional basis over a 10-day period to provide a 'snapshot'
Domiciliary Scheduling in the Community System (DominiC) (Dean, 2013; Bowers and Durrant, 2014)	Computer system collates prospective data that is entered at the point of referral; uses these data to produce a daily schedule for each team and allocate an appropriately skilled nurse to undertake the activity; a combined caseload, workload and workforce management tool	Yes	Yes Centrally held patients' details	Records patients' needs and predicted visit length	Added features include: Patient choice of timed visits; allocates work geographically and the same nurses for continuity of care; provides reminders for future visits; highlights risks; records patient quality data; records staff roster; identifies future service shortfalls; produces reports on service delivery and efficiency

Name of Tool	Key Features/Aims	Number of Visits	Type (Activity/Task or Diagnosis)	Duration; or Dependency	Other: e.g. The Number of Referrals, Admissions and Discharges; Non-Contact Time
Cassandra Matrix Workload Activity Tool (Leary, 2011; Jackson et al., 2015a,b)	Community nursing workload activity tool that provides a robust mechanism for collecting complex multi-dimensional workload activity; originally paper-based tool (now web-based) to capture what nurses do (interventions), where their actions occur (contexts), whom the work is done for (patients or carers), and what nurses do not have time to do (work left undone)	Yes	Interventions in four main groups: 1. Case management and administration 2. Physical 3. Psychological 4. Social	Context; where the care took place; a number of variables are recorded, rather than simple visit numbers or dependency	Current systems based on counting numbers of patients are inadequate, and new computerised solutions do not yet capture data about the amount of care left undone Tool has enabled more complex data to be collected that describes what people are doing and what breakdown of activity types is occurring within organisations and across NHS career grades within the workforce
Sheffield Community Caseload Classification System (Chapman et al., 2017)	Workload assessment tool that uses caseload classification (according to nursing need / care required) and dependency scoring to measure work-load. and skill mix requirements Agreed protocols developed.	Yes	Caseload Classification distinguishes between 12 domains or areas of care need	Dependency is measured as 'Levels of complexity'; 3 levels of complexity identified (routine, additional and significant); denotes acuity and dependency of the patient; includes the social situation	Data is uploaded to the electronic patient record; allows 'real-time' daily capture; enables timely deployment of appropriate staff with the correct skill mix
SystmOne, RIO, CHS, PARIS, ECR, Emis, Lorenzo	Many IT systems currently in use; mainly for patient records; to varying degrees, also provide the facility to allocate patients, categorise by task and run reports that reflect caseload and workload features				'The right staff, with the right skills, in the right place, at the right time to deliver high-quality community nursing care and services'

measuring the workload of community nurses is acknowledged, with a paucity of accurate measurement systems available (Byrne et al., 2007; Brady et al., 2007, 2008).

Reid et al. (2008) used systematic review methodology to identify four methods of workforce planning, including professional judgement, population-based health needs, caseload analysis and dependency acuity. The conclusion was that each of the techniques on their own was flawed in some way (Hurst, 2006; Reid et al., 2008), with mixed methods advocated as most useful for the purpose of developing services aimed at effectively meeting client need. These methods were then employed to successfully inform a major service redesign (Kane, 2008). The improved efficiency of the restructure was evident in the outcome of reduced administration and inappropriate referrals, along with very consistent caseload sizes. The 'eCAT' (Electronic Caseload Assessment Tool) model has been developed over a period of years and is being used by a number of health organisations (Kane, 2015). Also in line with the idea of mixed methods, the Scottish Community Nursing Workload Measurement Tool (SCNWM) advocates a triangulated approach to workload measurement (Grafen and MacKenzie, 2015). This uses three sets of measures including a specialty-specific workload measurement tool (e.g. the SCNWM); a professional judgment tool using the knowledge and experience of the lead nurse and quality data appropriate to specific areas (Grafen and MacKenzie, 2015).

The Community Client Need Classification System (CCNCS) also appears to be adaptable for measuring the workload of the range of community disciplines as it was developed in an area where public health nurse roles encompass all age groups, with no differentiation between health visitors, district nurses or school nurses (Brady et al., 2007). It demonstrated a direct correlation between measured client need in the older population and the amount of community nursing time required (Brady et al., 2007: 47) and has been found to be consistently reliable (Brady et al., 2008). However, the dependency classification may be perceived as too general and its transferability to other health service environments has not yet been evaluated (Brady et al., 2007, 2008).

Computer-based systems, such as SystmOne, RIO, CHS, PARIS, DominiC, ECR, Emis, Lorenzo, and so on, are becoming more widespread for managing and recording community nursing activity, although it was found that over a third of respondents indicated that they use a manual paper-based system for patient allocation (QNI, 2014b). Information technology (IT) systems are designed to provide a 'seamless' record of community nursing interventions, care plans, caseload data and other information such as prescriptions (TPP, 2016). It is suggested that using systems that are fully automated will negate human error and ensure data are trustworthy (Newland, 2014) while Griffith (2015: 512) reminds that district nurses 'must always approach their record keeping as if they will be relying on them as evidence in court'.

Advancing from the use of IT systems for allocation and record keeping, emerging models such as eCAT (Kane, 2014, 2015) have potential to help address the recognised need to capture some of the complexities within the community setting to inform service and workforce need. The eCAT model involves multiple types of data collection, for example, eight categories, such as 'demographics', 'caseload size', 'visiting patterns' and 'dependency', each with a number of variables (Kane, 2015). It produces instant access to information that can be easily displayed, interpreted and reflected upon or responded to by practitioners as well as provides data for all levels of an organisation (Kane, 2015).

For both primary care and community services, being able to clearly capture workload and workforce data would help quantify the benefits of changing skill-mix and could help reduce pressures on existing staff (Addicott et al., 2015). It is seen as important to map workload activity and workforce requirements within the local context as there is a risk that simplistic methods may 'underestimate and misrepresent the complexity and multiple dimensions of the community care episode, the time taken to provide it and the skill mix required to deliver it' (Jackson et al., 2015a: 128). This aim to more fully reflect and measure the multidimensional and sometimes less visible aspects of community nursing is seen in the 'Cassandra Matrix' capacity-and-demand model (Jackson et al., 2015a,b; Wright et al., 2015). Originally, the tool aimed to identify what specialist nurses do (interventions), in context (where) and to whom (patient/carer), as well as record work left undone (Leary, 2011). Findings on its adaptation to the community setting suggest that the tool would make the contribution of community nurses more visible, has potential be used to support integrated service delivery (Jackson et al., 2015a) and its use was recommended to 'provide big data that shows complexity of community nursing and broader care challenges for workforce planning... so that the future workforce is fit for future purpose' (Jackson et al., 2015b: 72).

One impact of the lack of reliable or robust measurement systems is in the slow recognition of concerns around workforce pressures, staffing shortages, skill-mix and caseload (Foot et al., 2014; Maybin et al., 2016). Addicott et al. (2015) indicate it is worrying that large gaps in data on the community workforce show it has not kept pace with the policy impetus and despite aims to raise the level and range of community services, there is no evidence of staffing increases to support this. In relation to workforce planning, systems such as the Domiciliary Scheduling in the Community, or DominiC (Dean, 2013) use a combination of features to assess workload and caseload, as well as highlighting staff requirements to assist with allocation and to identify gaps in staffing. While limitations are recognised, this clinician-led tool offers a 'dynamic and transparent system on which to measure ever-changing patient need' (Bowers and Durrant, 2014: 64) and has the potential to pre-empt workforce issues. In lieu of NICE guidance on safe staffing levels for community nurses it is suggested a focus on 'safe caseloads' better reflects the complexity of district nursing services (National Quality Board, 2017).

The role of community nurses in influencing service provision

It can be perceived that the continuum from 'everyday' prioritisation of care to the broader remit of service organisation is interrelated. The right staff, with the right skills, in the right place, at the right time are required in order to deliver high-quality community nursing care and services. Just as it is necessary for community nurses to be aware of the changing needs of their populations so as to influence the way services are organised, structural systems and staffing resources are an influence on the everyday practice of work organisation. With scant research evidence to support specific approaches for assessing and determining nursing staff requirements and/or skill mix (Fields and Brett, 2015; Jackson et al., 2016), team leaders are tasked with assuring safe and effective care using the tools adopted by their organisation and their own clinical judgment. Nurses are accountable for their own practice and as careers progress to higher levels such as specialist or advanced practice, this accountability extends beyond the confines of their individual competence towards their team, the populations they serve and in the need to influence services and resources (NMC, 2001, 2004, 2015a).

ACTIVITY 15.4

Reflection point

Kay is a health visitor based in a socio-economically deprived area. It is becoming an increasingly busy caseload, particularly in relation to safeguarding. She is the only qualified health visitor attached to this GP practice, working with one staff nurse health visitor and a nursery nurse. Because of the increase in the number of child protection cases, Kay has been unable to attend well-baby clinics or drop-in services for some time. Recently, several mums have contacted Kay to say they are not happy with the advice they have been given at the baby clinic.

• How would you approach these challenges?
• How might service redesign help address these problems?

Community caseloads comprise the most vulnerable members of society and practitioners must always consider potential safeguarding issues (DH, 2010a; NMC, 2010a), the centrality of the patient/client and the need for empowerment and advocacy. As a community practitioner, this accountability necessarily extends beyond the remit of individuals to the wider structures influencing service provision. The need for community practitioners has paradoxically not been aligned with the budget to support practitioner development, with a significant drop in the number of trained specialist community nurses (NHS Digital, 2017b; QNI, 2009a, 2014a,b).

Highly efficient ways of working are greatly needed, as is evidence of 'productivity', both of which are easier to achieve through service review. Access to and consistent use of reliable ICT systems that document client contact and other pertinent statistics also help provide the required evidence to demonstrate the quantity and breadth of work undertaken in the community setting. Another area where data collection and analysis may help improve services is in relation to evaluating service quality with a recognised need for national systems to be developed to meaningfully capture and reflect care quality (Maybin et al., 2016). It is recommended that national bodies should work with providers and researchers to radically improve quality measurement in community services and that 'Community Information Data Sets (CIDS) must be developed urgently' (Foot et al., 2014: 37). There is no available evidence about the cost-effectiveness of models of community services (Bramwell et al., 2014)

Table 15.4 GP attachment compared with geographical working/corporate caseload

GP Attachment	Geographical Working/Corporate Caseload
Care provision and documentation to all GP registered patients	Care provision for the whole population – no need for patients to be GP registered
A range of services integrated within one convenient and familiar setting	'A range of service models are challenging the central role of the GP and the practice' (Brocklehurst et al., 2003)
Close communication links with the GP; direct access to notes	Communication/documentation variable – not usually direct access to 'notes'
Potential for 'integrated' team working to meet a full range of needs of the practice population	Potentially greater autonomy/ability to balance GP requests with other work; negotiation of services
Ability to 'know the patient' with a more confined caseload; better continuity of care; less risk of communication issues; clearer lines of accountability	Potential for lack of continuity; serious concerns and safeguarding issues being missed; and lines of accountability becoming confused (DH, 2009c)

but the way services are structured, for example, whether services are GP attached or geographical, may impact on quality and staff engagement. While some benefits have been described by health visitors changing from GP attachment to corporate caseloads (Table 15.4), there has also been a reported need for further evaluation as initial research demonstrated no improvement in staff stress levels or the quality of client service or increase in public health nursing activity (Hoskins et al., 2007).

CONCLUSION

The safe, cost-effective and efficient management of care in the community setting is one of the many challenges nurses face on a regular basis. The practitioner's accountability for care delivery extends beyond daily patient prioritisation and work organisation to influencing the structures and systems within which care is delivered, measured and recorded. Integral to decision making is the evaluation of services and the skill mix of the team to ensure the needs of the population are identified and addressed with high-quality care provision.

REFERENCES

Addicott R, Maguire D, Honeyman M and Jabbal J (2015) *Workforce Planning in the NHS.* London: King's Fund. (Accessed 6 May 2016) www.kingsfund.org.uk/publications/workforce-planning-nhs.

Aldridge-Bent S, Fanning A and Potter K (2013) *Transition to Community Nursing Practice.* Queen's Nursing Institute (QNI).

Audit Commission (1999) *First Assessment: A Review of District Nursing Services in England and Wales.* London: Audit Commission.

Bain H (2015) The Unique Knowing of District Nurses in Practice. Thesis submitted for the degree of Doctor of Education.

Bain H and Baguley F (2012) The management of caseloads in district nursing services. *Primary Health Care* 22(4):31–7.

Baldwin M (2006) The Warrington workload tool: Determining its use in one trust. *British Journal of Community Nursing* 11:391–5.

Ball J, Philippou J, Pike G and Sethi G (2014) *Survey of District and Community Nurses in 2013: Report to the Royal College of Nursing.* London: NNRU.

Barrett A, Latham D and Levermore G (2007) Defining the unique role of the specialist district nurse practitioner. *British Journal of Community Nursing* 12:442–8.

Bentley J and Dandy-Hughes H (2010) Implementing KSF competency testing in primary care Part 1: Developing an appraisal tool. *British Journal of Community Nursing* 15:485–91.

Bentley J and Tite C (2000) Developing an activity measuring system in district nursing. *British Journal of Community Nursing* 9(18):2016–20.

Bowers B and Durrant K (2014) Measuring safe staff levels in the community: The 'DominiC' workforce management tool. *British Journal of Community Nursing* 19(2):58–64.

Brady A-M, Byrne G, Horan P et al. (2007) Measuring the workload of community nurses in Ireland: A review of the workload measurement systems. *Journal of Nursing Management* 15:481–9.

Brady A-M, Byrne G, Horan P et al. (2008) Reliability and validity of the CCNCS: A dependency workload measurement system. *Journal of Clinical Nursing* 17:1351–60.

Bramwell D, Checkland K, Allen P and Peckham S (2014) *Moving Services out of Hospital: Joining up General Practice and Community Services?* Policy Research Unit in Commissioning and the Healthcare System: PRU Comm.

Brewerton A (2015) Achieving equitable workloads. *Community Practitioner* 88(6):13.

Brewerton A (2015a) Lady in weighting. *Community Practitioner* 88(6):14–5.

Brewerton A (2015b) Part three: Caseloads special report. *Community Practitioner* 88(7):14–7.

Brocklehurst N, Heaney J and Pollard C (2003) GP attachment versus geographical working: What's best? *Community Practitioner* 76:81–2.

Buurtzorg Nederland (2011) 'A new perspective on elder care in the Netherlands'. (Accessed 1 August 2016) http://omahasystem.org/AARPTheJournal_Summer2011_deBlok.pdf.

Byrne G, Brady A, Horan P et al. (2007) Assessment of dependency levels of older people in the community and measurement of nursing workload. *Journal of Advanced Nursing* 60(1):39–49, CINAHL Plus, EBSCOhost, viewed 16 August 2015.

Care Act (2014) Legislation.gov.uk. N.p., 2014. (Accessed 7 April 2016).

Carers UK (2007) Valuing carers: Calculating the value of unpaid care. http://tinyurl.com/valuing-carers.

Chapman H, Kilner M, Matthews R, White A, Thompson A, Fowler-Davis S, and Farndon L (2017) Developing a caseload classification tool for community nursing. *British Journal of Community Nursing*, April 2017, 22 (4), 192–196.

Cook R, Sweeney K, Perkins L et al. (2009) The future of district nursing: The Queen's Nursing Institute debate. *British Journal of Community Nursing* 14:540–4.

Cowley S and Bidmead C (2009) Controversial questions (part three): Is there randomised controlled trial evidence for health visiting? *Community Practitioner* 82:24–8.

Dean E (2013) Technology streamlines district nursing work. *Nursing Management*-UK 19(10):8–9, CINAHL Plus, EBSCOhost, viewed 16 August 2015.

DH (2004) *The NHS Knowledge and Skills Framework and the Development Review Process.* London: DH.

DH (2006) *Caring for People with Long-Term Conditions: An Education Framework for Community Matrons and Case Managers.* London: The Stationary Office.

DH (2009) Healthy child programme: Pregnancy and the first five years of life (DH, 2009 – amended August 2010) (Accessed 25 April 2016) www.dh.gov.uk/publications.

DH (2009a) Transforming community services: Enabling new patterns of provision. (Accessed 25 September 2015) www.dh.gov.uk/publications.

DH (2009b) Transforming community services programme. Transformational reference guides (6 in total). (Accessed 25 September 2015) www.dh.gov.uk/publications.

DH (2009c) Unite the union, Community Practitioners' and Health Visitors' Association (CPHVA) *Action on Health Visiting Getting It Right for Children and Families 'Ambition, Action, Achievement'.* (Accessed 25 September 2015) www.dh.gov.uk/publications.

DH (2009d) Unite the Union, Community Practitioners' and Health Visitors' Association (CPHVA) *Action on Health Visiting Getting It Right for Children and Families: Defining Research to Maximise the Contribution of the Health Visitor.* (Accessed 2 May 2010) www.dh.gov.uk/publications Last.

DH (2010a) Equity and excellence: Liberating the NHS. (Accessed 2 January 2016) www.dh.gov.uk.

DH (2010b) Clinical governance and adult safeguarding—An integrated process. National 'No secrets' NHS Advisory Group Essex NHS Operational Leads Group. (Accessed 2 January) www.dh.gov.uk/.

DH (2010c) Advanced level nursing: A position statement. Chief Nursing Officer's Directorate. (Accessed 2 January) www.dh.gov.uk/cno.

DH (2011a) The Government's response to the recommendations in frontline care: The report of the Prime Minister's Commission on the Future of Nursing and Midwifery in England. Chief Nursing Officer's Directorate. (Accessed 31 August 2015) www.dh.gov.uk.

DH (2011b) Transforming community services: Demonstrating and measuring achievement: Community indicators for quality improvement. (Accessed 31 August 2015) www.dh.gov.uk.

DH (2011c) Health visitor implementation plan 2011–15. (Accessed 2 May 2016) www.dh.gov.uk.

DH (2013) Care in local communities: A new vision and model for district nursing. (Accessed 2 May 2016) www.gov.uk/government/uploads/system/uploads/attachment_data/file/213363/vision-district-nursing-04012013.pdf.

DH (March 2014c) NHS England's business plan 2014/15–2016/17: Putting patients first. (Accessed 2 May 2016) www.dh.gov.uk.

DH (2015a) Transfer of 0–5 children's public health commissioning to local authorities mandation factsheet 2: Commissioning the national healthy child programme: Mandation of universal healthy child programme assessments/reviews. (Accessed 2 May 2016) www.dh.gov.uk.

DH (2015b) The national health visitor plan: Progress to date and implementation from 2013 onwards. (Accessed 2 May 2016) www.dh.gov.uk.

DH and Public Health England (2014) Maximising the school nurse team contribution to the public health of school aged children. (Accessed 2 May 2016).

Drennan V, Goodman C and Leyshon S (2005) Supporting the expert nurse to work in community settings—Supporting experienced hospital nurses to move into community matron roles. Primary Care Nursing Research Unit. (Accessed 28 December 2010) www.dh.gov.uk/publications.

Ervin N (2008) Caseload management skills for improved efficiency. *Journal of Continuing Education in Nursing* 39:127–32.

Fields E, Brett A (2015) Safe staffing for adult nursing care in community settings. National Institute for Health and Care Excellence 2015. (Accessed 07 July 2017) https://www.nice.org.uk/media/default/news/safe-staffing-community-nursing-evidence-review.pdf.

Foot C, Sonola L, Bennett L et al. (2014) *Managing Quality in Community Health Care Services*. London: King's Fund. (Accessed 8 May 2016) www.kingsfund.org.uk/publications/managing-quality-community-health-care-services.

Frame G and O'Donnell P (1996) Weightlifter: How to measure community nursing workload. *Health Service Journal* 106:5524.

Gould J (2010) Autonomous District Nursing Service Review Report—An Evaluation (Unpublished Report).

Grafen M and MacKenzie F (February 2015) Development and early application of the Scottish Community Nursing Workload Measurement Tool. *British Journal of Community Nursing* 20(2):89–92.

Griffith R (2015) Understanding the Code: Keeping accurate records *British Journal of Community Nursing* October 20(10).

Haycock-Stuart E, Jarvis A and Daniel K (2008) A ward without walls? District nurses' perceptions of their workload management priorities and job satisfaction. *Journal of Clinical Nursing* 17:3012–20.

Health and Social Care Information Centre (HSCIC) (January 2017) NHS workforce statistics, provisional statistics. (Accessed 27 April 2016) http://www.hscic.gov.uk/.

Health Education England (HEE) (2015) District nursing and general practice nursing service education and career framework (Accessed 26 April 2016).

HM Government (Cross Government Publication) (2010) Recognised, valued and supported: Next steps for the Carers Strategy Crown. (Accessed 28 December 2015) www.dh.gov.uk/publications.

Hoskins R, Gow A and McDowell J (2007) Corporate solutions to caseload management—An evaluation. *Community Practitioner* 80:20–4.

Hurst K (2005) Relationships between patient dependency, nursing workload and quality. *International Journal of Nursing Studies* 42:75–84.

Hurst K (2006) Primary and community care workforce planning and development. *Journal of Advanced Nursing* 55:757–69.

Jackson C, Leadbetter T, Manley K et al. (March 2015a) Making the complexity of community nursing visible: The Cassandra project. *British Journal of Community Nursing* 20(3):126–33.

Jackson C, Leary A, Wright T, Leadbetter T, Martin A, Manley K (2015) *The Cassandra Project: Recognising the multidimensional complexity of community nursing for workforce development*. (Accessed 7 July 2017) https://create.canterbury.ac.uk/14360/1/CNWDP%20report%20FINAL%2016th%20April.pdf.

Jackson C, Wright, T, and Martin A (2016) *Safe Caseloads for Adult Community Nursing Services—An Updated Review of the Evidence* ©ECPD / NHS Improvement (Accessed

7 July 2017) https://improvement.nhs.uk/uploads/documents/Final_Version_
Managing_Safe_Caseloads.pdf

Jarvis A, Mackie S and Arundel D (2006) Referral criteria: Making the district nursing
service visible. *British Journal of Community Nursing* 11:17–22.

Jones A and Russell S (2007) Equitable distribution of district nursing staff and ideal team
size. *Journal of Community Nursing* 21:4–9.

Kane K (2008) How caseload analysis led to the modernization of the DN service. *British
Journal of Community Nursing* 13:11.

Kane K (2014) Capturing district nursing through a knowledge-based electronic caseload
analysis tool (eCAT). *British Journal of Community Nursing* 19(3):116–24. doi:10.12968/
bjcn.2014.19.3.116 (Accessed 26 April 2016).

Kane K. (2015) From problem to solution: Caseload analysis tool. *Independent Nurse*.
(Accessed 16 May 2016) http://www.independentnurse.co.uk/professional-article/
from-problem-to-solution-caseload-analysis-tool/64484/.

Kennedy C (2002) The work of district nurses: First assessment visits. *Journal of Advanced
Nursing* 40:710–20.

Kennedy C (2004) A typology of knowledge for district nursing assessment practice.
Journal of Advanced Nursing 45:401–9.

Kerr H (2004) *Adaptation of the Warrington Workload Tool*. North Wales: Conwy and
Denbighshire NHS Trust.

Kirby E and Hurst K (2014) Using a complex audit tool to measure workload, staffing and
quality in district nursing. *British Journal of Community Nursing* 19:219–23.

Kolehmainen N, Francis J, Duncan E and Fraser C (2010) Community professionals'
management of client care: A mixed-methods systematic review. *Journal of Health
Services Research and Policy* 15:47–55.

Leary A (2011) Proving your worth: Alison Leary has tips on how nurse specialists can
demonstrate added value. *Nursing Standard* 25(31):62–3

Lewis M and Pontin D (2008) Caseload management in community children's nursing.
Paediatric Nursing 20:18–22.

Lord Laming (2009) *The Protection of Children in England: A Progress Report*. London: The
Stationery Office.

Luker K and Kenrick M (1992) An exploratory study of the sources of influence on the
clinical decisions of community nurses. *Journal of Advanced Nursing* 17:457–66.

Maybin J, Charles A and Honeyman M (2016) *Understanding Quality in District Nursing
Services Learning From Patients, Carers and Staff*. London: King's Fund. (Accessed 1
September 2016) www.kingsfund.org.uk/publications/quality-district-nursing.

McDonald A, Frazer K, Cowley DS (2013) Caseload management: an approach to making
community needs visible. *British Journal of Community Nursing*; 2013 Mar;18(3):140–7.

National Institute for Health and Care Excellence (NICE) (2015) Safe staffing for adult nursing
care in community settings Evidence review. (Accessed 2 September 2016) https://www.
nice.org.uk/media/default/news/safe-staffing-community-nursing-evidence-review.pdf.

Newland R (2014) *The District Nursing Workforce Planning Project; Literature Review*;
London: Queen's Nursing Institute.

NHS Alliance and Queen's Nursing Institute (2009) Briefing No. 11. *Understanding
Commissioning and Providing*. London: QNI.

NHS Education for Scotland (2011) *Career and Development Framework for District
Nursing*. Edinburgh: NES.

NHS Employers (November 2006) *Briefing: from Hospital to Home—Supporting Nurses to Move from Hospital to the Community.* Issue 26. London: NHS Employers.

NHS Scotland (2010) *Route Map to the 2020 Vision for Health and Social Care.*

NHS Wales (2015) A planned primary care workforce for Wales approach and development actions to be taken in support of the plan for a primary care service in Wales up to 2018. (Accessed 2 May 2016).

NHS Digital (2017a) Children and Young People's Health Services Monthly Statistics, England - February 2017, Experimental statistics Publication date: June 9, 2017 (Accessed 07 July 2017) https://digital.nhs.uk/catalogue/PUB24164

NHS Digital (2017b) NHS Workforce Statistics—March 2017, Provisional statistics Publication date: June 21, 2017 (Accessed 07 July 2017) https://digital.nhs.uk/catalogue/PUB30003

NHS England (2014) *Five Year Forward View* (accessed 07 July 2017) http://www.england.nhs.uk/wp-content/uploads/2014/10/5yfv-web.pdf

NHS England (2015) *Framework for Commissioning Community Nursing.* London: NHS England. (Accessed 07 July 2017) https://www.england.nhs.uk/wp-content/uploads/2015/10/Framework-for- commissioning-community-nursing.pdf

NHS England (2017) *Next Steps on the NHS Five Year Forward View* (accessed 7 July 2017) https://www.england.nhs.uk/publication/next-steps-on-the-nhs-five-year-forward-view/

NHS Improvement and National Quality Board (2017) *Safe, Sustainable and Productive Staffing: An Improvement Resource for the District Nursing service* https://improvement.nhs.uk/resources/safe-staffing-district-nursing-services/

Nursing and Midwifery Council (NMC) (2001) *Standards for Specialist Education and Practice.* London: NMC. (Accessed 22 November 2010) www.nmc-uk.org.

NMC (2004) Standards of proficiency for specialist community public health nurses (Accessed 7 July 2017) www.nmc-uk.org

NMC (2009) Guidance for the care of older people. (Accessed 2 December 2015) www.nmc-uk.org.

NMC (2010a) Raising and escalating concerns: Guidance for nurses and midwives. (Accessed 7 March 2015) www.nmc-uk.org.

NMC (2010b) Standards for Pre-registration nursing education. (Accessed 7 October 2015) www.nmc-uk.org.

NMC (2014) Standards for competence for registered nurses (Accessed 7 July 2017) www.nmc-uk.org

NMC (2015a) *The Code: Professional Standards of Practice and Behaviour for Nurses and Midwives.* London: NMC. (Accessed 7 May 2016) www.nmc-uk.org.

NMC (2015b) Revalidation (Accessed 7 May 2016) www.nmc-uk.org.

Pollock J, Horrocks S, Emond A et al. (2002) Health and social factors for health visitor caseload weighting: Reliability, accuracy and current and potential use. *Health and Social Care in the Community* 10:82–90.

Queen's Nursing Institute (QNI) (2006) *Vision and Values—A Call for Action on Community Nursing.* London: QNI.

QNI (2009a) *2020 Vision Focusing on the Future of District Nursing.* London: QNI.

QNI (2009b) *Practice Based Commissioning—Briefing.* London: QNI.

QNI (2010) *Position Statement – Nursing People in their Own Homes – Key Issues for the Future of Care.* London: QNI.

QNI (2014a) DN Workforce Planning Project Report. (Accessed 26 April 2016) www.qni.org.uk.

QNI (2014b) 2020 Vision—5 years on (Accessed 26 April 2016) www.qni.org.uk.

QNI (2015) *The value of the district nurse specialist.* London: QNI.

QNI (2016) Discharge planning: Best practice in transitions of care. (Accessed 2 September 2016) www.qni.org.uk.

QNI and QNIS (2015) The QNI/QNIS voluntary standards for district nurse education and practice. (Accessed 26 April 2016) www.qni.org.uk.

Reid B, Kane K and Curran C (2008) District nursing workforce planning: A review of the methods. *British Journal of Community Nursing* 13(11).

Roberson C (2016) Caseload management methods for use within district nursing teams: a literature review. *British Journal of Community Nursing* 21(5): 248–55

Royal College of Nursing (RCN) (2003) *Developing Referral Criteria for District Nursing Services Guidance for Nurses.* London: RCN.

Royal College of Nursing (RCN) (2010) *Guidance on Safe Nurse Staffing Levels in the UK.* London: RCN.

Royal College of Nursing (RCN) (August 2015) Policy and International Department Policy Briefing 02/15. *The Buurtzorg Nederland (home care provider) model Observations for the United Kingdom (UK).* Updated edition. RCN Policy and International Department.

Scottish Government (2016) *A National Clinical Strategy for Scotland* (Accessed 07.07.17) http://www.gov.scot/Resource/0049/00494144.pdf

Skills for Health (SFH) (2010) Improve quality and productivity through workforce transformation. *How Skills for Health can Help You: A Summary of Tools, Products and Services.* (Accessed 3 December 2015) www.skillsforhealth.org.uk.

Speed S and Luker KA (2004) Changes in patterns of knowing the patient: The case of British district nurses. *International Journal of Nursing Studies* 41:921–31.

The Phoenix Partnership (TPP) (2016) SystmOne. (Accessed 31 January 2016) www.tpp-uk.com/systmone.

The Stationery Office (TSO) (2007) *Trust, Assurance and Safety—The Regulation of Health Professionals in the 21st Century.* London: The Stationery Office.

Thomas L, Reynolds T and O'Brien L (2006) Innovation and change: shaping District Nursing services to meet the needs of primary health care. *Journal of Nursing Management*, 14, 447–454.

Turnball A (2015) Increase in health visitor workloads despite Implementation Plan. *Independent Nurse.* www.independentnurse.co.uk/news/increase-in-health-visitor-workloads-despite-implementation-plan/88148.

Unite/Community Practitioners' and Health Visitors' Association (CPHVA) (2008) The Omnibus Survey, 2008. www.unite-cphva.org.

Wakefield S, Stansfield K and Day P (2010) Taking a solution-focused approach to public health. *British Journal of School Nursing* 5:7. (Accessed 20 November 2015) www.Internurse.com.

Willis (2013) Quality with Compassion: The Future of Nursing Education. Report of the Willis Commission on Nursing Education Published by the Royal College of Nursing on behalf of the independent Willis Commission on Nursing Education. (Accessed 26 April 2016) www.rcn.org.uk/williscommission.

Wright T, Jackson C, Manley K et al. (2015) Developing a caseload model to reflect the complexity of district and community nursing. *Primary Health Care* 25:7, 32–3. (Accessed 26 April 2016) http://dx.doi.org/10.7748/phc.25.7.32.e1057.

CHAPTER 16

Leading quality, person-centred care in the community

Caroline A.W. Dickson

LEARNING OUTCOMES

- Explore the concept of person-centredness.
- Critically discuss the role of clinical leadership in the delivery of quality person-centred care.
- Explain the practice development and consider its contribution to the wider clinical governance agenda.
- Reflect on enablers and barriers of getting evidence into practice.
- Consider means of achieving sustainable change.
- Examine quality measures and quality improvement processes.

INTRODUCTION

The only certainty within the health service today is that change is inevitable. Change is constantly occurring in response to new policy and changing demographics and to meet the needs of service users and their carers. More care is being delivered at home and in communities and there is an emphasis on avoiding unnecessary hospital admissions (NHS England [NHSE], 2014; Scottish Government [SG], 2013). This requires integrated working between health and social care. Community nurses have a key leadership role in this new health and social care landscape. Effective leadership is required to shape and develop practice to ensure that service delivery is based on best evidence, delivered in a manner acceptable to people being cared for, within a culture that values the participation and involvement of all stakeholders. The means of achieving this must fit within the framework of clinical governance where responsibility for providing quality person-centred healthcare lies with every member of an organisation, as well as the organisation itself. This chapter explores leading quality person-centred care and is intended to be useful for all community nurses in the belief we are all clinical leaders. The practice development model, adapted from seminal work by McCormack and Garbett (2002) is used as a conceptual framework. It is useful for clinical leaders to evidence and develop their practice, improve patient and carer experience, while developing teams and transforming the culture and context of care (Figure 16.1).

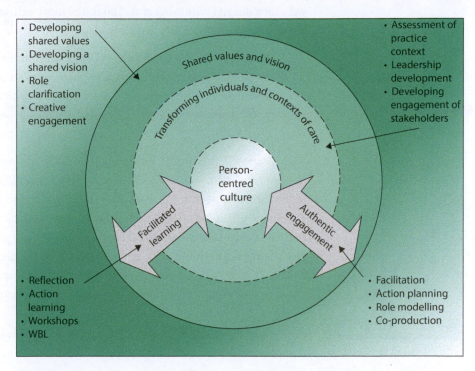

• Developing shared values
• Developing a shared vision
• Role clarification
• Creative engagement

• Assessment of practice context
• Leadership development
• Developing engagement of stakeholders

Shared values and vision

Transforming individuals and contexts of care

Person-centred culture

Facilitated learning

Authentic engagement

• Reflection
• Action learning
• Workshops
• WBL

• Facilitation
• Action planning
• Role modelling
• Co-production

FIGURE 16.1 A practice development conceptual framework. (Adapted from McCormack B and Garbett R, *Nursing Times Research*, 7[2], 87–100, 2002. With kind permission.)

To set the scene, the concepts of clinical governance, person-centredness and practice development are examined. Different approaches to leadership and facilitation, workplace cultures, active learning, getting evidence into practice, quality improvement processes, and approaches to sustaining change will be explored within the context of delivering quality, person-centred care in the community.

ACTIVITY 16.1

Take a few moments to consider your own knowledge on leading quality, person-centred care and questions you would like addressed as you proceed to read this chapter.

CLINICAL GOVERNANCE

During the mid-1990s, there was recognition of variance in the quality of care provided for patients/clients throughout the United Kingdom. Until the mid-1990s, National Health Service (NHS) Trusts were accountable for their financial expenditure, through corporate governance, but not for the quality of care provided within their organisations. Twenty years ago, policies such as *The New NHS Modern and Dependable* (Department of Health, 1998) and *Designed to Care* (Scottish Office, 1997) introduced clinical governance which placed responsibility and accountability for quality care on the shoulders of chief executives. In order to carry this obligation, shared responsibility was encouraged through working in open systems, formal standards, procedures, regular monitoring and reporting were introduced (Wilkinson et al., 2004). The most well-known definition of clinical governance is that of Scally and Donaldson:

> A framework through which NHS organisations are accountable for continuallyimproving the quality of their services and safeguarding high standards of care bycreating an environment in which excellence in clinical care will flourish.
>
> *(Scally and Donaldson, 1998: 61)*

They proposed this would be the main vehicle for continuously improving the quality of patient care and developing the capacity of the NHS in England. Since then, the addition of staff governance has led to the concept of healthcare governance. This includes all three aspects: corporate, clinical and staff governance. Practice development, key to addressing the clinical governance agenda enables practitioners to demonstrate accountability, although practice development is driven 'bottom-up', whereas clinical governance is 'top-down'. Both frameworks however aim to support safe, effective person-centred care.

ACTIVITY 16.2

You might like to take time to find out the clinical governance structures and support available in your organisation.

PERSON-CENTREDNESS

You will be very familiar with person-centredness as it underpins current healthcare policy (SG, 2010, 2014) and is reflected in *The Code* (Nursing and Midwifery Council [NMC], 2015). It is linked to the concept of co-production, anticipatory care and strengths-based approaches which are important in contemporary community nursing practice. They are equally important in terms of developing practice and the professional development of community nurses. The emphasis is on commitment to enable others to take responsibility for their own health and well-being. This challenges nurses and other practitioners to design and develop their services with patient and other service-user experience central (Freeth, 2006) and to reflect on their professional attributes (NMC, 2015).

According to McCormack and McCance person-centredness is

> an approach to practice established through the formation and fostering of healthful relationships between all care providers, service users and others significant to them in their lives. It is underpinned by values of respect for persons, individual right to self-determination, mutual respect and understanding. It is enabled by cultures of empowerment that foster continuous approaches to practice development.
>
> *(2010: 31–31)*

Person-centredness is concerned with all persons including those being cared for as service users, their supporters and colleagues. There are four constructs:

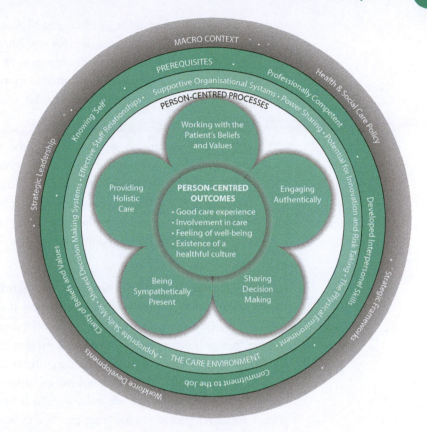

FIGURE 16.2 Person-centred practice framework. (From McCormack B and McCance T, eds., *Person-Centred Practice in Nursing and Health Care: Theory and Practice*, 2nd edn, Oxford: Wiley-Blackwell, 2016.)

pre-requisites, care environment, person-centred processes and outcomes. To achieve positive outcomes for service users and staff, McCormack and McCance (2016) suggest attention must be given to pre-requites and the care environment. This will in turn enable person-centred care processes (Figure 16.2). A particular challenge for community nurses in delivering quality person-centred care is the inter-agency nature of teams involved in care and service delivery, where practitioners may have differing values and beliefs. Cultures of health and social care are different which impacts on workplace cultures. Practice development is a means of achieving person-centred cultures and can achieve new ways of working.

PRACTICE DEVELOPMENT

Practice development was initially introduced as a means of developing evidence from practice to substantiate nursing as a profession in the early 1990s (Redfern and Stevens, 1996; Pearson, 1997) through the establishment of nursing and practice development units. Since then, theoretical understanding and the evidence to support practice development as a means of taking practice forward has grown considerably. In the early years, the purpose of practice development was advocated as good quality patient-focussed care achieved through the improvement of technical knowledge and skills (Garbett and McCormack, 2002), and through the dissemination of research into practice (Kitson, 2009). Although this approach was direct and effective in working to short-term goals, it was associated with top-down change and was often an ineffective sustainable approach. McCormack et al. (2007) and Dewing (2008) among others take a broader, transformational view of practice development:

> Practice development is a continuous process of developing person-centred cultures. It is enabled by facilitators who authentically engage with individuals and teams to blend personal qualities and creative imagination with practice skills and practice wisdom. The learning that occurs brings about transformations of individual and team practices. This is sustained by embedding both processes and outcomes in corporate strategy.
>
> *(Manley et al., 2008: 9)*

It is a systematic approach that aims to help practitioners and healthcare teams to look critically at their practice and identify how it can be improved (McCormack et al., 2009). Current thinkers in practice development however argue development occurs, not only within the confines of a project framework, but is also a means of scrutinising and developing workplace cultures to find new and improved ways of working. Cultures of practice where learning is encouraged and embraced are receptive to change, as are cultures which enable practitioners to consider issues for development arising from practice as well as development required by directives from policy makers. The approach is one where there is participation and involvement of all stakeholders – patients, clients, families and staff.

ACTIVITY 16.3   Is the culture where you work a person-centred culture? What do you think would make it a person-centred culture?

EFFECTIVE WORKPLACE CULTURE

The recent Francis Inquiry (2013) has had ramifications for healthcare services and practitioners across the United Kingdom. A key finding of the report was 'unhealthy cultures' which has resulted in growing attention in addressing cultures of organisations (King's Fund, 2013). This reflects current thinking which suggests workplace cultures have an impact on safe, effective, person-centred care (Manley et al., 2013). Negative cultures exist because of narrow, ritualistic practices which go unchallenged. Manley et al. (2013) suggest positive cultures have the potential to transform quality of care, patient experience, health outcomes, staff well-being and commitment, learning and evidence use in the workplace. Lord Francis advocated cultures based on positive values, including care and compassion. Shared values is one of the five attributes of effective workplace cultures identified by Manley (2004). They also identified that values are realised and experienced in practice through a shared vision which charges everybody to take individual as well as adopt collective responsibility for upholding these values. Manley et al. (2013) also identify adaptability, innovation and creativity as a third attribute which upholds workplace effectiveness. The fourth is maintaining the needs of patients/communities as the drive behind change and a fifth attribute the existence of formal systems that enable and evaluate learning performance and shared governance. Community nurses' contribution to developing positive organisational cultures is giving attention to workplace cultures or, 'the way things are done around here' (Dreenan, 1992: 3).

Example: During a project, developing person-centred cultures with Marie-Curie, values clarification of one hospice including families was achieved by adopting a number of steps. Adopting values clarification process identified by Manley (2004) individuals from across the hospice in the practice development group were asked to address the following:

I believe the purpose of a person-centred culture is...

I believe person-centred culture can be achieved by...

I believe the factors that will enable and inhibit a person-centred culture are...

Members of the practice development group then facilitated this exercise in their own workplace. Individuals engaged in this activity during meetings, using graffiti boards, as a 'time-out' exercise, during conversations, during meetings. All data were themed until the statements could be re-written using the prefix 'we believe.' This was ultimately used to form the hospice shared vision.

Active learning

Lord Rose's recent review, *Better Leadership for Tomorrow* (2015), challenges NHS staff to become the best versions of themselves at work. Life-long learning is supported by governmental policy and organisations have the responsibility within the clinical governance framework, to ensure there are systems in place to support this. Managers have a responsibility to ensure teams meet all statutory and professional requirements, although all professionals have a responsibility to ensure they continually grow and develop. Amy (2008) carried out survey research to identify the contribution of leaders to learning at individual and organisational levels. She identified the required behaviours as facilitation, problem solving and decision making, communication, relating and developing. Although attending courses, study days and conferences, are useful, there is little evidence to suggest the result is development of practice.

Practice development is achieved through challenging practice learning of individuals and teams (Manley and McCormack, 2003; Dewing, 2008). The facilitation of critical reflection, crucial in this type of learning occurs through critical questioning where enlightenment, empowerment and emancipation occur (Dewing, 2008; McCormack et al., 2009). Emancipation or liberation from old ways of thinking together with balanced participation is required to recognise areas of practice that require attention. Active learning is an approach discussed by Dewing (2008).

She advocates learning taking place in the workplace rather than being a separate activity in more didactic training study days. The purpose of active learning is action which contributes to transformation of workplace cultures. It involves the multiple use of the senses and intelligences, reflecting and engaging with an internal dialogue with self and an ongoing dialogue with others (Dewing, 2008). An active learning relationship is facilitated in practice through relationships that enable high support and high challenge. The relationship is based on facilitators and co-learners as the intention is for all of those involved to learn and learn about learning. Relationships may take the form of clinical supervision (Driscoll, 2007), critical companionship (Titchen, 2004) and action learning (McGill and Brockbank, 2003). Other relationships that support personal and professional development are preceptorship, mentorship and coaching. Preceptorship programmes are now more commonplace for newly qualified staff and offer support in the consolidation of their educational preparation programme. Examples of this are NHS Flying Start. The Northern Ireland Practice and Education Council for Nursing and Midwifery (www.nipecdf.org/) has a similar programme. Mentorship and coaching relationships however are less commonplace and appear to be confined to senior managers and leaders.

ACTIVITY 16.4

If you are in one of these relationships, do you consider you are engaging in active learning and mentorship? What does the facilitation of active learning look like?

MEASURING QUALITY

The Institute of Medicine's Six Dimensions of Quality Care (2001) (Figure 16.3) have been adapted in a number of policy documents.

Every practitioner is responsible for ensuring clinical effectiveness, managing risk and continuous quality improvement. Lord Darzi's Report *High Quality Care for All: NHS Next Stage Review* (Department of Health, 2008) outlined quality improvement as a core element of any approach to leadership and this has been cemented in current policy drivers. Healthcare governance and the drive to modernise the NHS has created a culture where clinical quality indicators, performance indicators and other targets have become part of the culture of healthcare. In England, the NHS Outcomes Framework (Department of Health, 2014b), the Public Health Outcomes Framework (Department of Health, 2015) and the Adult Social Care Outcomes Framework (Department of Health, 2014a) assure quality by assessing progress in five domains. These are scrutinised and quality assured by the Care Quality Commission by asking five key questions of services: Are they safe? Are they effective? Are they caring? Are they responsive to people's needs? Are they well-led? (www.cqc.org.uk/content/five-key-questions-we-ask).

In Scotland, Health Improvement Efficiency Access Treatment (HEAT) targets are implemented through each NHS Board's Local Delivery Plan as part of the national plan, Scotland Performs. While these targets are more acute care focussed, they now have an emphasis on both health and social care. The Quality Outcomes Framework, introduced in 2004, as part of the General Medical Services (GMS) contract

Safe	Avoiding injuries to patients from the care that is intended to help them
Effective	Providing services based on scientific knowledge to all who could benefit and refraining from providing services to those not likely to benefit (avoiding underuse and overuse); doing the right thing for the right person at the right time
Family-centred	Providing care that is respectful of and responsive to individual patient preferences, needs and values, and ensuring that patient values guide all clinical decisions
Timely	Reducing waits and sometimes unfavourable delays for both those who receive and those who give care
Efficient	Avoiding waste, in particular waste of equipment, supplies, ideas and energy
Equitable	Providing care that does not vary in quality because of personal characteristics such as gender, ethnicity, geographic location and socio-economic status

FIGURE 16.3 Six specific aims for improvement. (From Institute for Medicine, http://www.nationalacademies.org/hmd/~/media/Files/Report%20Files/2001/Crossing-the-Quality-Chasm/Quality%20Chasm%202001%20%20report%20brief.pdf Accessed 30th June 2017, 2001.)

(www.nice.org.uk/aboutnice/qof/qof.jsp) in England, Wales and Scotland is a framework of performance measures that benchmark activities within general practice. Although the NHS Boards and general practice are measured against these targets, teams are expected to contribute to their achievement and to use the targets to guide service delivery and development. Current NHS Scotland Improvement Priorities are

- Health inequalities and prevention
- Antenatal and early years
- Person-centred care
- Primary care
- Integration

QUALITY IMPROVEMENT

While examples such as Mid Staffordshire (Francis, 2013) highlight the perils of targets and performance indicators, practitioners can choose their response to such measures. Disastrous incidents are most often preceded by an incubation period where warning signs are ignored or misinterpreted, where false assumptions are made and misplaced optimism predominates (Macrae, 2014). Leaders can create culture and processes that ensure such warning signs are understood and addressed early. They can base their improvement efforts on empirically tested models for person-centred care that focus on the active engagement of practitioners in transforming the workplace and practices individuals and teams engage in (McCormack and Garbett, 2003). Rather than measure people and practice, leaders can work collaboratively to understand their practice contexts and create the conditions that make it possible for them to enhance their contexts such that practice and people flourish. An example of how a district nurse (DN) leader can use practice development principles in response to targets is provided in this case study.

The DN team leader receives communication that there are clinical quality and financial performance indicators required to be reported every quarter for their service.

In preparation for the next team meeting, targets that must be achieved are shared. The team leader asks that the team commit a half hour discussing these. At the meeting some members of the team express their disgust at imposed targets. Others express their concerns about being scrutinised while working in people's homes. Others debate the relevance and importance of the targets.

Previously, the team have identified and agreed and made explicit shared values and beliefs underpinning their practice. The team leader refers to these, 'We believe we should always strive to provide care that is safer, evidence-based, more effective and more person centred.' She then encourages dialogue by asking, 'How do we currently know we are achieving that?' The group discover 'proving' care is good is difficult because of the way they work and that much of what they do is crucial but not reflected in these current targets.

The group agreed it would be useful for them all to be involved in collecting data about their practice. This would include the specified targets, but also data on other aspects of practice deemed important by them and their client group. A member of staff agreed to run a short life working group to use the 'Good Enough' model of evaluation proposed by Wilson and McCance (2015) to identify appropriate indicators of quality for their service. They also sought to create a framework that ensured staff were involved in data collection, giving and receiving feedback and engaged in reflecting on practice in light of their data.

Over the next 6 months, the whole team collected data twice. This included the clinical quality and financial target data as well as performance data on wound management and quality of interactions with patients and their families. They used observation, records reviews and interviews with patients and families to understand the quality of care provided. Following their first data collection they commenced an active learning group where they looked at their collective performance and work on issues in practice. This led to two projects being commenced, one focusing on improving wound care and the other at exploring how access to social activities in the local community can be enhanced.

What evaluation methods have you come across in practice? What types of data were collected? How were the data used to evidence practice and evidence key targets set by the organisation?

LEADING PERSON-CENTRED PRACTICE

Within current healthcare, post–Francis Inquiry (2013), there is a recognition of the importance of effective leadership at all levels of organisations and across systems (King's Fund, 2013). Leadership theories are concerned with who the leader is, what the leader does and in what context. Old paradigm leadership models, according to Northouse (2010) view leadership as a process that involves influencing others, occurs within a group context and involves goal attainment. Limitations of these models lie in the emphasis on one aspect of leadership, often at the detriment of the others. Conversely, new paradigm models are seen as a process of social influence which deals with the realities of constant change, and place considerable emphasis on the power and importance of followers (Bass and Steidlmeir, 1999). One such model is transformational leadership. Wong and Cummings (2007) systematically reviewed studies examining the relationship between transformational leadership nursing and patient outcomes. The findings provide evidence supporting a positive relationship between transformational nursing leadership practices and improved patient outcomes. This theoretical perspective is linked in the literature to practice development and currently underpins the majority of development programmes used within the NHS. According to Barr and Dowding,

> transformational theories of leadership are based on the idea that leaders are people who motivate others to perform by encouraging them to see a vision which changes their perception of reality. Such leaders are seen as committed individuals with long term vision, a need to empower others and are interested in the consequences.
>
> *(2012: 62)*

Contemporary leadership theorists claim old paradigm models are in fact management rather than leadership (Figure 16.4). In addition, the evidence underpinning the new paradigm models, they claim is questionable (e.g. Alimo-Metcalfe and Alban-Metcalfe, 2005). These models are based largely on US studies of 'distant' leaders, top-level managers and chief executives, rather than those close to the realities of practice directly with their followers. An alternative model of transformational leadership was proposed by Alimo-Metcalfe and Albans-Metcalfe (2005, 2008) that examined the leadership interaction with followers. In this model of 'close' or 'nearby' leadership, there is a theme or ordinariness, rather than heroism. Follower engagement is placed at the heart of leadership and leaders are committed to building a shared vision through participation and inclusion of all stakeholders. They suggest leaders increase followers' self-efficacy and self-worth by communicating confidence and expectation to a mission of a better future. Alimo-Metcalfe and Albans-Metcalfe (2008) claim leaders who achieve high engagement are able to achieve high levels of motivation, job satisfaction and job commitment among their staff.

Models of leading person-centred practice are more participatory than old and new paradigm theories suggest. They are also value based, and the leader and follower have a more dynamic relationship. Participatory leadership is acknowledged by the King's Fund (2013). Their model of patient-centred leadership places core values of care and compassion at the heart of leadership practices. The purpose is focussing on patients' needs first and foremost and improving quality care. Stanley (2006, 2008) developed a model of congruent leadership by studying nurses in one NHS Trust. He concluded clinical leaders were found at all nursing levels and tended not to be at the most senior level. They are motivational, inspirational, organised, effective communicators and relationship builders. Their leadership approach is based upon

Old Paradigm	New Paradigm	Contemporary Leadership
Trait leadership Leaders are born, not made and possess such traits as self confidence, empathy, ambition, self-control, curiosity (Dawes and Handscomb, 2005).	**Transformational leadership** Individuals who stimulate and inspire followers to both achieve extraordinary outcomes and in the process develop their own leadership capacity. Transformational leaders help followers grow and develop into leaders by responding to individual followers' needs by empowering them and by aligning the objectives of the individual followers, the leader, the group, and the larger organisation (Bass and Riggio, 2006: 3).	**Close/nearby leadership** A 'nearby' transformational or engaging leader is someone who encourages and enables the development and well being of others, in the ability to unite different groups of stakeholders in articulating a shared vision, and in delegation of a kind that empowers and develops potential, coupled with the encouragement of questioning and of thinking which is critical as well as strategic (Amilio-Metcalfe and Albans-Metcalfe, 2008: 16).
Behavioural leadership From the studies of Lewin (1947), authoritarian, democratic and laissez-faire leadership styles were identified.	**Transactional leadership** The emphasis is on mutual agreement of goals. Transactional leaders clarify the role of subordinates, show consideration to them, initiate structure, reward and punish and attempt to meet social needs. Motivate by appealing to self-interest via pay or motivation (Bass, 1985).	**Congruent leadership** Leadership is a match (congruence) between the activities, actions and deeds of the leader and the leader's values, vision and beliefs (Stanley, 2006b: 132).
Situational leadership Leaders employ different leadership styles for different situations (Bourmans and Londerweerd, 1993). Leaders vary the level of guidance, direction and support depending on the followers' maturity and level of development, i.e. enthusiastic beginner, disillusioned learner, capable but cautious contributor and self-reliant achiever (Hersey and Blanchard, 1993).	**Charismatic leadership** Charismatic leaders are often found in the highest level of society and organisations. They transform followers' needs, values, preferences and aspirations and motivation is driven by a need to serve the collective (Michaelis et al., 2009).	**Action-centred leadership** The group or functional approach where the role of leader is to address the needs of the task, the team and the individual. He/she achieves this through different functions: planning, initiating, controlling, supporting, informing, evaluating. While responsible for addressing the three areas of need, the leader would not be expected to perform all the functions, rather distribute them appropriately throughout the team (Adair, 2005).

FIGURE 16.4 Key leadership theories from old and new paradigms.

a foundation of care that is fundamental to their values and beliefs of nursing care. Stanley identified the attributes of clinical leaders as clinical competence, clinical knowledge, approachability, motivation, empowerment, decision making, effective communication being a role model and visibility.

Figure 16.4 provides an overview of some key theories. Please see additional leadership literature for a more in-depth study of leadership theory.

Lynch (2015) and Cardiff (2014) have developed Hersey and Blanchard's model of situational leadership (1993) as a means of leading person-centred cultures in practice. The model proposed by Lynch (2015) of 'partnering for performance' suggests that while leaders adapt their leadership style from delegating, supporting, coaching and directing as advocated by Hersey and Blanchard, the aim of leadership is to enable followers to assess their practice using McCormack and McCance's person-centred practice framework (2016). Partnering will enable followers to move along a continuum to achieve person-centred practice. It is achieved by transformational learning (Meizerow, 1981), facilitating critical reflection, engaging in critical dialogue and using such evaluative tools as the workplace culture critical analysis tool (McCormack et al., 2009). Cardiff (2014) developed a conceptual model of person-centred leadership which he suggests enables leaders to base their leadership practices on person-centred values. This model is relational, involving leader and *associate* rather than *follower* or *subordinate*, indicating the continually changing relationship for which he represents in the metaphor of the Argentine tango. The purpose of leadership for Cardiff (2014) is enabling empowerment and well-being, allowing associates to 'come into their own'. This is achieved by *sensing* where the other is at, enabling *reflexivity, balancing* their needs, *contextualising* or helping the associate make sense of their social world, *presencing* and *communing* or reaching shared visions or decision making. Leaders respond to individuals in different situations by *stancing*. Cardiff (2014) acknowledges the effect culture and context on leadership and vice versa. He suggests systems of evaluation and availability of safe, critical and creative spaces and the needs of the associate all have a significant impact on person-centred leadership.

ACTIVITY 16.6

Is there someone you can think of you consider to be a good leader? They do not necessarily have to work in healthcare. What is it you admire about them? In relation to this, what are your strengths and what are your areas for development? Who and where will you get help in order to develop these skills?

GETTING EVIDENCE INTO PRACTICE

We know from our professional code that decisions made in practice and advice given by nurses must be evidence based (NMC, 2015). Implementation and utilisation of evidence are not straightforward. They require leadership and are essential for developing practice. Evidence is drawn from practice and research and drives the need for practice development. Practice development also generates evidence which can show performance and achievement of targets and outcomes. Evidence is readily available in different formats, for example, guidelines, protocols and best practice statements, and there are many means available to evidence practice, for example, audits, questionnaires and other feedback mechanisms. However, the process of getting evidence into practice is complex. As discussed earlier, clinical leaders have a role in developing cultures where individuals and teams are open to challenge, are actively seeking the best ways of doing things, a culture where practitioners are keen to demonstrate clinical effectiveness. They also have a role in facilitation. Rycroft-Malone (2004, 2013) offers a practical framework, Promoting Action on Research Implementation in Health Services (PARIHS) which helps the implementation of evidence. This has been developed and tested since the seminal work by Kitson et al. (1998). She asserts clinical effectiveness is more than the availability of robust evidence, it is also concerned with effective facilitation and a receptive context. She identifies these aspects as being on a continuum from high to low. These are the areas therefore that require attention.

ACTIVITY 16.7

Consider how the core components of the PARIHS framework could be applied in a community setting to get evidence into practice.

Evidence

The changing context of healthcare delivery means community nurses need knowledge and the skills to retrieve data, critique the quality of evidence. They must consider how to use the evidence most effectively to improve patient care and ways of dissemination of best practice. However, gold standard evidence does not necessarily take into account person-centredness, evidence from practice or the uniqueness of the practice context. Patients are people with individual needs and decisions about care must be based on these needs. Workplace cultures vary in their receptiveness to change and development. Many areas of nursing practice do not lend themselves to randomised controlled trials; thus the PARIHS framework considers other types of evidence. Rycroft-Malone (2013) includes evidence from clinical experience, patients and local information or data relevant to the context. This should be considered and critiqued in the same way as research evidence. Figure 16.5 identifies the types of knowledge required to support clinical effectiveness.

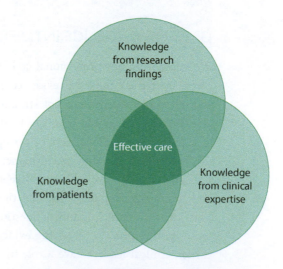

FIGURE 16.5 Knowledge to support effective care. Three overlapping spheres with effective care in the centre, knowledge from research findings; knowledge from clinical expertise/practice data; knowledge from patients in each circle.

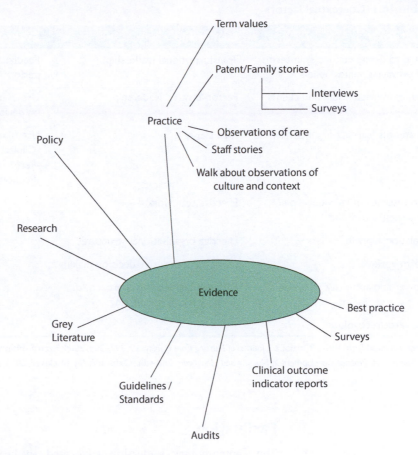

FIGURE 16.6 Types of evidence.

ACTIVITY 16.8

Figure 16.6 identifies some of the available types of evidence to inform practice. Can you identify what evidence is being collected in your clinical area and how it is being used to inform, develop and evaluate practice?

Context

Context is the environment or practice setting, broken down into culture, leadership and evaluation in the PARIHS framework. Leadership and culture have been discussed earlier in this chapter. Process and outcome evaluation are of equal importance in practice development. Practice developers use creative means of engaging with stakeholders to gain evaluation data. While the data may be numbers achieved against targets identified through audits, they also emerge through exercises like values clarification (Manley, 2004), visioning, observations of care and practice and patient stories. The dimensions of context are outlined in Table 16.1.

ACTIVITY 16.9

Consider the context of practice you are familiar with. Where do you think it is on the continuum from high to low context?

Table 16.1 Contextual factors

Culture	Leadership	Evaluation
Able to define culture(s) in terms of prevailing values/beliefs	Transformational leadership	Feedback on individual, team and system performance
Values individual staff and clients	Person-centred leadership	Use of multiple sources of information on performance
Promotes learning organisation	Role clarity	Use of multiple methods of evaluations: -Clinical -Performance -Economic
Consistency of individual role/ experience to value	Effective teamwork	
Relationship with others	Effective organisational structures	
Teamwork	Democratic inclusive decision making	
Power and authority	Enabling/empowering approach to learning, teaching/managing	
Rewards/recognition		

Source: Adapted from Rycroft-Malone J, *Journal of Nursing Care Quality,* 19, 297–304, 2004; Rycroft-Malone J, in McCormack B, Manley K, and Titchen A, eds., *Practice Development in Nursing and Healthcare,* 2nd edn., Oxford: Wiley-Blackwell, 2013, pp. 146–68.

Facilitation

The contemporary leadership advocated in healthcare policies is based on facilitation (NHS Scotland, 2008) and is ideal for addressing the current changing context in healthcare. Facilitation, advocated in practice development, is the process of valuing a nurturing critical questioning environment that allows a team to learn and develop together (Huber, 2010; Shaw et al., 2008). Heron (2002) identifies modes of facilitation as planning interventions (setting goals for the group); giving meaning (helping the group to make sense of experience); confronting (raising the group's awareness of the gap between saying and doing and tackling resistances); structuring (choosing which methods of learning are best suited to the event) and valuing (creating a climate which gives people recognition). The characteristics of facilitation in practice development and the attributes of effective leaders and practice developers are outlined in Table 16.2.

Change models

The literature abounds with change models. While they can be valuable, unlike practice development, they do not have person-centredness, transforming cultures and contexts and active learning as explicit intentions. Models of planned change help to structure the process of change and assist with transition, although are criticised as being too linear and simplistic. Probably the best known model of change was developed in 1951 by Kurt Lewin. He said that in order to prepare a team

Table 16.2 Characteristics of facilitation in practice development

Simmons five facilitation characteristics (simmons, 2004)	Attributes of effective clinical nurse leaders (cook and leathard, 2004)	Attributes of practice developers (garbett and mccormack, 2003)
Critical thinking	Creativity	Values and beliefs: commitment to improving patient care, enabling not telling
Shared decision making	Highlighting	Facilitative skills
Making things easier	Influencing	Energy and tenacity
Leadership of change	Respecting	Flexibility, sensitivity and reflexivity
Equity	Supporting	Knowledge
		Creativity
		Political awareness (being in the middle)
		Credibility

for change, the status quo must be de-stabilised to increase the sense of discontent with current practice. To assist with this process he recommended carrying out a force-field analysis where the driving and restraining forces of the intended change are identified by the team. The 'unfreezing' process, he argued would increase the perceived need for change and involve stakeholders. He then identified the 'moving' stage where the change is implemented and established. The 're-freezing' stage was the change being imbedded into the organisation.

Kotter identified eight steps to successful change in his emergent model of change (Kotter, 2012: 54). The steps he identified are establishing a sense of increased urgency, creating a guiding coalition, developing a vision and strategy, communicating the change vision, empowering broad-based action and generating short-term 'wins'. Finally he identified, consolidating gains and producing more change. The DICE mode, currently being used within the health service, was developed by Sirkin et al. (2005). They stated duration (of the project), integrity (of the team), commitment (by both management and employees) and effort (demands made of employees), determine the outcome of any transformation initiative. If the project is long term, short milestones and regular evaluation are advocated. The integrity of the team relates to the ability of the team to deliver the project successfully; commitment, to the support from senior management as well as 'buy-in' from those affected by the change. Saskin and his colleagues considered employees could not be expected to make more than 10% increased effort above their current workload. These aspects are important to be considered when supporting teams through change.

TOOLS TO DEVELOP PRACTICE

The tools you would use to develop practice may depend on whether you are adopting a practice development or change management approach. You will remember that important in practice development is the identification of vision and values, involvement and participation, facilitation and evaluation of the context. An example of values clarification has already been given. The following is an example of creating a safe environment and visioning.

Example: Creating a safe environment. CHOICE: Connecting Health and Social Care to Offer Individualised Care at End of Life was a project developing integrated ways of working for people being cared for at home at end of life. This was funded by the Queen's Nursing Institute Scotland. The purpose of the project was to test out a model of integrated working between community nurses and social care workers caring for people at end of life at home. The process of creating a safe environment was enabled by connecting together, establishing ways of working and checking in before the end of the session. We aimed to create an environment that involved all participants, encouraging everyone to contribute. First we used imagery to ask participants to share how they were feeling about being part of the project. In future sessions we used tools including the 'blob tree' (www.blobtree.com/pages/frontpage). This helped us all to be aware of each other and the energies in the room and be respectful accordingly. Highlighting terms of engagement, similar to setting ground rules was enabled with increased involvement with the group. At the end of the session the facilitator used imagery to check how everyone was feeling and if they were happy to leave the group. It was also used in ongoing process evaluation. Participants were asked for one word to describe how they felt. An example from the close of one early session is shown in Table 16.3.

Example: Creating a shared vision. Images were also used to create a shared vision in the CHOICE project (Figure 16.7). These images represented…

Two groups that then engaged in dialogue and presented the other group with a vision statement. Together the group turned the two statements into a shared vision statement:

Integrated person-centred end-of-life care at home is…

'*Skilled health and social care staff working together, supporting each* other to build a relationship with the 'cared-for person' and family and/or significant others to provide holistic care where everyone feels valued, has choice and

Table 16.3 Team process evaluation

Comforted, supported, reassured and positive	Beginning to reach goals
The team is coming together	Getting to know each other and appreciate each other's roles
Helping each other	Know where to reach out for support
Role appreciation	Joint working
Reaching to others to get answers	Look what we can achieve together
Increasing knowledge	Very supportive to each other

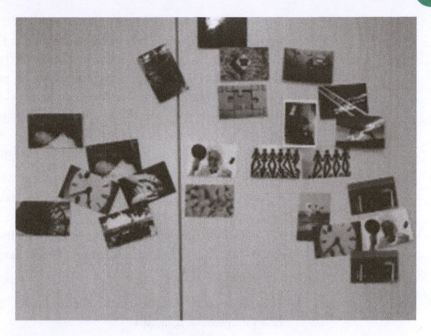

FIGURE 16.7 Creating a shared vision.

dignity through open communication. We will work together with 'cared for persons' to asses, plan and evaluate care of their choice giving sufficient time to give streamlined, co-ordinated care with staff continuity to achieve a dignified death'.

The National Institute for Health and Care Excellence (NICE) have produced guidance, How to Change Practice Guide (https://www.nice.org.uk/process/pmg30/chapter/introduction-and-background). The barriers to change in healthcare are identified as awareness and knowledge of the required change, motivation of individuals and teams, skills required to make change happen, acceptance and beliefs of the quality of current practice and the proposed change and practicalities in terms of resources and organisational structures.

Other models to guide quality improvement are widely available. Audit is a crucial component of most processes and helps monitor improvements in the quality of patient care (Patel, 2010). To be helpful, however, it must be an ongoing dynamic process that supports the constant reviewing of practice standards (McSherry and Pearce, 2011). Steps in the audit cycle are outlined in Box 16.1.

Box 16.1

1. Evaluate clinical practice against standards.
2. Identify areas requiring change.
3. Evaluate standards for practice set informed by evidence.
4. Evaluate practice and identify variations.
5. Implement change (development of action plan).

(Adapted from Bryar and Griffiths, 2003)

The National Patient Safety Programme in NHS Scotland makes use of the Improvement Model. The 'Plan-Do-Study-Act' or PDSA cycle. A key component in this model focuses on persistent improvement throughout the process of change. It also encourages teams to constantly review their practice through the use of evaluation to shape the ongoing development (Nelson et al., 2007). Although the emphasis of this quality improvement tool is less on transforming culture and context and more on testing new ways of working on a small scale within short time frames, evaluation within it allows effectiveness to be demonstrated.

- *Plan* – Plan the change to be implemented and its evaluation criteria.
- *Do* – Implement the change.
- *Study* – Evaluate the data from before and after the change.
- *Act* – Act upon information gained from change and plan further changes necessary.

NHS Institute for Healthcare Improvement (www.ihi.org/resources/Pages/HowtoImprove/default.aspx)

ACTIVITY 16.10

Consider an issue in practice where you have identified evidence development is needed. Using one of the quality improvement tools, develop an outline plan indicating how it could be addressed.

LEADERSHIP DEVELOPMENT

As developing leadership across organisations is a key priority in the NHS there are lots of resources available to help you in your leadership development. There is a particular drive for community nurses to increase their leadership and management capacity as more people are being cared for in their own homes and communities. The challenging context of the community, where nurses practice autonomously at all levels means leadership is essential for safe, effective, person-centred care. Continuous improvement and development of services requires everyone to play their part across organisations, at strategic level and at the clinical interface. Attributes of effective nurse leaders have been highlighted in the literature as stewardship, respect, caring, advocacy, honesty, confidentiality and initiating a values programme by Jooste (2004). Cook and Leathard (2004) advocated creativity, highlighting, influencing, respecting and supporting.

The need to develop leadership has been recognised in the emergence of the NHS Leadership Academy (www.leadershipacademy.nhs.uk/) providing programmes for different stages of development, discussion boards and interactive activities. There have also been a range of frameworks developed to guide professional growth, for example, the Clinical Leadership Competency Framework (NHS Leadership Academy, 2011 available at www.leadershipacademy.nhs.uk/wp-content/uploads/2012/11/NHSLeadership-Leadership-Framework-Clinical-Leadership-Competency-Framework-CLCF.pdf). This is centred on five pillars, demonstrating personal qualities, working with others, managing services, improving services and setting direction. In Scotland, NHS Education for Scotland has established a National Leadership Unit and provides resources for developing leaders (www.nes.scot. nhs.uk/education-and-training/by-theme-initiative/leadership-and-management. aspx). In Scotland, Leading Better Care (LBC) (SG, 2008) is a role framework which provides senior charge nurses and community team leaders with support to meet Knowledge and Skills Framework profile (www.evidenceintopractice.scot.nhs.uk/ leading-better-care.aspx). The aim of LBC is to help in the achievement of high-quality, person-centred safe and efficient care for every patient the first time and every time. This is achieved by ensuring there are better processes, effective ways of working, efficient and person-centred care that result in more effective use of all resources.

ACTIVITY 16.11

Access one of the leadership frameworks above. Take a look at the resources available to support leadership development. Identify the qualities you would like to develop. Design your own personal development plan indicating how you will develop, who will help you and the resources you need.

SUMMARY

The practice development conceptual framework (Garbett and McCormack, 2002) and the Person-Centred Practice Framework (McCormack and McCance, 2016) provide useful frameworks to consider leading quality, person-centred care in community nursing practice. Practice development is everybody's concern and therefore an understanding of the purpose and processes involved is essential for all practitioners. The essential elements of leadership, person-centredness, quality and evidence-based practice together with process to achieving change have been discussed within the context of the clinical governance agenda. After reading the chapter and undertaking the activities, it is hoped you will develop an understanding of, not only the context of their practice, but of yourselves as leaders of quality, person-centred community nursing practice.

FURTHER RESOURCES

www.fons.org – Foundation of Nursing Studies
www.leadershipfoundation.no – Leadership Foundation
www.realworld-group.com – Real World Group: Engaging Leadership
McCormack B, Dewar B, Wright J et al. (2006) *A Realist Synthesis of Evidence Relating to Practice Development: Final Report to NHS Education for Scotland and NHS Quality Improvement*. Scotland: Quality Improvement Scotland.

REFERENCES

Adair J (2005) How to Grow Leaders: *Seven Key Principles of Effective Leadership Development*. London: Kogan-Page.
Alimo-Metcalfe B and Alban-Metcalfe J (2005) Leadership: Time for a new direction?

Alimo-Metcalfe B and Alban-Metcalfe J (2008) Engaging Leadership: Creating organisations that maximise the potential of their people.

Amy AH (2008) Leaders as facilitators of individual and organisational learning. *Leadership and Orgsanisational Development Journal* 29(2):212–34.

Barr J and Dowding L (2012) *Leadership in Healthcare*, 2nd edn. London: Sage Publications.

Bass BM and Steidlmeir P (1999) Ethics, character and authentic transformational leadership behaviour. *Leadership Quarterly* 10(2):181–217.

Bass MB and Riggio EG (2006) *Transformational Leadership* (2nd ed.). Mahwah, NJ: Lawrence Erlbaum Associates.

Bryar RM and Griffiths JM (2003) *Practice Development in Community Nursing: Principles and Process*. London: Arnold.

Cardiff S (2014) Person-centred Leadership: A Critical Participatory Action Research Study Exploring and Developing a New Style of (clinical) Nurse Leadership (Unpublished Thesis). (Accessed 2 October 2015) http://ethos.bl.uk/OrderDetails.do?did=1&uin=uk. bl.ethos.625505.

Cook MJ and Leathard HL (2004) Learning for clinical leadership. *Dimensions of Critical Care Nursing* 24(1):32–4.

Dawes D and Handscombe A (2005) A literature review on team leadership. The European Nursing Leadership Foundation. Available at: http://www.nursingleadership.org.uk/ publications/teamreport.pdf (Accessed 30th June 2017).

Department of Health (1998) *The New NHS: Modern and Dependable*. London: The Stationery Office.

Department of Health (2008). *High Quality Care For All: NHS Next Stage Review Final Report*. London: The Stationery Office. Cm 7432. Available at: www.dh.gov.uk/en/ Publicationsandstatistics/Publications/PublicationsPolicyAndGuidance/DH_085825 (Accessed 30th June 2017).

Department of Health (2014a). *The Adult Social Care Outcomes Framework 2014–2015*. London: DH.

Department of Health (2014b) *The NHS Outcomes Framework 2015-16*. London: DH.

Department of Health (2015) *Public Health Outcomes Framework 2013-2016*. London: DH.

Dewing J (November 2008) Implications for nursing managers from a systematic review of practice development. *Journal of Nursing Management* 16(2):134–40.

Dreenan D (1992) *Transforming Company Culture*. London: McGraw-Hill.

Driscoll J (2007) *Practical Clinical Supervision: A Reflective Approach for Health Care Professionals*. London: Balliere Tindall.

Francis R (2013) *Report of the Mid Staffordshire NHS Foundation Trust Public Inquiry*. London: The Stationery Office. (Accessed 20 September 2015) http://webarchive.nationalarchives. gov.uk/20150407084003/http://www.midstaffspublicinquiry.com/report.

Freeth R (2006) Person-centred or patient-centred? *Healthcare Counselling & Psychotherapy Journal* 6(3):36–9.

Garbett R and McCormack B (2002) A concept analysis of practice development. *NT Research* 7:87–99.

Garbett R and McCormack B (2003) The qualities and skills of practice developers. *Journal of Clinical Nursing* 12(3):317–25.

Heron J (2002) *The Facilitator's Handbook*. London: Koganpage.

Hersey P and Blanchard KB (1993) *Management of Organization Behavior Utilizing Human Resources* (8th. ed.). Englewood Cliffs, NJ: Prentice Hall.

Huber D (2010) *Leadership and Nursing Care Management*, 4th edn. Philadelphia, PA: Saunders Elsevier.

Institute of Medicine (2001) *Crossing the Quality Chasm*. http://iom.nationalacademies.org/Reports/2001/Crossing-the-Quality-Chasm-A-New-Health-System-for-the-21st-Century.aspx?_ga=1.266239047.915440910.1443970951. Accessed 30th June 2017

Jooste K (2004) Leadership: A new perspective. *Journal of Nursing Management* 12:217–23.

King's Fund (2013) *Patient-Centred Leadership: Rediscovering Our Purpose*. London: King's Fund.

Kitson A (2009) The need for systems change: Reflections on knowledge translation and organisational change. *Journal of Advanced Nursing* 65(1):217–28.

Kitson A, Harvey G and McCormack B (1998) Enabling the Implementation of evidence based practice: A conceptual framework. *Quality in Healthcare* 7:149–58.

Kotter JP (2012) Leading change. *Harvanrd Business Review Press*.

Lewin K (1947). Frontiers in group dynamics. In Cartwright D (Ed.), *Theory in Social Science*. London: Social Science Paperbacks.

Lewin K (1951) *Field Theory in Social Science*. New York, NY: Harper.

Lord Rose (2015) Better Leadership for Tomorrow. (Accessed 20 September 2015) https://www.gov.uk/government/uploads/system/uploads/attachment_data/file/445738/Lord_Rose_NHS_Report_acc.pdf.

Lynch B (2015) Partnering for performance in situational leadership: A person-centred leadership approach. *International Practice Development Journal* 5: 1–10. (Accessed 25 September 2015) http://www.fons.org/library/journal/volume5-person-centredness-suppl/article5.

Macrae C (2014) Early warnings, weak signals and learning health care disasters. *British Medical Journal Quality and Safety* 23:440–5.

Manley K (2004) Transformational cutlure: A culture of effectiveness. In McCormack B, Manley K, and Garbett R (eds) *Practice Development in Nursing*. Oxford: Blackwell Publishing.

Manley K and McCormack B (2003) Practice development: Purpose, methodology, facilitation and evaluation. *Nursing in Critical Care* 18(1):22–9.

Manley K, McCormack B and Wilson V. (2008) Introduction. In Manley K, McCormack B, and Wilson V (eds) *Practice Development in Nursing: International Perspectives*. Oxford: Blackwell Publishing Ltd, pp. 1–16.

Manley K, Solman A and Jackson C (2013) Working towards a culture of effectiveness in the workplace. In McCormack B, Manley K, and Titchen A (eds) *Practice Development in Nursing and Healthcare*, 2nd edn. Oxford: Wiley-Blackwell, pp. 146–68.

McCormack B, Dewing J, Breslin L et al. (2009) Practice development: Realising active learning for sustainable change. *Contemporary Nurse* 32(1–2):92–104.

McCormack B and Garbett R (2002) A concept analysis of practice development. *Nursing Times Research* 7(2):87–100.

McCormack B and Garbett R (2003) The characteristics, qualities and skills of practice developers. *Journal of Clinical Nursing* 12(3):317–25.

McCormack B and McCance T (eds) (2010) *Person-centred Nursing: Theory and Practice*. Oxford: Wiley-Blackwell.

McCormack B and McCance T (eds) (2016) *Person-Centred Practice in Nursing and Health Care: Theory and Practice*, 2nd edn. Oxford: Wiley-Blackwell.

McCormack B, Wright J, Dewar B et al. (2007) A realist synthesis of the evidence relating to practice development: Findings from telephone interviews and synthesis of the data. *Practice Development in Healthcare* 6(10):56–73.

McGill I and Brockbank A (2003) *Action Learning Handbook Powerful Techniques for Education, Training and Professional Development*. London: Routledge Falmer.

McSherry R and Pearce P (2011) *Clinical Governance: A Guide to Implementation for Healthcare Professionals*, 3rd edn. Chichester: Wiley Blackwell.

Meizerow J (1981) A critical theory of adult learning and education. *Adult Education Quarterly* 32(1):3–24.

Michaelis B, Stegmaier R, and Sonntag K (2009). Affective commitment to change and innovation implementation behavior: The role of charismatic leadership and employees' trust in top management. *Journal of Change Management* 9(4): 399–417.

National Institute for Clinical Excellence (2007) *How to Change Practice* http://www.nice.org.uk/media/D33/8D/Howtochangepractice1.pdf.

Nelson E, Batalden P and Godfrey M (2007) *Quality by Design: A Clinical Microsystems Approach*. San Francisco, CA: Jossey-Bass.

NHS England (2014) *The Five Year Forward View*. London: NHS England.

NHS Leadership Academy (2011) Healthcare Leadership Model. http://www.leadershipacademy.nhs.uk/wp-content/uploads/2014/10/NHSLeadership-LeadershipModel-colour.pdf Accessed 30th June 2017

NHS Scotland (2008) *Leading Better Care, Report of the Senior Charge Nurse Review and Clinical Quality Indicators Project*. Edinburgh: The Scottish Government.

Northouse PG (2010) *Leadership: Theory and Practice*, 5th edn. London: Sage.

Nursing and Midwifery Council (2015) *The Code for Nurses and Midwives*. London: Nursing and Midwifery Council. (Accessed 21 September 2015) http://www.nmc.org.uk/standards/code/.

Patel S (2010) Achieving quality assurance through clinical audit. *Nursing Management* 17(3):28–34.

Pearson A (1997) An evaluation of the King's Fund Centre Nursing Development Unit network 1989–91. *Journal of Clinical Nursing* 6:25–33.

Redfern S and Stevens W (1996) Nursing development units: Their structure and orientation. *Journal of Clinical Nursing* 7:218–26.

Rycroft-Malone J (2004) The PARIHS framework—A framework for guiding the implementation of evidence-based practice… Promoting Action on Research Implementation in Health Services. *Journal of Nursing Care Quality* 19(4):297–304.

Rycroft-Malone J (2013) How you might use PARIHS to deliver safe and effective care. In McCormack B, Manley K, and Titchen A (eds) *Practice Development in Nursing and Healthcare*, 2nd edn. Oxford: Wiley-Blackwell, pp. 146–68.

Scally G and Donaldson LJ (1998) The NHS's 50th anniversary. Clinical governance and the drive for quality improvement in the new NHS in England. *BMJ* 217(7150):61–5.

Scottish Government (2008) *Leading Better Care: Report of the Senior Charge Nurse Review and Clinical Quality Indicators Project*. Scottish Government. http://www.scotland.gov.uk/Publications/2008/05/30104057/0.

Scottish Government (2010). *The Healthcare Quality Strategy for NHS Scotland*. Scottish Government. http://www.gov.scot/Resource/Doc/311667/0098354.pdf Accessed 30th June 2017.

Scottish Government (2013) A routemap to the 2020 vision for health and social care. http://www.gov.scot/Resource/0042/00423188.pdf Accessed 30th June 2017.

Scottish Office (1997) *Designed to Care.* The Stationery Office Edinburgh.

Simmons M (2004) 'Facilitation' of practice development: A concept analysis. *Practice Development in Health Care* 3(1):36–52.

Shaw T, Dewing J, Young R, Devlin M, Boomer C, and Legius M (2008) Enabling practice development: Delving into the concept of facilitation from a practitioner perspective. In Manley, K., McCormack, B. and Wilson, V. (eds), *International Practice Development in Nursing.*

Oxford: Blackwell Publishing. pp 147–169.

Sirkin H, Keenan P and Jackson A (2005) The hard side of change management. *Harvard Business Review* 83(10):108–18. (Accessed 20 September 2015) http://www.ncbi.nlm.nih.gov/pubmed/16250629.

Stanley D (2006) Recognising and defining clinical nurse leaders. *British Journal of Nursing* 15(2):108–11.

Stanley D (2008) Congruent leadership: Values in action. *Journal of Nursing Management* 16(5):519–24.

Titchen A (2004) Helping relationships for Practice Development: Critical companionship. In McCormack B, Manley K, and Garbett R (eds) *Practice Development in Nursing*, Chapter 7. Oxford: Blackwell Publishing.

Wilkinson J, Rushmer R and Davies H (2004) Clinical governance and the learning organisation. *Journal of Nursing Management* 12(2):105–13.

Wilson V and McCance T (2015) Good enough evaluation. *International Practice Development Journal* 5(Suppl) [10]: 1–9. http://www.fons.org/library/journal.aspx.

Wong C and Cummings G (2007) The relationship between nursing leadership and patient outcomes: A systematic review. *Journal of Nursing Management* 15(5):508–21.

CHAPTER 17

eHealth

Heather Bain

LEARNING OUTCOMES

- Explore the meaning of eHealth including the associated terminology of telehealth and telecare.
- Appraise the suitability of eHealth for use within community nursing practice.
- Explore the professional and ethical issues in the use of technology within community nursing.
- Discuss the educational needs of the future eHealth community nurse.

INTRODUCTION

One of the most significant developments in health and social care in recent years has resulted from the increased use of information technology (IT), in particular the Internet and the World Wide Web. Accelerating the uptake of digital technologies and providing support for its implementation was identified as one of the recommendations to address the nine characteristics of good quality care in district nursing (Maybin et al., 2016). Considering the changing demographics of society and the fact that advances in technology can save time and money, national strategies have identified eHealth as an approach to improve healthcare (Cruickshank et al., 2010; Department of Health, 2014; Scottish Government, 2015; Welsh Government, 2015; Health and Social Care Board, 2016).

All four UK countries have identified national IT programmes which support the diverging health policies in the UK countries. Northern Ireland, Scotland and Wales all have identified specific strategies to address eHealth development, whereas England have introduced it in the 'Five Year Forward View' (Department of Health, 2014) and have developed supporting work-stream road maps (National Information Board, 2015) and a resource for commissioners (NHS England, 2015). eHealth is about improving health outcomes, the safety of care and providing efficient care; it is not just about technology (NHS England, 2015; Scottish Government, 2017; Welsh Government, 2015; Health and Social Care Board, 2016). However, it is also important to note the strategic direction in the four countries towards the provision of integrated health and social care and this will be reflected in future developments where organisational boundaries are not a barrier to care in the community (Scottish Government, 2015; Welsh Government, 2015; Gilbert, 2016). It is therefore clear that eHealth needs to be an integral part of nursing practice, and it is important that community nurses have the underpinning knowledge relating to this technology and can use it effectively to meet the healthcare needs of individuals, families and communities.

This chapter therefore aims to explore eHealth within community nursing. First, the associated terminology will be examined, then the evidence base to support its use will be explored. Finally, some professional, ethical and contemporary issues will be considered specific to nursing in the community.

ACTIVITY 17.1

Action point

Before reading this chapter, draw a concept map/mind map/spider diagram outlining what you think eHealth is. Include in your map not only what you think eHealth is, but also its main features and the infrastructure that needs to be in place in order to effectively implement it in community nursing. You may wish to use this concept map to inform Activity 17.5.

THE TERMINOLOGY

eHealth

The term *eHealth* first appeared in the literature in the 1990s (Booth, 2006) but has since been increasingly and inconsistently used. The widespread use of the term suggests it is a significant concept that is commonly understood despite the lack of a precise definition. Oh et al. (2005) undertook a systematic review of definitions and identified 51 unique definitions with no clear consensus. However, they did identify two universal themes, health and technology, and six less mentioned themes of commerce, activities, stakeholders, outcomes, place and perspectives. Therefore, it can be concluded that the various definitions reflect different perspectives, settings and contexts where technology is used to support healthcare needs. The World Health Organisation (2016), which was not included within this systematic review, encompasses the two universal themes and defines eHealth as 'the use of information and communication technologies for health to, for example, treat patients, pursue research, educate students, track diseases and monitor public health.' The Scottish Government (2015) suggests eHealth is an umbrella term with wide parameters and is defined as 'the use of information, computers and telecommunications to meet the needs of individuals and improve the health of citizens'.

Within this definition of eHealth it is recognised that there are many evolving terms encompassed, such as health informatics, nursing informatics, information communication technology, assistive technology, telemedicine, telenursing, telecare, telehealth, electronic patient record, and they are often used interchangeably (Cowie and Bain, 2011). It is not possible to cover them all in depth here; however, it is important that there is an understanding of the broad principles of the key terms, in order that technology can be used appropriately within the community.

Health and nursing informatics

Health informatics is generally defined as 'the knowledge, skills and tools which enable information to be collected, managed, used and shared to support the delivery of healthcare and to promote health' (Department of Health, 2002). Despite this definition being dated it is still regularly cited today (Health Education England, 2017). Nursing informatics is similar in that it is the collection of data and use of information to support nursing practice. This encompasses the electronic patient record. The development of infrastructures to support health and nursing informatics is a priority within national policy (Department of Health, 2014; Scottish Government, 2017; Welsh Government, 2015; Health and Social Care Board, 2016).

Electronic patient record

Record keeping is an essential element of nursing practice and includes all records that are relevant to your scope of practice (NMC, 2015a). The electronic patient record is, as it sounds, an electronic copy of a person's nursing or medical record. The aim within the NHS is for a single integrated electronic health record to be available to authorised users, including the service user (RCN, 2012b). In the United Kingdom, the development of the healthcare record is at varying stages, with some general practice (GP) surgeries having used electronic records for many years. However, the challenge is for the record to cross primary and secondary care boundaries, and to be a fully integrated health and social care record, allowing access to authorised individuals while safeguarding patient confidentiality (Department of Health, 2014; Scottish Government, 2017; Welsh Government, 2015; Health and Social Care Board, 2016).

CASE STUDY

Mrs A is an 83 year old who lives alone in her own home. She has rheumatoid arthritis, chronic obstructive pulmonary disease and type 2 diabetes. Mrs A has been assessed on numerous occasions by various health and social care professionals including the occupational therapist, social workers, the district nurse, the diabetes specialist nurse, and is also under the care of a hospital consultant for her rheumatoid arthritis, and her general practitioner. Until recently, Mrs A has had to repeat her story every time she was assessed by a new professional. Now, using a shared electronic care record all the professionals involved in her care have access to share information and co-ordinate care, and if she has an exacerbation of any of her co-morbidities out of hours there is adequate information to manage her care in a timely manner and ideally avoid hospital admission.

Telehealth

Telehealth is the provision of health services at a distance using a range of digital technologies and mobile technologies (Scottish Government, 2012; Telecare Services Association, 2016). This can be to promote self-care, for example, to enable a patient to monitor their own vital signs such as blood pressure, or from a monitoring perspective, physiological data could be transferred to a remote monitoring centre to allow for health professionals to intervene if measurements fall outside of expected parameters. The RCN (2012c) suggests telehealth is not a new technology or branch of health care, but should be integrated within existing healthcare infrastructures. The services could involve consultation, patient monitoring, diagnosis, prescriptions or treatment and can be done in real time or delayed through media such as teleconferencing, videoconferencing or the Internet. It should be a targeted approach to enhance service delivery focused around the service user, enabling a more efficient and effective use of clinical resources (Cruickshank et al., 2010; RCN, 2012a, c; Telecare Services Association, 2016).

CASE STUDY

Mrs B is a 31 year old who has recently been diagnosed with type 1 diabetes. She has been commenced on twice-daily insulin and has received education from the diabetic clinic at her local hospital, and has been followed up by her practice nurse. Her blood glucose levels remain unstable.

She is therefore identified as suitable for the telehealth programme until her blood glucose stabilises. A telehealth monitor is installed in her home and she is shown how to connect her glucometer to the telehealth monitor.

Mrs B then carries out a monitoring session using the telehealth monitor daily. The monitor gathers her blood pressure, heart rate, oxygen levels and weight, and some data from prescribed questions. Finally, she connects her glucometer to the monitor and the readings from the past 24 hours are transmitted.

Her data are then analysed by a triage nurse at the local community hospital. The triage nurse then contacts her to discuss the readings that are outside of normal limits and provides the relevant education and support. A weekly report is then sent to the diabetic clinic.

Following 8 weeks of this high intervention, Mrs B's blood sugars stabilise and she is confident to self-care for her condition.

Telecare is defined as the use of communications technology to provide health and social care direct to the patient (Barlow et al., 2007). Earlier development of telecare also referred to assistive technology and smart homes or smart technology (Sergeant, 2008). Assistive technology is another collective term for devices for personal use to enhance people's functional ability. It may include fixed assistive technologies such as stair lifts or portable devices such as bath seats. Therefore, this can include telecare, but is not limited to the kind of technology normally considered within eHealth. Telecare Services Association (2016) summarise the definition of telecare as 'support and assistance provided at a distance using information and communication technology. It is the continuous, automatic and remote monitoring of users by means of sensors to enable them to continue living in their own home, while minimising risks such as a fall, gas and flood detection and relate to other real time emergencies and lifestyle changes over time'.

Telecare has now become an umbrella term for all assistive and medical technology that enables people to maintain their independence in their own environment (Doughty et al., 2007; Telecare Services Association, 2016), which is more commonly their own home but it can be in any care setting. The Audit Commission (2004) identified three components of telecare: providing information, monitoring the environment and monitoring the person. Telecare was then categorised into three generations (Brownsell et al., 2008):

- First-generation telecare refers to equipment found in most community alarm schemes. It involves user activation, for example, a cord is pulled which triggers an alarm at a control centre where someone can organise a response of some kind. They have the benefit of providing 24-hour care; however, a major limitation is the reliance on the user to raise the alarm.

- Second-generation telecare is based on first generation but provides a more sophisticated and comprehensive support to managing risk and is less reliant on the user. It involves sensors to collect and transmit information, such as a door opening, movement within the home and bathwater running.

- Third-generation telecare is based on the automatic detection of the second generation, but with the increased availability of broadband, wireless and audiovisual technology it offers the potential for virtual or teleconsultations between the service user and the health professional or support worker. This has the potential to reduce home visits or hospital appointments and provides more opportunities for people unable to leave their own homes.

While the 'generation terms' are still used by some in the literature, they are becoming increasingly redundant as technology continues to evolve. Recent strategy documents and organisations such as Telecare Services Association and Joint Improvement Team no longer make reference to these categories within telecare.

CASE STUDY

Mrs B is an elderly lady living in sheltered accommodation. She has a medical history of rheumatoid arthritis, angina, deafness and a history of falls.

Following discharge from hospital after a fall, she was assessed by a district nurse who arranged for care workers to attend four times a day to meet her personal needs. However, Mrs B became increasingly confused and was getting out of bed and wandering through the sheltered housing complex at night.

Mrs B was then referred for a telecare assessment to identify the risks and to see if there were any interventions that could manage these risks. This resulted in the property being fitted with an activity monitor which is used to monitor movements within the home, flood detectors, a gas sensor and a bed sensor, which will detect if Mrs B has failed to return to bed in the time set. This ensures that if she gets out of bed and falls the warden can intervene accordingly.

mHealth and mCare

mHealth or mCare refers to mobile health or mobile care and uses mobile devices to extend the principles of telecare and telehealth (Telecare Services Association, 2016). This technology has made significant advances in recent years and continues to evolve from both a practice and education perspective. One key feature of mobile technology is the use of apps, which are software applications. While currently there has been limited evaluation of the use of mHealth, Guo et al. (2015) in their literature review identified that mobile technologies can potentially improve access to information, enhance productivity of care, reduce errors, increase engagement with learning and support evidence-based decision making at the point of care delivery. Clearly, within community nursing the advances in mHealth have great potential from both a professional and service user perspective to support self-care. The activity below will allow you to explore the potential usage of mHealth within community nursing.

ACTIVITY 17.2

Action point

Access a mobile app of your choice related to your role as a nurse working in the community. Critique it using the following questions adapted from the European Commission (2017):

Is the app primarily for health or social care purposes?

What category does the app fit into:
• Patient decision making and self-management
• Clinical decision-making support tool
• Behaviour change support
• Diagnostic or monitoring function
• Electronic health records access
• Medical devices control
• Documentation function
• Tracking device
• Other

Who are the principal beneficiaries of the app?

Is there a cost?

Are there any risks in its use such as safety or data protection?

Is the app usable and accessible?

Is the app desirable?

Is the app credible and supported by an evidence base?

Is the app reliable?

Has the app been validated by a group or organisation?

Does the app use language suitable to its target audience?

Does the app have longevity?

Telehealthcare

Considering all the definitions above, it is evident that there are interrelationships between all the terms. Doughty et al. (2007) have reviewed the terminology used and acknowledge it will evolve as technology develops, although to avoid confusion the term *telehealthcare* may be more appropriate as it clearly integrates both telehealth and telecare. However, they suggest this does not necessarily include traditional forms of assistive technology. NHS 24 and Scottish Centre for Telehealth (2010) also acknowledge this. Although there will be parallel developments between telecare and telehealth, as technology develops there will be the convergence of telecare and telehealth to provide effective high-quality healthcare, particularly around services delivered in the community. The key terms within eHealth are conceptualised in Figure 17.1.

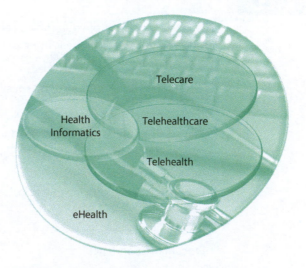

FIGURE 17.1 Diagram conceptualising eHealth.

ACTIVITY 17.3

Discussion point

Considering the terminology of eHealth and areas of telehealth and telecare convergence, reflect on how eHealth can support your role as a community nurse:

• What are the challenges?

• What are the opportunities?

Taking into account all the various concepts within eHealth, it is clear that there are many overlaps and all have a potential use within community nursing. The opportunities and challenges are summarised in Table 17.1. There are also many ways that eHealth can be used by a variety of methods, some of which are identified in Table 17.2.

There have been several projects across the United Kingdom to ensure that eHealth becomes an integral part of community care provision. However, one of the challenges has been to accurately quantify the benefits, due to the small scale of the projects and the differing methods of evaluation. To further confirm the contribution of eHealth to healthcare, evaluation needs to integrate monitoring, outcomes and personalised feedback (Flodgren et al., 2015; Verhoeven et al., 2007; Fatehi et al., 2016).

Table 17.1 Summary of opportunities and challenges of eHealth

Strengths	Challenges
Reinforces existing advice	May be expensive to develop
Overcomes challenges of distance	Lack of access to software and hardware
Addresses needs of remote and rural areas	Lack of consistency across services and interoperability
Reduces unnecessary outpatient appointments	Technical problems and compatibility
Out-of-hours access	Relies on technical competence of staff and service users
Quicker access to specialist advice	Potential health and safety risk with equipment
Improved safety because of up-to-date recording of information	Maintaining confidentiality
	Usability for people requiring reasonable adjustments
	Reliability of evidence within apps
Improved continuity of care	
Portable information	
Improved health outcomes	
Early diagnostic capability	
Evidence-based healthcare accessible to all 24 hourly	

Table 17.2 Examples of how eHealth can be used

Method	Example	Uses
Telephony	Mobile phones: calls and text	Message delivered via text to reinforce health education; phone applications to monitor health status
Videoconferencing	Patient monitoring	Remote advice from specialists
Internet/World Wide Web	Use of search engines and touch-screen Internet kiosks	Accessing clinical decision support systems Provide healthcare advice and education
Digital imagery	Digital cameras, webcams, podcasts	Image of wound of housebound patient can be shared with specialist
Gaming	Games consoles	Interactive games can provide education
Email	Communication at a distance	Referral between health professionals
eHealth record	Patient-held medical record	Care pathways can be shared among professionals
Sensors	Fall detectors, flood detectors, smoke detectors, bed occupancy detectors	Allow high-risk people to stay in their own homes
Electronic databases	Caseload management	Audit practice and aid planning
eRostering M Apps	Use of apps	Access to health information, self-tracking fitness, fall detection, self-management of long-term conditions
ePrescribing	Generation of electronic prescription	Easier management of statistics to identify trends and variations Quicker access to medicines
Self-check in kiosks	Appointments and repeat prescriptions	Quick check-ins at doctors' surgery
Social media	Twitter online chats	Peer support

eHEALTH TECHNOLOGY WITHIN COMMUNITY NURSING

The evidence to support the use of eHealth and in particular telehealthcare by community nurses to manage individuals in the community is increasing. However, as new technology develops and eHealth is integrated within everyday practice the evidence base at the highest levels of reliability remains variable. This can provide a dilemma for the practitioner, who until the evidence gap is addressed faces difficult decisions about adopting such concepts into their practice. However, current government policy does support the development of using technology in practice as discussed previously, and it is clear that eHealth has huge potential, particularly in the management of long-term conditions (Cruickshank et al., 2010; Healthcare Improvement Scotland, 2016a).

The evidence base

There is literature that does explore the clinical effectiveness of the use of telehealthcare to support the management of many long-term conditions such as diabetes, mental health, high-risk pregnancy monitoring, dermatology, heart failure and cardiac disease (Bensink et al., 2006; Barlow et al., 2007; Healthcare Improvement Scotland, 2015, 2016a, b). However, there is consensus that more robust evaluations and research are required to address the limitations of the current evidence (Davies and Newman, 2011).

In reviewing the literature it is important to consider the hierarchy of evidence (Aveyard et al., 2016). There are many hierarchies of evidence available, however, some are more suitable for specific different research questions (Davies and Newman, 2011). The hierarchy of evidence best suited for determining the effectiveness of an intervention is most commonly developed from Sackett et al's. (1996) work. This hierarchy identifies systematic reviews of randomised controlled trials at the top with anecdotal evidence being at the bottom. This hierarchy is illustrated in Figure 17.2.

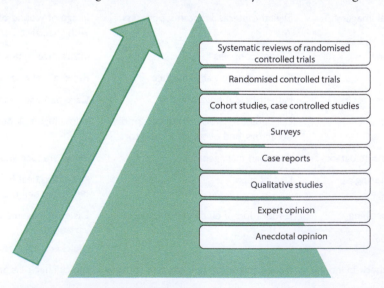

FIGURE 17.2 Hierarchy of evidence.

Fatehi et al. (2016) acknowledge that research methods specific to telehealth will depend on the maturity of the intervention. To address this, they proposed a five-stage model as a framework to support research within eHealth: concept development, service design, pre-implementation, implementation and post-implementation. While this framework could equally be applicable to other areas of service evaluation, it is useful as an additional tool to appraise research and its applicability and validity relating to the development of emerging technology to address healthcare needs from various perspectives.

ACTIVITY 17.4

Action point

Identify an area of practice relevant to your role, and then undertake a small literature review to examine the evidence base to support the use of telehealthcare to manage healthcare needs in your chosen area.

From undertaking Activities 17.3 and 17.4, you will have recognised that integrating telehealthcare within your nursing practice requires different clinical skills and approaches to care. The following practice recommendations can be made:

- Practitioners must assess the suitability of telehealthcare to manage healthcare needs on an individual basis.
- The use of telecommunications is feasible for the motivation and management of patients with long-term conditions, and can be cost-effective and reliable.
- Telehealthcare is feasible and acceptable for educating patients, monitoring and assessing clinical outcomes.
- Telehealthcare is more meaningful to service users if delivered by specialised nurses and prescribers.
- More complex systems such as web-based medical records and permanent healthcare professional support can achieve significant benefits in improving clinical outcomes.
- Effective management and improved clinical outcomes in the management of long-term conditions involves medicines management.

PROFESSIONAL AND ETHICAL ISSUES

A comprehensive understanding of professional and ethical issues is a fundamental part of community nursing and is discussed more fully in Chapter 3. This section therefore focuses on some of the main issues related to eHealth. Baker et al. (2007) explored professional and ethical issues that have emerged with the use of technology and articulated a gap between the potential of eHealth as positively perceived by eHealth leaders and the reality experienced by nurses in clinical practice. However, all respondents clearly identified the global eHealth future. Nearly a decade later, it is still recognised that strong professional leadership is essential to enhance the provision of health and social care through eHealth (Raeve et al., 2016).

Professional and ethical issues of eHealth can all be directly mapped to the Nursing and Midwifery Council's (NMC, 2015a) *Code: Professional Standards of Practice and Behaviour for Nurses and Midwives*, and in particular to the following clauses:

2.2 Recognise and respect the contribution that people can make to their own health and well-being

3.3 Act in partnership with those receiving care, helping them to access relevant health and social care, information and support when they need it

5.2 Make sure that people are informed about how and why information is used and shared by those who will be providing care

5.4 Share necessary information with other healthcare professionals and agencies only when the interests of patient safety and public protection override the need for confidentiality

5.5 Share with people, their families and their carers, as far as the law allows, the information they want or need to know about their health, care and ongoing treatment sensitively and in a way they can understand

6.1 Make sure that any information or advice given is evidence-based, including information relating to using any healthcare products or services

8.6 Share information to identify and reduce risk,

10.1 Complete all records at the time or as soon as possible after an event, recording if the notes are written some time after the event

10.4 Attribute any entries you make in any paper or electronic records to yourself, making sure they are clearly written, dated and timed, and do not include unnecessary abbreviations, jargon or speculation

13.5 Complete the necessary training before carrying out a new role.

19.2 Take account of current evidence, knowledge and developments in reducing mistakes and the effect of them and the impact of human factors and system failures

21.6 Co-operate with the media only when it is appropriate to do so, and then always protecting the confidentiality and dignity of people receiving treatment or care

In reality, many of the professional and ethical issues are not different from other areas of nursing practice, but because of the evolving nature of eHealth the issues are perceived to be more challenging to address.

While undertaking Activity 17.5, many professional and ethical issues will have been identified. You may also have considered the following issues.

ACTIVITY 17.5

Reflection point

Reflect on the case examples of telehealth and telecare provided in this chapter, or examples of the use of eHealth available in your area of practice, and consider the following:

• What are the professional and ethical issues?

• How can eHealth support you to manage healthcare needs in the community in a more effective and timely manner?

Access to information

Assessment of individuals, families, carers and communities as identified in Chapters 1, 7, 8 and 9 is a core skill in community nursing to address healthcare needs. However, often the first assessment of a change in health status is not undertaken by a health professional, but by the individual. In 2006, the Picker Institute estimated that a third of the 80% of people actively accessing information about their health first do it through the Internet. Ten years later in 2016, 89% of households have Internet access; 82% of adults access the Internet on a daily basis; and 70% of adults access the Internet on a mobile phone (Office for National Statistics, 2016). While the use of technology is perceived by many to be a generational issue for both healthcare professionals and service users, one must be careful not to make assumptions on this. Institute for the Future (2016) in their international poll identified that 79% of people 55 years and over regarded technology as important to improve healthcare, compared to 69% of those aged 18–34.

Information is most often accessed via a search engine on the Internet. Although there are many benefits to this, such as quicker access to information, there is the danger that service users can access incorrect information or it can be of variable quality (Aveyard et al., 2016). However, the NHS in the United Kingdom provides much credible information to the public via the Internet promoted through media campaigns. For example, NHS Inform online allows users to check their symptoms online and provides advice accordingly, and similarly there are many mobile apps which provide access to health information. This technology is changing the balance of power between health professional and the public. However, it provides nurses with the opportunity to empower and enable people (National Information Board, 2014), which has always been a key concept within nursing practice (NMC, 2001, 2004, 2015a).

Decision making

When an individual chooses to consult with a community nurse or is referred to a community nurse, eHealth can play a supportive role in the decision-making process of the assessment. Clinical decision support systems can be utilised for this purpose (Stacey et al., 2017). Increasingly, these clinical decision systems are being integrated with electronic patient records or are applications that can be downloaded onto tablets, mobile phones and potentially smart watches and are therefore a useful tool for the community nurse, who is often working in people's homes. However, as with all expert systems, they should be seen as tools and not as a replacement to clinical judgement.

ACTIVITY 17.6

Reflection point
Reflect on your experience of computerised decision support systems. How do they enhance your practice? What are the challenges in their use? How does it impact on your ability to make a decision? What is the evidence base behind the system?

Equity and access to services

A major challenge in addressing healthcare needs within the community is the concept that everyone should have equal access to services regardless of where they live, which has been a core concept of the NHS since its inception. This can be considered on two levels: first, access to clinical services and, second, equity of access to eHealth services (Audit Scotland, 2011). However, often there is a sound reason for unequal approaches to addressing healthcare needs. For example, third-generation telecare relies on the availability of broadband; however, in some areas of the United Kingdom this may be limited, or patients may not have the ability to adapt to such technology. This is when the concepts of telehealthcare need to be embedded into care pathways, and, following the assessment of the service user, have suitable exit criteria for its use (Cruickshank et al., 2010) and the use of ethical frameworks by the practitioner needs to accompany this process (Eccles, 2010).

Social media

The use of social media is another development within ehealth. Social media tools include social networking platforms such as Twitter and Facebook, blogs, microblogs, wikis, virtual reality and gaming environments. There are many different uses of social media tools from the patient's, the carer's and the professional's perspective. Social media can be used in the promotion of health, and support of those with long-term conditions and their carers, as well as practitioners using them to keep up to date and share the latest evidence (Moorley and Chinn, 2014).

As a professional, it is essential that you are aware of professional and personal boundaries within online practices. The NMC (2015b) has produced additional guidance which underpins *The Code* (NMC, 2015a) that it is essential you are aware of. A term that has been emerging in recent years is *digital professionalism* that supports the professional/personal boundaries when engaging online. Ellaway (2010: 706) identified seven principles of digital professionalism:

Establish and sustain an online professional presence that befits your responsibilities while representing your interests. Be selective in which channels and places you establish a profile.

Use privacy controls to manage more personal aspects of your online profile and do not make anything public that you would not be comfortable defending as professionally appropriate in a court of law.

Think carefully and critically about how what you say or do will be perceived by others and act with appropriate restraint in online communications.

Think carefully and critically about how what you say or do reflects on others, both individuals and organisations, and act accordingly.

Think carefully and critically about how what you say or do will be perceived in years to come; consider every action online as permanent.

Be aware of the potential for attack or impersonation, and know how to protect your online reputation and what steps to take when it is under attack.

An online community is still a community and you are still a professional within it. The call for 'is there a doctor. . .' may come online as well as on a 'plane or in a theatre'.

ACTIVITY 17.7

Reflection point

Reflect on the social media tools that you are aware of. If you are unfamiliar with any you may choose to access http://wecommunities.org/ which is a website that supports the use of Twitter to connect professionals and share information through online chats. What are the benefits of social media to support nursing in the community? What are the challenges?

eRostering and workforce planning

The principles of caseload management and workforce planning are discussed in detail in Chapter 15. However, it is well recognised that the use of technology to support rostering, workforce planning and caseload management are not consistent across the United Kingdom. Maybin et al. (2016) identified the potential for technologies to enable remote working and to improve efficiency and productivity with timely access to, for example, patient's records and to support caseload management. This in turn would release more time for professionals to deliver quality services.

ACTIVITY 17.8

CASE STUDY

Action point

There are many case studies available online illustrating the benefits from eRostering.

www.rotamaster.co.uk/case-studies/case-study-lcwucc/

www.ehealthireland.ie/Case-Studies-/eRostering/

www.nhsemployers.org/case-studies-and-resources/2012/02/case-studies-five-high-impact-actionswww.skillsforhealth.org.uk/services/item/16-realtime-rostering

Please access a selected case study or reflect on a case example from your own area. What are the challenges of implementing electronic packages to support rostering, caseload management and workforce planning? What are the advantages?

It is clear from considering the above that the professional and ethical issues in the use of eHealth are similar to other areas of nursing practice and many of the skills are transferable. However, the focus can be different and there is a need to develop new approaches and additional knowledge to use eHealth efficiently and effectively to address healthcare needs in the community.

EDUCATING THE FUTURE eHEALTH COMMUNITY NURSE

It is evident that technology will not address healthcare agendas unless practitioners are provided with the education (Booth, 2006) to use it effectively. Up until recent years the emphasis in nurse education has been on computer literacy rather than information literacy and eHealth. However, it is evident that community nurses need to understand the technology and be confident in its use to adequately address healthcare needs (RCN, 2012a) and this requires more than information literacy. It is suggested that particularly undergraduate nursing must take a proactive approach to integrating eHealth within the curriculum, and educators should take a leading role in this (Booth, 2006).

In recent years educational programmes have embedded the principles of eHealth within curriculum in both undergraduate and postgraduate studies. Additionally national career frameworks have been explicit in that community nurses must be able to use a range of technology to support patient care (Health Education England, 2015; NHS Education for Scotland, 2016). In the Queen's Nursing Institute/Queen's Nursing Institute Scotland (2015: 3) *Voluntary Standards for District Nurse Education and Practice*, the following competence was developed:

> Source and utilise eHealth technology and technology assisted learning systems to support self-care and improve efficiency and effectiveness of the district nursing service.

Clearly, eHealth education is an essential requirement to address both the theoretical foundations of integrating technology within healthcare and to provide the practical skills of using technology. While tomorrow's educated nurses may have these skills, the needs of experienced practitioners who have not accessed formal education in recent years must also be considered. The RCN (2012d) in their eHealth survey identified that two-thirds of respondents had received training in their workplace to support their use of information technology. UK governments acknowledge the importance of training and identify the development of their workforce as a key priority (Scottish Government, 2015).

ACTIVITY 17.9

Training need analysis

Reflect on your role. Make a self-assessment on your knowledge and skills by considering some of the concepts you have explored in this chapter. You may have a tool in your local area that you can access or you may wish to develop a tool such as in the table shown that can be used within your team. Consider any supporting evidence to demonstrate your knowledge and skills, and then identify any areas where you would benefit from further training, education and development.

Outcome:	I	2	3	Evidence
1. Demonstrate understanding of how and why information technology is able to support clinical practice and ways of working.				
2. Demonstrate understanding of how electronic health records are used in your practice.				
3. Demonstrate understanding of assessment tools used to assess the use of telecare as a nursing intervention.				
4. Demonstrate understanding of the key NHS national initiatives to support eRostering.				
5. Describe the principles of digital professionalism.				

1. I require training and development in most or all of this area.
2. I require training and development in some aspects of this area.
3. I am confident I already do this competently.

CONCLUSION

This chapter has provided an overview of eHealth considering some of the key terminology. The suitability of its use has been briefly explored within community nursing and some of the associated professional and ethical issues have been highlighted. It is recognised that eHealth is not just about technology, it is about using technology more effectively to address healthcare needs. Although eHealth is becoming an integral part of government policy, applying the principles in practice can be a challenge, and it is therefore essential that healthcare professionals are provided with appropriate education and training to prepare them for the development of eHealth.

FURTHER RESOURCES

www.ehealthnurses.org.uk – Health Nurses Network
http://sctt.org.uk – Scottish Centre for Telehealth and Telecare
https://digital.nhs.uk – NHS Digital
http://www.ehealth.nhs.scot/ – eHealth

REFERENCES

Audit Commission (2004) *Implementing Telecare: Strategic Analysis and Guidelines for Policy Makers, Commissioners and Providers*. London: Audit Commission.

Audit Scotland (2011) *A Review of Telehealth in Scotland, Project Brief.* Edinburgh: Audit Scotland.

Aveyard H, Payne S and Preston N (2016) *A Post-graduate's Guide to Doing a Literature Review.* Maidenhead: McGrawHill.

Baker B, Clark J, Hunter E et al. (2007) *An Investigation of the Emergent Professional Issues Experienced by Nurses When Working in an eHealth Environment.* Bournemouth: Bournemouth University.

Barlow J, Singh D, Bayer S and Curry R (2007) A systematic review of the benefits of home telecare for frail elderly people and those with long term conditions. *Journal of Telemedicine and Telecare* 13:172–9.

Bensink M, Hailey D and Wotton R (2006) A systematic review of successes in home telehealth: Preliminary results. *Journal of Telemedicine and Telecare* 12:8–16.

Booth R (2006) Educating the future eHealth professional nurse. *International Journal of Nursing Education Scholarship* 3: Article 13.

Brownsell S, Blackburn S and Hawley M (2008) Evaluating the impact of 2nd and 3rd generation telecare services in older people's housing. *Journal of Telemedicine and Telecare* 14(1):8–12.

Cowie J and Bain H (2011) Development and implementation of policy–communities and health. Scottish perspective. In Porter E and Coles L (eds) *Policy and Strategy for Improving Health and Wellbeing.* Exeter: Learning Matters.

Cruickshank J, Beer G, Winpenny E and Manning J (2010) *Healthcare Without Walls, A Framework for Delivering Telehealth at Scale.* London: 2020health.

Davies A and Newman S (2011) *Evaluating Telecare and Telehealth Interventions.* London: King's Fund.

Department of Health (2002) *Making Information Count: A Human Resources Strategy for Health Informatics Review.* London: DH.

Department of Health (2014) *Five Year Forward View.* London: DH.

Doughty K, Monk A, Bayliss C et al. (2007) Telecare, telehealth and assistive technologies: Do we know what we are talking about? *Journal of Assistive Technologies* 1:6–10.

Eccles A (2010) Ethical considerations around the implementation of telecare technologies. *Journal of Technology in Human Services* 28:44–59.

Ellaway R (2010) Digital professionalism. *Medical Teacher* 32(8):705–7.

European Commission (2017) Report of the Working Group on mHealth Assessment Guidelines. https://ec.europa.eu/digital-single-market/en/news/report-working-group-mhealth-assessment-guidelines (accessed 14/6/17).

Fatehi F, Smith A, Maeder A et al. (2016) How to formulate research questions and design studies for telehealth assessment and evaluation. *Journal of Telemedicine and Telecare,* pp. 1357633X16673274.

Flodgren G, Rachas A, Farmer AJ, Inzitari M, and Shepperd S (2015) Interactive telemedicine: Effects on professional practice and health care outcomes. *Cochrane Database of Systematic Reviews* Issue 9. Art. No.: CD002098. doi: 10.1002/14651858.CD002098.pub2.

Gilbert H (2016) *Supporting Integration through New Roles and Working Across Boundaries.* http://www.kingsfund.org.uk/publications/supporting-integration-new-roles-boundaries (accessed 14/6/17).

Guo P, Watts K and Wharrad H (2015) An integrative review of the impact of mobile technologies used by healthcare professionals to support education and practice. *Nursing Open.* 3(2):66–78. http://onlinelibrary.wiley.com/doi/10.1002/nop2.37/abstract.

Health and Social Care Board (2016) *eHealth and Care Strategy for Northern Ireland.* Belfast: Health and Social Care Board.

Health Education England (2015) *District Nursing and General practice Nursing Service Education and Career Framework.* London: HEE.

Health Education England (2017) *An Online Introduction to the Use of Informatics in Healthcare.* http://www.e-lfh.org.uk/programmes/health-informatics/. (accessed 14/6/17).

Healthcare Improvement Scotland (2015) *Is Patient Self-Monitoring of Oral Anticoagulant Therapy Safe, Efficacious and Cost Effective?* http://www.healthcareimprovementscotland. org/our_work/technologies_and_medicines/shtg_-_evidence_notes/evidence_note_57. aspx (accessed 14/6/17).

Healthcare Improvement Scotland (2016a) *What Is the Clinical Effectiveness and Cost Effectiveness of Home Health Monitoring Devices Compared with Usual Care for Patients with Hypertension.* http://www.healthcareimprovementscotland.org/our_ work/technologies_and_medicines/shtg_-_evidence_notes/evidence_note_59.aspx. (accessed 14/6/17).

Healthcare Improvement Scotland (2016b) *What Is the Clinical Effectiveness, Cost Effectiveness and Safety of Home Health Monitoring Compared with Usual Care for Patients with Moderate to Severe Chronic Obstructive Pulmonary Disease.* http://www. healthcareimprovementscotland.org/our_work/technologies_and_medicines/shtg_-_ evidence_notes/evidence_note_60.aspx. (accessed 14/6/17).

Institute for the Future (2016) *Future Health Index 2016.* https://s3-eu-west-1.amazonaws.com/ philips-future-health-index/report/2016/Future_Health_Index_Report_2016_FULL.pdf. (accessed 14/6/17).

Maybin J, Charles A and Honeyman M (2016) *Understanding Quality in District Nursing Services.* London: King's Fund.

Moorley C and Chinn T (2014) Using social media for continuous professional development. *Journal of Advanced Nursing* 71(4):713–7.

National Information Board (2015) *National Information Board's Workstream Roadmaps.* https://www.gov.uk/government/publications/national-information-boards-workstream- roadmaps. (accessed 14/6/17).

National Information Board (2014) *Using Data and Technology to Transform Outcomes for Patients and Citizens.* https://www.gov.uk/government/uploads/system/uploads/ attachment_data/file/384650/NIB_Report.pdf. (accessed 14/6/17).

NHS 24 and Scottish Centre for Telehealth (2010) *Scottish Centre for Telehealth Strategic Framework 2010–2012.* Aberdeen: Scottish Centre for Telehealth.

NHS Education for Scotland (NES) (2016) *Career Development Framework for Nurses, Midwives and Allied Health Professionals.* http://www.careerframework.nes.scot.nhs.uk/. (accessed 14/6/17).

NHS England (2015) *Technology Enabled Care Services: Resource for Commissioners.* https:// www.england.nhs.uk/wp-content/uploads/2014/12/TECS_FinalDraft_0901.pdf. (accessed 14/6/17).

Nursing and Midwifery Council (2001) *Standards for Specialist Education and Practice.* London: NMC.

Nursing and Midwifery Council (2004) *Standards of Proficiency for Specialist Community Public Health Nurses.* London: NMC.

Nursing and Midwifery Council (2015a) *The Code: Professional Standards of Practice and Behaviour for Nurses and Midwives.* London: NMC.

Nursing and Midwifery Council (2015b) *Social Media Guidance.* https://www.nmc.org.uk/standards/guidance/social-media-guidance/. (accessed 14/6/17).

Office for National Statistics (2016) *Internet Access: Households and Individuals.* http://www.ons.gov.uk/peoplepopulationandcommunity/householdcharacteristics/homeinternetand socialmediausage/bulletins/internetaccesshouseholdsandindividuals/2016. (accessed 14/6/17).

Oh H, Rizo C, Enkin M and Jadad A (2005) What is eHealth: A systematic review of published definitions. *Journal of Medical Informatics* 7(1).

Picker Institute (2006) *Assessing the Quality of Information to Support People in Making Decisions About their Health and Healthcare.* (Accessed 8 April 2011) www.pickereurope.org/page.php?id=48.

Queen's Nursing Institute/Queen's Nursing Institute Scotland (2015) *The QNI/QNIS Voluntary Standards for District Nurse Education and Practice.* London: QNI.

Raeve P, Gomez SM, Hughes P et al. (2016) Enhancing the provision of health and social care in Europe through eHealth. *International Nursing Review.* http://onlinelibrary.wiley.com/doi/10.1111/inr.12266/full.

Royal College of Nursing (2012a) *Putting Information at the Heart of Nursing Care.* London: Royal College of Nursing.

Royal College of Nursing (2012b) *Nursing Content of eHealth Records.* London: Royal College of Nursing.

Royal College of Nursing (2012c) *eHealth the Future of Health Care.* London: Royal College of Nursing.

Royal College of Nursing (2012d) *Positioning Nursing in a Digital World.* London: Royal College of Nursing.

Sackett D, Rosenberg W, Muirgray J et al. (1996) Evidence based Medicine: What it is and what it isn't. *British Medical Journal* 312:71–2.

Scottish Government (2012) *A National Telehealth and Telecare Delivery Plan for Scotland to 2015.* Edinburgh: Scottish Government.

Scottish Government (2015) *eHealth Strategy 2014–2017.* Edinburgh: Scottish Government.

Scottish Government (2017) *Digital Health and Social Care Strategy 2017–22 – Development.* http://www.ehealth.nhs.scot/strategies/the-person-centred-ehealth-strategy-and-delivery-plan-stage-one/. (accessed 14/6/17).

Sergeant E (2008) *Aberdeenshire Council Telecare Project.* (Accessed 8 November 2010) www.aberdeenshire.gov.uk/about/departments/AberdeenshireTelecareProjectEvaluationReport.

Stacey D, Légaré F, Lewis K et al. (2017) Decision aids for people facing health treatment or screening decisions. *Cochrane Database of Systematic Reviews* 4. Art. No.: CD001431. doi:10.1002/14651858.CD001431.pub5.

Telecare Services Association (2016) *Health and Social Care* https://www.tsa-voice.org.uk/health-social-care. (accessed 14/6/17).

Verhoeven F, van Gemert-Pijnen L, Dijkstra K et al. (2007) The contribution of teleconsultation and videoconferencing to diabetes care: A systematic literature review. *Journal of Medical Internet Research* 9:5.

Welsh Government (2015) *Informed Health and Social Care: A Digital Health and Social Care Strategy for Wales.* Cardiff: Welsh Government.

World Health Organisation (2016) *eHealth.* www.who.int/topics/ehealth/en.

CHAPTER

18

Development of community nursing in the context of changing times

Anne Smith and Debbie Brown

LEARNING OUTCOMES

- Identify the key policy drivers that impact on delivering effective healthcare.
- Examine the new roles and ways of working that are emerging in response.
- Analyse personal skills development that may enable practitioners to contribute more effectively.
- Explore the impact of enhanced skills such as non-medical prescribing on the delivery of services.

INTRODUCTION

It is important to have a working understanding of health policy in order to contextualise the changes that are occurring in commissioning, managing and delivering community services. The four nations of the United Kingdom are responsible for managing their own National Health Service (NHS) services (The Health Foundation and Nuffield Trust, 2014). This is achieved in different ways according to the priorities set by each one, but the principles are common to all. There is a commitment across the four nations to integrate primary and secondary care provision, aiming for a smoother transition for patients between the two, but more importantly trying to reduce hospitalisation by anticipating potential problems and providing support services to prevent admission. There is an increasing emphasis on public health, health promotion and self-care. It is recognised that with the changing demographics in the population, with life expectancy now extended, services must be reconfigured to respond. A higher percentage of the population is now living with long-term conditions or terminal illnesses, increasing the challenges on health and social care services. The nations face similar issues trying to devise a workable framework on which to base their service delivery. These will be explored further within this chapter.

Since its inception, the NHS has been a service free to all, but there has been a conceptual shift away from illness orientation and paternalism to a more egalitarian approach, with the user taking interest and responsibility for making decisions about their care. The language has changed from that of 'patient', suggesting dependency, to that of 'client', 'consumer' or 'service user', all of which suggest a partnership approach (Hinchliff et al., 2008). The 'Expert Patient' programmes (DH, 2001) were a catalyst for this shift of emphasis. These programmes were designed to enable people to become more confident in making educated decisions about their condition and their care. This approach continues to be a central tenet of the government's ideal (DH, 2012a) reflected in publications such as 'No Decision about Me without Me' (DH, 2012b).

This chapter first briefly examines the ways in which healthcare is managed by the devolved governments of the United Kingdom. The Conservative Government returned to power in 2015 and are keen to progress with reforms initiated prior to the General Election. Practitioners will be required to respond in real time to changing needs employing scarce resources more productively. The whole infrastructure of primary care will change dramatically according to the latest projections (NHS England, 2014a, 2016a). While there is a dearth of general practitioners (GPs) to deliver care, new roles are being designed and training put in place. There is a radical change required to manage the changing demography and changing health needs of the population as we move forwards to 2020 and beyond. Community nursing services are central to the management of the health needs of an ageing population within primary care. One of the considerations within this chapter is to examine how the four countries have equipped themselves to undertake this task.

KEY POLICY DRIVERS THAT IMPACT ON DELIVERING EFFECTIVE HEALTHCARE

England

The Francis Report (2013) and the Willis Report (2015) were influential in changing policy. The Francis Report was scathing regarding the treatment of patients in North Staffordshire and this prompted a rapid response from across the whole of the NHS in the United Kingdom. Willis was instrumental in setting the direction for the education of nurses and care assistants in response to some of these recommendations which clearly identified the need for a much more rigorous educational system for those providing the care.

In October 2014, the Chief Executive of the NHS announced the publication of 'The Five Years Forward View' (FYFV) (NHS England, 2014a) and the impact has been visible across all sectors. The 'Shape of Caring Review' (Willis, 2015) was concerned with shaping the way the workforce developed educationally with new roles being configured to support the qualified workforce. The creation of Health Education England (HEE, 2012) has provided a national body to oversee education and training (E&T) of the nursing workforce. Their purpose is to ensure that the health workforce has the appropriate training to develop the skills to support the delivery of excellent healthcare and health improvement. Significant publications

(HEE, 2016a) that followed the Willis review have outlined the framework of the future workforce and how the education for these roles will be achieved. Emphasis has been placed on recruiting and educating care assistants to be 'nursing associates' in order to expand the capacity to care within the workforce.

Primary care is in the process of undergoing very radical reform outlined in the 'GP Forward View' document (NHS England [NHSE], 2016b). Ongoing difficulty recruiting doctors to work in primary care has proved challenging, especially as the Health Secretary has been promising better access to primary care services, particularly out of hours (Roberts, 2015). Various initiatives have enabled a growth in the number of full-time GPs over the past 10 years but further recruitment is crucial to push forward these reforms. It is imperative that a whole new framework is developed to enable 24-hour access to services. There has been serious consideration of how this can be supported. Making more effective use of the multi-disciplinary team is paramount. The introduction of a Multi-Specialty Provider Model (MCP) is part of the wider plan. This will create a new clinical and business model (NHS England, 2016b). One initiative is the training of physicians' associates. The education of these practitioners is based on an American model. Until recently very few training centres offered this pathway but there are now more courses being set up. The intention is to recruit individuals who would not normally be employed in the NHS rather than to draw practitioners from other healthcare specialisms, such as nurse practitioners, to fulfil the role. Likewise an extended role for pharmacists is being devised, as the plan is to engage and extend the role of all clinicians allied to medicine (Royal College of Physicians, 2014). Non-clinical roles are also being developed such as health navigators and patient liaison officers. The National Association of Primary Care (NAPC) established the role of the primary care navigator (PCN). By training front-line non-clinical staff, who already deal with patients and carers on a day-to-day basis, the PCN is empowering people to identify their own needs. With support, encouragement and localised navigation tools a more effective self-management approach is achieved (NAPC, 2015). This is an evolving role and so inevitably at this time each area appears to be interpreting the role differently.

A radical change took place in primary care in 2012 as a result of the Health and Social Care Act (2012), which included the formation of clinical commissioning groups (CCGs). This introduced practice-based commissioning (PBC) with the GP taking responsibility for 80% of the NHS budget. The commissioning and budgeting aspects are still contentious and the latest publication (GP Forward View) aims to prioritise funding for primary care services. Important changes also related to the strengthening of inspection and audit of services. The role of the Care Quality Commission (CQC) and other quality assurance bodies were amalgamated under one umbrella organisation in 2016. The NHS Trust Development Authority has been formed to provide support oversight and governance for all NHS Trusts.

The consequences surrounding the proposal about commissioning have been immense, and the plan to combine the management of service provision across the acute and primary care sectors has been challenging for all staff. New providers such as private sector companies have emerged following competitive tendering. The CCGs are functioning more effectively as members become more conversant with their roles and the expectations of how they will organise and commission care. The Five Years Forward View has endorsed the need to utilise devolved budgets efficiently (NHS England, 2014a). The GP Forward View (2016b) has sought to extend these ideals and promotes the view that if GP fails we will lose the foundation on which the NHS is built. There is still a great deal of uncertainty but those who can embrace the new world and work with uncertainty will be the main drivers of the new agenda.

An innovation reported in February 2015 was the plan to devolve the budget for health and social services in Manchester making it autonomous in managing its care needs. There was divided opinion as to the merits of such a system especially as opponents suggested it would lead to a fragmentation of the NHS making it no longer a national service. However other commentators remarked that the NHS as it stood was no longer fit for purpose and so this could herald a much needed modernisation (Grice and Cooper, 2015). This initiative became a reality in April 2016.

The Royal College of Nursing (RCN), Association of District Nurse Educators (ADNE) and Queens Nursing Institute (QNI) have continuously responded on behalf of the nursing profession to the Department of Health's agenda in relation to primary care. In its position statement (RCN, 2010) the RCN recognised that practitioners are operating in a rapidly changing landscape. The document stresses the importance of nurses' role in shaping and delivering services. There is concern over the increasing use of skill mix within nursing teams, with healthcare assistants (HCAs) being employed and educated to adopt roles previously undertaken by qualified nurses. However, their role is not regulated and the RCN has identified their vulnerability. The position of unregulated staff was brought more sharply into focus by the findings of the Francis Report (Francis, 2013) as within the recommendations comment was made about their roles and accountability. The Willis review (Willis, 2015) examined the training and development of all nursing and support staff and recommended a more robust framework for educating the workforce with national standards to adhere to. HEE and the NMC have responded proposing ways in which these recommendations can be achieved (HEE, 2016a).

Meanwhile, the QNI promoted a campaign, 'Right Nurse, Right Skills' (QNI, 2010) which highlighted the necessity to ensure that nurses working in the community are appropriately educated to undertake their roles, as often they are working alone and unsupervised in patients' homes. This campaign underpinned the emphasis within the Five Year Forward View (NHS England, 2014a) that endorsed the principle of caring for people in their own homes and avoiding hospital admissions. The chief executive of the QNI commented, 'We are delighted too with the change in focus to delivering care, when safe to do so, where people live their lives – in the homes and communities in which they live' (Oldman, 2014).

The QNI have previously been instrumental in highlighting the disinvestment in appropriately qualified nurses in the community (QNI, 2014a). This report demonstrated that the numbers of staff with the specialist district nurse qualification had vastly decreased. Community nursing services generally were fragmented with no standard framework for calculating workload or caseload allocation. The QNI have recently undertaken a review commissioned by the Department of Health (QNI, 2014b) examining a planning tool for district nurse (DN) workload allocation. In recent years, the lack of investment in qualified district nurses working in the community has led to poorer quality of leadership and care. Commissioners have recognised the issues associated with this and currently there is evidence that more DNs are being educated to take up senior roles in community care (QNI, 2014c).

The QNI examined discharge planning as this has a particular impact on caseload and workload management. A vital element of this process concerns the leadership and management of the team when organising scarce resources to manage this process. The recommendations echoed the sentiments of all the work on integration of services, namely the need for improved communication, collaboration and co-ordination (QNI, 2016). Lord Rose's recent review of the NHS (Rose, 2015) also drew the conclusion that leadership was lacking across the whole organisation although he commented that there were many committed and talented people employed in the NHS. Since the publication of that review a career framework has been published for district nursing and practice nursing that emphasises key characteristics of the role in driving the strategic direction in primary care (HEE, 2015). The QNI and QNIS have also published voluntary standards for tutors to use to underpin their programmes when educating district nurses which are more contemporary and reflective of practice than those standards produced by the NMC dating back to 2001 (QNI/QNIS, 2015). The recurrent theme recognises the need for senior staff to be effective leaders and budget managers.

The requirement to move care closer to patient's homes has been further endorsed by guidelines published by the National Institute for Health and Care Excellence (NICE, 2015) on the best practice for providing care to older people in their own homes. This guidance only serves to strengthen the ideal of home being the preferred place of care. It establishes priorities related to individualised person-centred care. This agenda can only be implemented with appropriately qualified leaders in community care.

ACTIVITY 18.1

Discussion point
Examine the framework document at https://hee.nhs.uk/2015/10/27/new-nursing-framework-supports-delivery-of-care-closer-to-home/. Think about how this may affect your role.

Scotland

In Scotland, there has also been progress in responding to the primary care agenda in relation to managing the demands placed upon it from the increasing number of older people in the population. Projections made in 2013, indicated that over the next 20 years demography alone could increase expenditure on health and social care by over 70% (Scottish Government, 2013). Social care has been free in Scotland since 2002. This has huge implications as the elderly population increases, because the financial burden of such a policy could well become unsustainable. The emphasis continues to be focused on integration of services, which became a reality in April 2016, and on anticipatory care rather than reactive treatment options. Scotland has the same issues to contend with as the other countries in devolving budgets from acute care to community. The publication of a national clinical strategy in 2016 (Scottish Government, 2016) has provided a strategic paradigm that builds on the 2020 vision outlined in 2013. The Route Map 2020 (Scottish Government, 2013) was a visionary document that focused on proactive care aimed at keeping people healthy. It also acknowledged that invariably primary care professionals are pivotal to enabling individuals with health challenges and long-term conditions to maintain their health. Its principles include enabling people to live at home in a fully supported environment. Scotland has a particular issue associated with delivering care because of the remote and rural distribution of their client group.

Major strategies have also been developed, for example, to assist with caring for patients with dementia, as estimates suggest that the number of people with dementia is set to rise from 71,000 to 127,000 within the next 20 years (Scottish Government, 2013). This is set against the background of the modernisation programme which commenced with the introduction of the Modernisation Community Nursing Board in December 2009 (RCN, 2010). The board's main aim was to provide a more cohesive approach to the delivery of community services across Scotland. The 'Remote and Rural Healthcare Action Plan' (Scottish Government, 2008) identified that 79% of the Scottish population live in remote or rural locations and life expectancy in these areas is the third worst in Scotland. The Scottish Government commissioned the development of a toolkit to support the work of the Modernisation Board. They have continued with the vertical integration of services first conceived 15 years ago and which culminated in implementation in April 2016 (Scottish Government, 2016). The CNO for Nursing and Midwifery has undertaken an educational review and set out six strategic aims with an implementation programme and action plan for nursing (Scottish Government, 2014b). This provided an educational bridging between the career framework (NES, 2012) and the route map to a 2020 vision (Scottish Government, 2013). The latter provides a futuristic perspective of how nursing can contribute to the strategic vision for health and social care. More recently a career framework has been published that determines developmental paths for all specialisms (NHS Education for Scotland, 2016).

Initiatives that have already been developed working towards this vision include the Intermediate Care framework (Scottish Government, 2012) which contributes to the idea that care is geared towards offering solutions other than hospital admission. The Reshaping Care for Older People Programme 2011–21 provides a jointly compiled framework (Scottish Government, 2011) whose central aim is to focus their approach around personalised outcomes for older people rather than to fit them into the service. It also seeks to be more creative when examining the support network available to older people. The Change Fund has been established to make this possible and to support preventative and anticipatory care.

In order to initiate the changes the eHealth strategy is a critical element and the investment in this will be the catalyst for the other changes to be effective. The eHealth Strategy 2011–17 (NHS Scotland, 2011) is progressing well with development of the patient identifier, more sharing of patient information between professionals and better organisation and access to NHS 24 and OOH facilities. It has since been refreshed and updated which according to the Scottish Government aims to develop 'an interoperable and clinically rich eHealth ecosystem' (Scottish Government, 2014a: 5). The Integrated Resource Framework (IFR) (NHS Scotland, 2012) is responsible for monitoring the costs and activities associated with this. In 2014 the Health and Social Care information sharing strategy framework (Scottish Government, 2014a) was published projecting activity until 2020. This acknowledges and seeks to overcome perceived barriers to the integration of care that may arise from the lack of a cohesive IT strategy to aid communication.

All the themes discussed above related to providing a streamlined and cost-effective service have been examined further within the National Clinical Strategy (Scottish Government, 2016). It sets strategic aims rather than describing the detail of how services will be adapted to achieve the outcomes. These aims encompass all the considerations with regard to providing care that is proportionate and relevant for the individual. Integrated care became a reality in April 2016. A fundamental aspect of such a strategy is more timely discharge linked to providing a more responsive approach in primary care.

Wales

The Welsh Government has taken a radical approach by removing the 'internal market' and implementing an integrated organisational structure. The detail concerning this was set out in *Setting the Direction* (WAG, 2010: 6). The reorganisation took place in 2009, creating seven single health organisations responsible for all aspects of healthcare in their area. The purpose of this strategy was to improve the delivery of community-based services in Wales by adopting a more integrated approach between the sectors that offer support. Interestingly, a primary principle of this strategy is to encourage 'citizens' to 'develop confidence in their ability to manage their own health'. 'Together for Health' (WAG, 2011) outlined the challenges to be overcome in Wales in order to provide a world-class service and set a 5-year action plan in place. 'Prudent Health care' (WAG, 2015) is a more recent initiative adopted by Welsh Government to endeavour to prevent over diagnosis and medical management of people. It is based on similar principles to the 2010 strategy. It is a term harnessed by Welsh Government defining an approach to healthcare that highlights the importance of demand management and involving the public in healthy behaviours and self-management of their health, rather than over management by health professionals. It advocates using a 'nudge' principle to motivate individuals to be proactive in managing their health. It is primarily focused on managing the ever-increasing demand with finite resources.

Since the findings of the Francis Report were published (DH, 2013) the Welsh government commissioned the 'Trusted to Care' Report (Andrews and Butler, 2014) examining care issues for the frail elderly in two hospitals in Wales. It made 18 recommendations which related to establishing a change in culture, better training of staff and more concern for the patient and carers' views. The seven Local Health Boards across Wales work autonomously and even before the publication of the Andrews report the Betsi Cadwaladwr Local Health Board in North Wales had independently published a statement of intent with regard to caring for older people with complex needs in the community (2014). This articulates the necessity to follow a framework of integrated care management but recognising the culture shift required to enable this. Governance priorities had already been defined in the government's delivery plan for 2013–16 in a document entitled 'Delivering Safe Care Compassionate Care' (WAG, 2013).

The Welsh Audit Office has undertaken individual district nursing audits for the specific Health Boards in Wales. The audits have served to raise the profile of district nursing and have encouraged a reassessment of service delivery. At the time of this writing, the Wales Audit Commission is in the process of preparing a document for publication to raise the profile of district nursing further. It is intended to take a comprehensive yet succinct approach to identifying the current status of the district nursing service throughout Wales; it will examine variations and explore potential ways to move district nursing forward in Wales.

Northern Ireland

Health and social care in Northern Ireland are more integrated than in the other countries of the United Kingdom. Responsibility for healthcare has been devolved from central government at Westminster to the Northern Ireland Assembly. However it is difficult to draw analogies or seek to replicate their approach as the situation in Northern Ireland is unlike the other UK countries, in its demography and geography. It is also unique in that since 2009 there has been only one commissioning body for the whole province (Ham et al., 2013). The basic principles associated with NHS care delivery remain the same, but across Northern Ireland it is suggested that there is inconsistency around how it is interpreted. Another fundamental issue that has to be addressed is the fact that Social Services consider themselves the poor relation with regard to providing an integrated approach to care. Their perspective is that it is not a marriage of equal partners. Coupled with the view that financial investment continues to be poured into the acute sector there is still some way to go in providing integrated community care (Sprinks, 2015).

Community nursing services came under the spotlight in June 2011 with the publication of a consultation document reviewing the District Nursing Service (Department of Health Social Services and Public Safety) (DHSSPSNI, 2011a).

Key messages that emerged from this related to the pivotal role of the district nurse in providing person-centred care in the community. The document advised that care management must include a proactive and anticipatory approach rather than a reactive one. The need to move funding across to community services from the hospital sector was highlighted and a model of 'outreach' and 'in reach' suggested (p. 55). This was further supported by the intention for district nurses to facilitate discharge planning and thus enable a more seamless approach to patient care. It also identified that patients with long-term conditions would benefit from a care management approach (p. 52).

The number of DNs in the workforce has dropped from 7% to 6% since 2010. In line with the national picture, there has been much disillusionment across the DN service with the current staff shortages but there is also optimism as the DHSSPS have increased the numbers of DN training places, and DNs are becoming more involved in the strategic development of the service. Currently, work is being undertaken to review the DN services in Northern Ireland.

During the past 5 years, other documents have been influential in shaping services with a common theme of moving care away from hospitals and also with the intention to move budgets. Transforming Your Care (TYC) (DHSSPSNI, 2011b) otherwise known as the Compton Review identified key changes in the arrangements for care provision including the establishment of Integrated Care Partnerships (ICPs) but the Health and Social Care Trusts have not demonstrated consistency in their approach towards implementation. Age UK NI published a report in 2014 which argued that people were being assessed differently according to where they lived and which Health and Social Care Trust they resided within. In 2015 the departments of Health and Justice published a joint document regarding the safeguarding of adults at risk which will also have implications for community teams and the population they serve (DHSSPS and Department of Justice [DOJ], 2015).

The TYC document focused on providing care for an ageing population but NI has not been able to transfer services from hospital to community. A first contact single assessment tool (NISAT) has been developed to enable any member of the integrated care team to undertake a first assessment and share that information with other members of the team (Regulation and Quality Improvement Authority, 2012). While the tool has many benefits, it is however unwieldy in practice and not always available electronically. In some areas further nursing assessments have been developed by community nurses, therefore inconsistency in practices is evident. DNs are working with commissioners and colleagues from across primary care to implement the vision of TYC. This is evident from the use of an electronic caseload analysis tool (eCAT) which examines individual caseloads and allows for comparison of these (Yarra Software, 2010). This tool has since been piloted by a community team in England with a view to implementation (Bhardwa, 2015).

The Northern Ireland Practice and Education Council (NIPEC, 2015) has published its Annual Business Plan for 2015/16. Their mission is to provide a 'beacon' of good practice to aid nurse and midwife development in order that safe and effective care can be delivered across the Province. Key priority 2D in this report demonstrates their commitment to work with the NMC and QNI in developing educational standards for Specialist District Nursing programmes that truly reflect the complexity of the DN role. This is a comprehensive and timely document.

Digital solutions such as telehealth are becoming more widely available although, not surprisingly, these have not been embraced and used to their full potential by DNs. The development of the caseload and workload analysis tools and the single assessment document are reliant on communication technology which was a theme highlighted in the Donaldson Report (DHSSPS and DOJ, 2015). The report took an overview of the whole of NHS delivery in Northern Ireland and concluded that there needed to be a culture change across the whole organisation. It focused on serious case reviews but the recommendations were concerned with standardisation of best practice across all areas, citing examples from other regions where this approach has had a favourable impact. The report also highlighted the need for the implementation of robust and joined up IT systems which had been found lacking to date. This is a recurring theme across the United Kingdom in respect of community nursing where further investment is needed to provide nurses with the technology to support their role.

ACTIVITY 18.2

Discussion point

What is the impact of technology on your area of work? Consider how changes in your workplace have been influenced by the availability of IT devices and resources at the local level.

All four countries recognise the benefits of shifting the balance of care from the acute sector to the community. While there are differing opinions on how to develop health services, all the nations are challenged with the same issues associated with the changing demographics of the population. People are living longer, but associated with this is the potential for ill health and compromised quality of life. It is clear that one approach to coping with the increased demand on services is to proactively seek out and support the highest users of services. However, in tandem with this there is the need to actively promote a healthy lifestyle for individuals, families and communities.

NEW WAYS OF WORKING

It is clear that all nations of the United Kingdom are examining how the workforce can be organised to promote efficiency and effectiveness. Employers are being urged to consider deploying resources (including staff) in new ways. The latest vision within the Five Year Forward View (NHS England, 2014a) echoes this theme with a strong commitment to integrated care and the formation of multi-specialist community providers in primary care. A DN career framework has been published which highlights the contribution the DN can make to integrated care and provides a formal route for career progression in this role (HEE, 2015).

Proactive rather than reactive care was the ideal behind the introduction of the role of the community matron in England (DH, 2005). Community matrons were to adopt a case finding and case management approach to offer holistic care to vulnerable older people in the community with long-term conditions. The role and status of community matrons has undergone many changes since they were first introduced. Some continued to work autonomously while others merged with the DN team. In some places their role disappeared while other areas recruited nursing consultants as an extension of this role. In other organisations they were re-branded as neighbourhood nurse leads (NNLs). As the emphasis shifts towards an integrated approach to care it is imperative that key professionals such as matrons or their equivalent work across professional boundaries to provide a truly joined up service.

Example 18.1

In south London, health and social services are providing a co-ordinated approach to enable older people to remain in their homes with extra assessment and support. Southwark and Lambeth Integrated Care is a partnership that spans the Foundation hospitals, GP practices and social care agencies. They make use of technology to enhance communication both with the clients and colleagues within the team. They are able to rapidly access specialist advice and they also have support from voluntary agencies such as Age UK (Benison, 2015).

Audit and community (or practice) profiling are useful tools with which to examine the uptake and the success of services, as previously discussed in Chapters 1 and 7. In order to provide cost-effective, appropriate care, audit and evaluation are essential (Jack and Holt, 2008). Without such data it is difficult to justify changing services. Historically, the community nursing workforce have not been actively promoting their expertise or publishing good practice which makes it difficult to appraise the evidence. Front-line practitioners should be proactively involved in this process, and should be contributing to the decision on changes. The QNI (2010) has cautioned that nurses may well end up as merely the 'passengers' as the governmental reforms take place. However, there are opportunities for staff to contribute to the agenda. Burke and Sheldon (2010) describe the benefits of using such information-gathering models as the 'World Café' model. This is an exercise organised at local or national level in which groups of practitioners meet in a relaxed café-style environment in order to network and share ideas about new ways of working and innovative approaches. This model was utilised to explore the 'Transforming Community Services' (TCS) initiative in England (DH, 2011), a programme with a variety of work streams examining the Quality Innovation, Productivity and Prevention agenda (QUIPP). This calls for practitioners to be personally equipped with the skills to engage with the vision which aims to transform services in the community in several key areas.

The whole idea of nurses being at the forefront of service redesign can seem daunting but with enthusiasm and tenacity it can be achieved.

Example 18.2

An excellent example is provided by two nurses who worked in general practice. When both GPs left their surgery simultaneously and they were unable to recruit to the vacancies, the nurses decided to tender to run the surgery. Nine years later, they have just moved into new premises as their enterprise has been so successful, demonstrated by the fact that they received an outstanding result in their CQC visit (Bhardwa, 2014). The concept of new business approaches such as creating a social enterprise is alien to many nurses. Rather than being viewed as passengers (QNI, 2010), the community nursing workforce remains central to the implementation of these far-reaching reforms.

It is pertinent to explore other factors that will determine the efficiency of the community workforce. The chief executive of the NHS has pointed out (NHS England, 2014a) that we are being confronted with an 'information revolution' that will affect our lives just as significantly as the agricultural and industrial revolutions did in their time. The use of technology to support nurses to work more effectively has been promoted for a long time, but organisations have been slow to engage with the concept or the opportunities. There are fundamental barriers to be overcome such as poor Internet connections. However, in the future practitioners will be reliant on mobile devices to access notes and communicate when the majority of their work is done in isolation.

'Agile working' is a term adopted by various organisations to describe the use of a flexible approach to working (enei, 2013: 3) They define it as 'based on the concept that work is an activity we do, rather than a place we go'. Increasingly the community workforce has abandoned the regular morning meetings for work allocation and has taken to working remotely. In this way, caseload and workload management have moved from the traditional allocation style. District nursing historically has been managed in a fragmented way and there has been a dearth of research to inform practice. However, the QNI have recently provided a report for the Department of Health (NHSE/QNI, 2014) that explores how a more robust system may be implemented that will ultimately assist commissioners of services to definitively measure the workload pressures associated with delivering services and to allocate resources appropriately.

SOCIAL ENTERPRISE AS AN EMERGING RESPONSE

Social enterprise is not a new term and is closely linked to the concept of social marketing. Social marketing (Lefebvre, 2003) is a concept underpinned by empowerment, with the focus on the service user taking responsibility for their well-being. This is an ideal which many community nurses already promote in their current day-to-day practice, for example, promoting an egalitarian approach when managing long-term conditions such as diabetes. However, Lefebvre (2003) also suggests, that social marketing is 'a problem solving process that may suggest new and innovative ways to attack health and social problems' (2003: 220) and this is where social enterprise may be a useful concept to consider.

Social entrepreneurs have a social rather than business focus (Leadbetter, 1997), tending to reinvest profits into the enterprise rather than take it for themselves. Motivation to become a social entrepreneur may be due to what are traditionally described as 'push' or 'pull' factors, for example, community nurses may be 'pushed' into entrepreneurial activity due to unemployment, or 'pulled' by the attraction of greater independence (Granger et al., 1995). Indeed, independent nurse practitioners can now find themselves in the position of employing salaried general practitioners (Baraniak and Gardner, 2001) in deprived communities, pulled by the opportunities to develop healthcare in these areas as in Example 18.2.

Nurses may perceive that they do not have the relevant skills or knowledge to be able to set up a social enterprise (Dawes, 2009). Traynor et al. (2007) suggest factors such as lack of mentorship and business support for entrepreneurs, the need to combine family and business responsibilities, and lack of self-belief and self-confidence as being prohibitive factors. Indeed, it could be suggested that nurses are not prepared during their undergraduate pre-registration education to even consider this sort of activity as a future option. The move to an all-graduate profession may have some impact on this perception and educational curriculum should provide some aspects of business studies to make nurses more confident in this area. However, it may be difficult for nurses to know where to start and the barriers to starting a social enterprise may seem too great. The RCN (2007) has published supportive guidance aimed at nurse entrepreneurs who are looking to set up their own enterprise, exploring issues such as becoming self-employed and providing advice on costs and cash flow, for example. The Department of Health has published a further guide for those wanting to learn more (DH, 2008a).

ACTIVITY 18.3

Discussion point
Read the DH publication (2008) *Social Enterprise, Making a Difference* in more detail. Then consider this approach and apply it using a scenario related to an area of personal interest.

Another emerging model is provided by the private sector. Since the Labour Government initiated the idea of competitive tendering for some primary care services in 2004, organisations such as Virgin Care have been entering the marketplace. The delivery of care by these alternative providers of medical services is centred on a business model driven by profit margins. Greaves et al. (2015) examined the impact of these organisations and found they performed poorly in comparison with the traditional GP service. This was partly due to the fact that they mostly served a non-traditional population. While they were able to provide a more flexible service with extended opening hours, for example, they were more likely to refer clients on to secondary care services. Greaves et al. (2015) suggest that when profit is a driver then the contact is important but the outcome is often influenced by moving the patient on rather than seeking a treatment option. They caution against the competitive market being introduced. This business model does not always sit comfortably alongside the values instilled in nurses associated with the 6Cs (DH/NHS, 2012) such as compassion, which are not possible to measure. The more aesthetic values encompassed by the 6Cs provide a benchmark for good nursing care, but the time needed to give quality care is not always appreciated by providers driven by targets of numbers treated. In 2016, a national framework with 10 'commitments' was published as a guide for all nursing, midwifery and care staff

(NHS England, 2016b). It discussed the 'triple aim measures' highlighted in the Five Years Forward View (2014a) and incorporated these themes with the 6Cs to provide a framework that encouraged all levels of staff to work towards providing the best experiences for patients while within the constraints of finite resources. It also reinforced the need for a whole population approach to enabling people to enhance their health and well-being.

Example 18.3

It is interesting to examine an international perspective such as the model provided by Buurtzorg Nederland (2011) which is a unique district nursing system and entirely nurse-led and cost effective. Buurtzorg is Dutch for 'Neighbourhood Care'. The King's Fund in its analysis of Buurtzorg (2013) has reached a similar conclusion. While extolling the model's virtues, it recognises that Buurtzorg's approach 'may not be right for all health systems but it highlights the potential benefits of taking a fresh look at professional roles.' The RCN in 2016 has also observed and critiqued the approach. It has candidly discussed the merits but is cautious about the transference of such a system to a country with a different healthcare economy and other significant issues. However, Buurtzorg is being piloted in several centres in the United Kingdom (RCN, 2016).

It is described as patient centred with highly skilled staff who offer a compassionate, innovative and synergistic approach to care. Jos de Blok and three other entrepreneurial nurses first created this concept in the Netherlands in 2006. They developed their own enterprise centred on a mission to provide holistic patient-centred care for their clients within their own homes. The Buurtzorg nurse acts as 'a navigator' for the patient and family, advising on innovative solutions to receiving the best care at home. This model has the potential to be replicated into primary care, enabling teams of healthcare workers to offer support for patients within a locality by navigating the patients' journey with other professionals. They are empowered and autonomous and their approach has been replicated and adopted across other countries such as Sweden, Japan and the United States. While the costs per hour are greater, fewer hours have been needed for care in total. Buurtzorg has accomplished a 50% reduction in hours of care, improved quality of care and raised work satisfaction for their employees.

ACTIVITY 18.4

Before you consider the next section on personal skills that you bring to the workforce, reflect on your personal strengths by doing a short exercise that assesses your personality type. Find the Myers Briggs Inventory at www.16personalities.com/free-personality-test and see what type of personal attributes you have.

PERSONAL SKILLS DEVELOPMENT AND MANAGING CHANGE

In order to work in an arena that is constantly changing and manage services effectively, it is imperative for practitioners to develop personal skills in managing and coping with change. They must be able to critically reflect on their current roles and have the appropriate skills in leadership and management to effect change, whatever their role. The morale of the workforce is dependent on the motivation and enthusiasm that can be generated, despite the regular requirement to implement and adjust to change. However, it could be argued that the expectation that practitioners can adjust, frequently not knowing what the system is about, and then provide high-quality outcomes, is unrealistic. There is a personal cost related to instability which may manifest itself either physically or psychologically (Nazarko, 2007). Individuals may feel a sense of loss or feel uncertain about their future in the new system. Transition has to be managed carefully and for change to be successful all parties need to understand and sign up to the vision. Leadership is a crucial aspect of the change process and much has been written about how to develop leadership potential among staff (Taylor, 2010). Clinical leadership is discussed in Chapter 15. Interestingly, while leadership is a quality frequently defined and discussed it is equally important for that leader to be supported by a good follower. As Whitehead et al. (2007) suggest, 'followership' is not a passive role but requires the individual to display active participation towards achieving the common goal. The follower is there to support the leader and to provide critical feedback on the progress of the change. The leader is reliant on the advocacy of their colleagues. Although not everyone is able to perform the leadership role, the supporting cast has a vital part to play in ensuring that change is implemented effectively and sustained. Maintaining a balanced approach is conducive to reducing the stress that inevitably accompanies change. It has been suggested that emotional intelligence (Goleman, 1998) is a quality that helps leaders and followers to manage the uncertainties often associated with the change process. If the practitioner has a range of coping strategies he or she will be better placed to manage the demands of the constantly fluctuating environment. An interesting perspective is presented in the document *Building and Strengthening Leadership* (NHS England, 2014b).

There is a wide range of models that can be of assistance when examining the process of change within the organisation, which also explore the rationale for change. Theoretical frameworks can be helpful in determining the forces that will impact on the change process. The Department of Health published a document in 2001 (Iles and Sutherland, 2001) called *Managing Change in the NHS* in which it proposed a variety of models that may provide frameworks for underpinning the change process at organisational level. It identified models such as 'PESTELI' and the '5 whys', both of which could be applicable in certain situations. These models are still applicable and relevant.

The PESTELI model is defined in Box 18.1.

Box 18.1 PESTELI model

P – Determine any political factors influencing the need to change

E – Economic constraints impacting on the process

S – Social determinants such as the changing demographics of the population or cultural changes

T – Technological changes or aspirations can be either a help or hindrance to change and innovation

E – Environmental issues including moving workplace bases may provoke anxiety

L – Legal aspects of any change must be carefully considered

I – A recent addition to the model has been a consideration of the 'industry'

As the NHS is increasingly becoming a business environment, with Foundation Trusts, GP consortia and other business models emerging for the commissioning and delivery of services, this will influence the change arena.

Another less well-known model is The D.I.C.E. Framework for Change (Sirkin et al., 2005) which is a tool for assisting in examining whether a change will be implemented successfully. This is an adapted version.

D – Duration of time in which the change programme is to be completed if it is a short target time; otherwise the time between reviews

I – Integrity of th project team's performance; i.e. ability to complete the initiative on time; calculated in respect of the members' ability

C – Commitment to change displayed by other influential players such as top management (C1) and staff (C2) affected by the change

E – Effort over and above the usual work that the change initiative demands of staff; linked to motivation levels

Different models are more applicable to certain circumstances One size does not fit all.

DEVELOPING ENHANCED SKILLS TO CONTRIBUTE TO THE NEW AGENDA

Different ways of delivering care are emerging in all areas of the NHS. Some quite radical changes were generated as a result of the Darzi Report (DH, 2008). It contained a range of ideas including the move for nursing to become a graduate profession which has since been instigated. One initiative that had national interpretation was the introduction of 'Darzi centres', which basically were offering a multitude of services under one roof, a 'one stop shop'. There was a commitment to enabling the general public easy access to care without the need to book a doctor's appointment. 'Darzi centres' were also to stay open for longer hours than surgeries and were intended also to reduce the pressure on A&E departments. The employers mainly relied on nurse practitioners to staff these centres. It was imperative therefore that practitioners were able to operate autonomously for these centres to achieve their targets. Other services that have developed over recent years are telephone support systems such as NHS 111 in England (which has replaced NHS Direct) and NHS 24 in Scotland. Again, the intention was to divert patients from attending A&E unnecessarily. However, as Matthews-King asserted, of 450,000 extra attendances in 2013–14, 220,000 were advised by NHS 111 to attend the emergency department. And 222,000 calls resulted in an ambulance being dispatched to them by NHS 111 (Matthews-King, 2014).

There is an abundance of examples of new and innovative ways of working but in order for these to have an impact it is essential that the workforce is appropriately trained. Within general practice various services managed by nurses, such as telephone triage, minor illness clinics and disease-specific clinics have been available. However, as there is a shift in care closer to home, making every contact count, nurses need to deliver and support self-care and personalised care planning, using generalised expertise in long-term conditions, with an holistic approach, for prevention and health and well-being, ideally using motivational interviewing techniques (Rollnick et al., 2013). One example by NHS England (2016) to demonstrate this approach is the 'House of Care' (NHS England, 2016c). As stated in the FYFV, training hubs such as that of Community Educational Provider Network (CEPN) are ideally placed to ensure appropriate, effective training and learning is provided and, tailor-made for each locality/federated model (HEE, 2016b). As previously discussed, technology is being embraced increasingly to supplement face-to-face care (see Chapter 17). Telehealth is now much more common and patients are managing their own monitoring rather than booking appointments at the surgery. Practitioners are therefore adapting to assessing and treating clients other than by face-to-face contact. These services are heavily reliant on having the right nurse with the appropriate skills to manage them.

One aspect of skills development that has now become more firmly established is non-medical prescribing. This has had a huge influence on the roles adopted by nurses. As independent prescribers are legally able to prescribe from the whole British National Formulary (BNF) their roles have also extended to take over certain roles previously only undertaken by doctors (Brookes and Smith, 2007). The NMC issued the Standards for Prescribing (NMC, 2006) but the devolved governments in the United Kingdom have been responsible for the development of prescribing within their own country and the governance issues surrounding it. Services have been transformed through this extension of the nurse's role, with the evolution of services such as Walk-In Centres and Out of Hours rapid access centres. The NMC has also expanded the use of the Community Nurses Formulary (NMC, 2009) to enable appropriately qualified community staff nurses to prescribe. Independent prescribing has been an important factor in expanding the nurse's role and has been the trigger for the introduction of a variety of services, which continue to evolve. Currently, the Standards for Prescribing are under review as they have not been updated since their introduction in 2006. The NMC are considering that prescribing may become an integral part of pre-registration education in the future.

As the requirement increases for nurses to expand their skills base to undertake the roles that are being demanded within the new agenda, the existing educational standards (UKCC, 2001) with which approved specialist practitioner courses must comply are outdated and do not adequately prepare students for these roles. The QNI and QNIS in partnership with the ADNE have launched voluntary standards (QNI/QNIS, 2015) that provide a more contemporary set of outcomes for educating the district nurses of the future, which in turn should make these programmes more attractive to commissioners. These standards for example refer to the advanced clinical assessment skills that are an integral part of being an independent prescriber. These standards acknowledge the complex and pivotal role of the district nurse as part of the multi-disciplinary team whose remit is to enable people to be cared for in their own homes and communities.

CONCLUSION

The NHS and primary care continue to undergo radical change. The Francis Report (DH, 2013) has influenced policy and practice as all the countries of the United Kingdom have responded by tightening their governance arrangements and providing transparency regarding their systems. The use of IT has the capacity to transform processes and care management although as yet this has not achieved its full potential. Professional nursing organisations are campaigning throughout the UK nations to ensure that standards of care are not compromised by the new agenda. All the countries of the United Kingdom are examining and promoting the district nurse and general practice nurse roles; these specialist generalists are seen as the lynchpin of the integrated team. Community nurses must ensure that they are involved in the decisions about how services will be developed at the strategic level. The future is going to involve working across community and acute care to offer a more seamless service. Integrated teams will be a critical factor in managing the complex needs of the ageing population. It is imperative that practitioners prepare to assert themselves as key members of the team, demonstrating the range of skills that they bring to contribute to the emerging landscape.

FURTHER READING

It is important to be familiar with any new government document that impacts on service delivery. The reference list contains many references to recent publications concerned with shaping services in primary care.

DH (2013) *Vision and Strategy: An Approach to District Nursing.* http://www.england.nhs. uk/wp-content/uploads/2012/12/6c-dist-nurse.pdf (accessed 17/6/17).

Welsh Assembly Government (2015) *Making Prudent Healthcare Happen.* http://www. prudenthealthcare.org.uk/ A useful resource that examines different ways of working in community (accessed 17/6/17).

Willis P (2015) *Raising the Bar Shape of Caring: A Review of the Future Education and Training of Registered Nurses and Care Assistants.* London: HEE.

REFERENCES

Andrews J and Butler M (2014) *Trusted to Care. An Independent Review.* (Accessed 3 August 2015) http://gov.wales/docs/dhss/publications/140512trustedtocareen.pdf.

Baraniak C and Gardner L (2001) Nurse-led general practice for nurses, doctors and patients. In Lewis R, Gillam S, and Jenkins C (eds) *Personal Medical Service Pilots.* London: King's Fund, pp. 75–87.

Benison L (2015) Health and social care partnership improves lives. *Practice Nursing* 26(2):60.

Bhardwa S (2014) A model for nurse led care. *Independent Nurse* 21: 32–33.

Bhardwa S (2015) First implementation in England of Northern Irish workforce planning tool. *Independent Nurse*. http://www.independentnurse.co.uk/news/first-implementation-in-england-of-northern-irish-workforce-planning-tool/75576 (accessed 17/6/17).

Brookes D and Smith A (eds) (2007) *Non-Medical Prescribing in Healthcare Practice. A Toolkit for Students and Practitioners.* Basingstoke: Palgrave.

Burke C and Sheldon K (2010) Encouraging workplace innovation using the 'world cafe' model. *Nursing Management* 17:14–9.

Buurtzorg Nederland (2011) *A New Perspective on Elder Care in the Netherlands.* (Accessed 18 July 2015) http://omahasystem.org/AARPTheJournal_Summer2011_deBlok.pdf.

Dawes D (2009) How nurses can use social enterprise to improve services in health care. *Nursing Times* 105:1, 22–5.

Department of Health (2001) *The Expert Patient: A New Approach to Chronic Disease Management in the 21st Century.* London: HMSO.

DH (2005) *Supporting People with Long Term Conditions.* London: Department of Health.

DH (2008) *Social Enterprise Making a Difference.* (Accessed 3 August 2015) http://www.socialenterprise.org.uk/uploads/files/2011/11/social_enteprise_making_a_difference_guide.pdf.

DH (2011) *Transforming Community Services.* (Accessed 3 August 2015) https://www.gov.uk/government/uploads/system/uploads/attachment_data/file/215624/dh_126111.pdf.

DH (2012a) *Health and Social Care Act.* (Accessed 3 August 2015) http://www.legislation.gov.uk/ukpga/2012/7/pdfs/ukpga_20120007_en.pdf.

DH (2012b) *Liberating the NHS: No Decision About Me, Without Me—Further Consultation on Proposals to Secure Shared Decision-making.* (Accessed 8 August 2016) https://consultations.dh.gov.uk/choice/choice-future-proposals/supporting_documents/Choice%20consultation%20%20No%20decison%20about%20me%20without%20me.pdf.

DH (2013) *Vision and Strategy: An Approach to District Nursing.* (Accessed 25 July 2015) http://www.england.nhs.uk/wp-content/uploads/2012/12/6c-dist-nurse.pdf.

Department of Health, Social Services and Public Safety (DHSSPSNI) (2011a) *A District Nursing Service for Today and Tomorrow. Consultation Document. Supporting People at Home.* Belfast: DHSSPSNI.

Department of Health, Social Services and Public Safety (DHSSPSNI) (2011b) *Transforming Your Care. A Review of Health and Social Care in Northern Ireland.* http://www.transformingyourcare.hscni.net/wp-content/uploads/2012/10/Transforming-Your-Care-Review-of-HSC-in-NI.pdf.

Department of Health, Social Services and Public Safety (DHSSPS) and the Department of Justice (DOJ) (2015) *Adult Safeguarding: Prevention and Protection in Partnership.* (Accessed 22 November 2015) https://www.dhsspsni.gov.uk/sites/default/files/publications/dhssps/adult-safeguarding-policy.pdf.

DH/NHS Commissioning Board (2012) *Compassion in Practice. Nursing, Midwifery and Care Staff. Our Vision and Strategy.* London: Crown Copyright.

Employers Network for Equality and Inclusion (enei) (2013) *Agile Working. A Guide for Employers.* (Accessed 8 August 2015) http://www.nhsemployers.org/~/media/Employers/Documents/SiteCollectionDocuments/Agile%20Working%20Guide.pdf.

Francis R (2013) *The Report of the Mid Staffordshire NHS Foundation Trust Public Enquiry.* London: The Stationary Office.

Goleman D (1998) *Working with Emotional Intelligence*. New York, NY: Bantam Books.

Granger B, Stanworth J and Stanworth C (1995) Self employment career dynamic: The case of the 'Unemployment Push' in United Kingdom book publishing. *Work, Employment and Society* 9:499–516.

Greaves F, Laverty A, Pape U et al. (2015) Performance of the new alternative providers of primary care services in England: An observational study. *Journal of the Royal Society of Medicine* 108(5):171–83.

Grice A and Cooper C (2015) NHS Devolution plan hands over £6bn budget for health and social care. *Independent i* 11.03.2015 4–5.

Ham C, Heenan D, Longlet M and Steel D (2013) *Integrated Care in Northern Ireland, Scotland and Wales. Lessons for England*. London: King's Fund. (Accessed 8 August 2015) www.integrated-care-in-northern-ireland-scotland-and-wales-kingsfund-jul13%20(1).pdf.

Health Education England (2012) *National Health Service England. The Health Education England Directions 2012*. https://www.gov.uk/government/uploads/system/uploads/attachment_data/file/212796/HEE-Directions-2012.pdf.

Health Education England (2015) *Our Leaders Our Structure*. (Accessed 18 July 2015) http://hee.nhs.uk/about/our-leaders-and-structure/.

Health Education England (HEE) (2016a) *Building Capacity to Care and Capability to Treat*. https://www.hee.nhs.uk/sites/default/files/documents/Response%20to%20Nursing%20Associate%20consultation%2026%20May%202016.pdf.

Health Education England (2016b) *Developing Community Education Providers Network*. https://hee.nhs.uk/sites/default/files/documents/2-Developing-CEPN.pdf.

Hinchliff S, Norman S and Schrober J (2008) *Nursing Practice in Health Care*, 5th edn. London: Hodder Education.

Iles V and Sutherland K (2001) *Managing Change in the NHS: Organisational Change: A Review for Healthcare Managers, Professionals and Researchers*. London: National Co-ordinating Centre for NHS Delivery and Organisation R and D.

Jack K and Holt M (2008) Community profiling as part of a health needs assessment. *Nursing Standard* 22:51–6.

King's Fund (2013) *Buurtzorg Nederland Presentation*. (Accessed 19 July 2015) http://www.kingsfund.org.uk/sites/files/kf/media/jos-de-blok-buurtzorg-home-healthcare-nov13.pdf.

Leadbetter C (1997) *The Rise of the Social Entrepreneur*. London: Demos.

Lefebvre C (2003) Social marketing and health promotion. In Bunton R and Macdonald G (eds) *Health Promotion. Disciplines, Diversity and Developments*, 2nd edn. London: Routledge.

Matthews-King A (2014) *Pulse*. (Accessed 18 July 2015) http://www.pulsetoday.co.uk/commissioning/commissioning-topics/urgent-care/nhs-111-putting-disproportionate-pressure-on-gps-and-ae/20008774.article#.VappY6TbLL9.

National Association of Primary Care (NAPC) (2015) *Primary Care Navigators Training Programme for Dementia: Evaluation of its Impact*. (Accessed 4 August 2015) https://www.evidence.nhs.uk/document?ci=http%3a%2f%2farms.evidence.nhs.uk%2fresources%2fHub%2f1045445&returnUrl=Search%3fq%3d%2522care%2bnavigator%2522&q=%22care+navigator%22.

Nazarko L (2007) Primary care reconfiguration: Managing the transition. *Primary Health Care* 17:14–6.

NHS Education for Scotland (2016) *Career Development Framework for Nurses, Midwives and Allied Health Professionals*. Edinburgh: NES. (Accessed 4 August 2016) http://

www.careerframework.nes.scot.nhs.uk/media/32227/nesd0057_postregistrationcareer framework_f.pdf.

NHS Education for Scotland (NES) (2012) *Careers and Development Framework for District Nursing.* (Accessed 4 August 2015) http://www.nes.scot.nhs.uk/media/834542/ district_nursing_career_framework_fsec.pdf.

NHS England (2014a) *Five Years Forward View.* (Accessed 4 August 2015) https://www. england.nhs.uk/wp-content/uploads/2014/10/5yfv-web.pdf.

NHS England (2014b) *Building and Strengthening Leadership. Leading with Compassion.* (Accessed 3 August 2015) http://www.england.nhs.uk/wp-content/uploads/2014/12/ london-nursing-accessible.pdf.

NHS England (2016a) *General Practice Forward View.* https://www.england.nhs.uk/ wp-content/uploads/2016/04/gpfv.pdf.

NHS England (2016b) *Leading Change Adding Value.* (Accessed 6 August 2016) https:// www.england.nhs.uk/wp-content/uploads/2016/05/nursing-framework.pdf.

NHS England (2016c) *Enhancing the Quality of Life for People with Long Term Conditions. The House of Care.* https://www.england.nhs.uk/house-of-care/.

NHS Scotland (2011) *Ehealth Strategy 2011-17.* (Accessed 3 August 2015) http://www.gov. scot/resource/doc/357616/0120849.pdf.

NHS Scotland (2012) *Integrated Resource Framework.* (Accessed 27 July 2015) www. shiftingthebalance.scot.nhs.uk/initiatives/sbc-initiatives/integrated-resourceframework/.

NHSE/QNI (2014) *Developing a National District Nurse Workforce Planning Framework.* London: QNI, NHSE.

NICE (2015) *Home Care: Delivering Personal Care and Practical Support to Older People Living in their Own Homes NICE Guidelines (NG21).* (Accessed 14 November 2015) http://www.nice.org.uk/guidance/ng21.

Northern Ireland Practice and Education Council for Nursing and Midwifery (NIPEC) (2015) *Annual Business Plan 2015/16.* (Accessed 26 November 2015) http://www.nipec. hscni.net/Image/SitePDFS/NIPEC%20%20Business%20Plan%202015-2016.pdf.

North Wales (2014) *Statement of Intent. A Framework for Delivering Care for Older People with Complex Needs.* (Accessed 3 August 2015) http://www.dvsc.co.uk/en/services/ partnerships/health-and-social-care/statement-of-intent-a-framework-for-delivering- integrated-health-social-care/.

Nursing and Midwifery Council (NMC) (2006) *Standards of Proficiency for Nurse and Midwife Prescribers.* London: NMC.

NMC (2009) *Standards of Education for Prescribing from the Nurse Prescribers Formulary for Community Practitioners for Nurses Without a Specialist Practitioner Qualification— Introducing Code V150.* London: NMC.

Oldman C (2014) Statement *to Political Parties.* (Accessed 3 August 2015) http://www.qni. org.uk/campaigns/policy_statements.

Queen's Nursing Institute (QNI) (2010) *Position Statement March 2010. Nursing People in their Own Homes—Key Issues for the Future of Care.* London: QNI.

Queen's Nursing Institute (QNI) (2014a) *2020 Vision Five Years on. Re-assessing the Future of District Nursing.* http://www.qni.org.uk/ docs/2020_Vision_Five_Years_On_Web1.1.pdf.

Queen's Nursing Institute (2014b) *Developing a National D/N Workforce Planning Framework. A Report Commissioned by NHS England.* Publications Gateway Reference 01518. (Accessed 3 August 2015).

Queen's Nursing Institute (2014c) *Report on District Nurse Education in the UK*. http://www.qni.org.uk/docs/District_Nurse_Education_Report_2014_web.pdf.

Queen's Nursing Institute (2016) *Discharge Planning. Best Practice in Transitions of Care*. London: QNI.

Queen's Nursing Institute and Queen's Nursing Institute Scotland (QNI/QNIS) (2015) *The QNI/QNIS Voluntary Standards for District Nurse Education and Practice*. London: QNI.

Royal College of Nursing (RCN) (2007) *Nurse Entrepreneurs. Turning Initiative into Independence*. London: RCN.

RCN (2010) *Pillars of the Community. The RCN's UK Position on the Development of the Registered Nursing Workforce in the Community*. London: RCN.

RCN (2016) *RCN Briefing. The Buurtzorg Nederland (Home Care Provider) Model. Observations for the UK*. London: RCN. (Accessed 5 August 2016) https://www.rcn.org.uk/about-us/policy-briefings/br-0215.

Regulation and Quality Improvement Authority (2012) *Review of the Implementation of the Northern Ireland Single Assessment Tool*. (Accessed 3 August 2015) http://www.rqia.org.uk/cms_resources/NISAT%20Overview%20report%20Final%20for%20publication%20(3).pdf.

Roberts N (2015) *Jeremy Hunt to Lead Seven Day Revolution After Tory Election Win*. (Accessed 3 August 2015) http://www.gponline.com/new-deal-gps-means-seven-day-services-jeremy-hunt-confirms/article/1352203.

Rollnick W, Miller R and Butler C (2013) *Motivational Interviewing in Health Care: Helping Patients Change Behaviour*. London: Guildford Press.

Rose S (2015) *Better Leadership for Tomorrow. NHS Leadership Review*. (Accessed 14 November 2015) https://www.gov.uk/government/uploads/system/uploads/attachment_data/file/445738/Lord_Rose_NHS_Report_acc.pdf.

Royal College of Physicians (2014) *Joint Statement on the Announcement of More Physician Associates*. (Accessed 4 August 2015) https://www.rcplondon.ac.uk/press-releases/joint-statement-announcement-more-physician-associates.

Scottish Government (2008) *Delivering for Remote and Rural Healthcare*. Edinburgh: Scottish Government. (Accessed 3 August 2015) www.scotland.gov.uk/Resource/Doc/222201/0059769.pdf.

Scottish Government (2011) *Re-shaping Care for Older People*. (Accessed 3 August 2015) http://www.gov.scot/Resource/0039/00398295.pdf.

Scottish Government (2012). *Maximising Recovery and Promoting Independence: Intermediate Care's contribution to Reshaping Care—An Intermediate Care Framework for Scotland*. Edinburgh: Scottish Government.

Scottish Government (2013) *A Route Map to the 2020 Vision for Health and Social Care*. (Accessed 3 August 2015) http://www.gov.scot/Resource/0042/00423188.pdf.

Scottish Government (2014a) *Health and Social Care Information Sharing. A Strategic Framework*. 2014–2020. (Accessed 3 August 2015) http://www.gov.scot/Resource/0046/00469375.pdf.

Scottish Government (2014b) *Setting the Direction for Nursing & Midwifery Education in Scotland*. (Accessed 3 August 2015) http://www.gov.scot/Publications/2014/02/4112.

Scottish Government (2016) *A National Clinical Strategy for Scotland*. (Accessed 4 August 2016) http://www.gov.scot/Publications/2016/02/8699.

Sirkin H, Keenan P and Jackson A (October 2005) The hard side of change management. *Harvard Business Review* 83(10):108–18. (Accessed 17 February 2015) http://unpan1.un.org/intradoc/groups/public/documents/unssc/unpan022087.pdf.

Sprinks J (2015) District nursing reaches crisis point in Northern Ireland. *Primary Health Care* 25(3):8–9.

Taylor R (2010) Leadership theories and the development of nurses in Primary Care. *Primary Care Nursing* 19:40–5.

The Health Foundation and Nuffield Trust (2014) *The Impacts of Asymmetric Devolution on Healthcare in the Four Countries of the UK.* (Accessed 14 November 2015) http://www.health.org.uk/sites/default/files/TheImpactsOfAsymmetricDevolutionOnHealthCareInFourCountriesUK.pdf.

Traynor M, Davis K, Drennan V et al. (2007) *The Contribution of Nurse, Midwife and Health Visitor Entrepreneurs to Patient Choice: A Scoping Exercise.* London: NCCSDO.

United Kingdom Central Council (UKCC) (2001) *Standards for Specialist Education and Practice.* London: UKCC.

Welsh Assembly Government (WAG) (2010) *'Setting the Direction'. Primary and Community Services Strategic Delivery Programme.* Cardiff: Welsh Assembly Government. (Accessed 3 August 2013) http://gov.wales/docs/dhss/publications/100727settingthedirectionen.pdf.

Welsh Assembly Government (2011) *Together for Health.* (Accessed 24 August 2016) http://www.wales.nhs.uk/sitesplus/documents/829/togetherforhealth.pdf.

Welsh Assembly Government (2013) *Delivering Safe Care, Compassionate Care.* (Accessed 3 August 2015) http://gov.wales/docs/dhss/report/130710safecarefen.pdf.

Welsh Assembly Government (2015) *Making Prudent Healthcare Happen.* (Accessed 3 August 2015) http://www.prudenthealthcare.org.uk/.

Whitehead D, Weiss S and Tappen R (2007) *Essentials of Nursing Leadership and Management*, 4th edn. Philadelphia, PA: F.A. Davis.

Willis P (2015) *Raising the Bar Shape of Caring: A Review of the Future Education and Training of Registered Nurses and Care Assistants.* London: HMSO.

Yarra Software (2010) *ecat Caseload Analysis and Activity Tool.* http://www.innovations.hscni.net/wp-content/uploads/2010/12/E-CAT_flyer_Yarra.pdf.

INDEX